Mental Health in Historical Perspective

Series Editors
Catharine Coleborne
School of Humanities and Social Science
University of Newcastle
Callaghan, NSW, Australia

Matthew Smith
Centre for the Social History of Health and Healthcare
University of Strathclyde
Glasgow, UK

Covering all historical periods and geographical contexts, the series explores how mental illness has been understood, experienced, diagnosed, treated and contested. It will publish works that engage actively with contemporary debates related to mental health and, as such, will be of interest not only to historians, but also mental health professionals, patients and policy makers. With its focus on mental health, rather than just psychiatry, the series will endeavour to provide more patient-centred histories. Although this has long been an aim of health historians, it has not been realised, and this series aims to change that.

The scope of the series is kept as broad as possible to attract good quality proposals about all aspects of the history of mental health from all periods. The series emphasises interdisciplinary approaches to the field of study, and encourages short titles, longer works, collections, and titles which stretch the boundaries of academic publishing in new ways.

More information about this series at
http://www.palgrave.com/gp/series/14806

Claire Hilton

Civilian Lunatic Asylums During the First World War

A Study of Austerity on London's Fringe

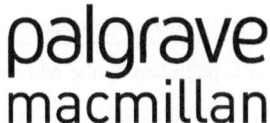

Claire Hilton
Centre for the History of Emotions
Queen Mary University of London
London, UK

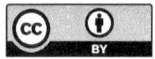

Mental Health in Historical Perspective
ISBN 978-3-030-54870-4   ISBN 978-3-030-54871-1   (eBook)
https://doi.org/10.1007/978-3-030-54871-1

In memoriam
Professor Tom Arie CBE (1933–2020)
A psychiatrist who led the way in humanising mental health services
and inspired others to do likewise

May his memory be for a blessing

Foreword

I am delighted to provide a foreword for this detailed and insightful book exploring the life of London's asylums during the First World War. It is a compelling but also harrowing read for all those interested in the history of psychiatry and mental health services. The book explores the structural, legal, relational and procedural side of asylum life in the First World War with a particular emphasis on the experience of patients. It draws on a breadth of source material reflecting their experiences.

In England and Wales there were 100,000 patients in asylums and whilst it might be tempting to think, when exploring the horrors of military life, that asylum life might be a welcome respite, the experiences of patients were quite the opposite. The book shows us that mental health care never existed outside the context of culture, politics and world events and was particularly prone to adversity when resource and workforce pressures abounded. There were huge staff shortages and general goods were in short supply but what was particularly obvious was the deficit in terms of innovation that had made some headway prior to the First World War.

There were some enlightened voices urging a focus on what would benefit patients, but treatment could be harsh and there was disregard for personal dignity along with poor hygiene and high death rates. It did make me feel grateful for our safeguarding procedures, mental health law that prioritises and protects patients and for regulators with real teeth, along with encouraging the externalising of complaints and concerns, rather than suppressing them.

An important reason to explore the past is to learn lessons for the future and Claire Hilton's book does that. Some challenges are still very much present 100 years on: stigma, human rights, power imbalances, resources, workforce, research, regulation and organisational structure remain part of our current discourse.

Read on with an open mind, a thirst for knowledge and with gratitude for what we can do for our patients. Continued self-reflection and challenge are vital. We could still do so much more.

Dr. Adrian James
President of the Royal College of Psychiatrists
London, UK

PREFACE

Bombarded by historical analyses of First World War "shell shock" and the suffering of military casualties left me wondering how 100,000 "pauper lunatics" fared in the wartime civilian lunatic asylums. Asylum patients were low priority on the scale of social welfare, regarded as a burden on the economy and unable to contribute to the war effort. Standards of care and treatment fell, discharge rates plummeted, and death rates due to infectious diseases escalated far in excess of those in the community. The neglect was particularly disturbing because the asylum leadership knew what should be done in the interests of the patients, but too often failed to act on that knowledge.

This book centres round the patients who were the *raison d'être* of the asylums. It explores how individuals helped them and hindered them and how the system let them down. It is an un-told story, about real people, which deserves to be heard.

London, UK   Claire Hilton

ACKNOWLEDGMENTS

Many people have helped, cajoled, criticised, supported and guided the research and writing of this book. Librarians and archivists, particularly at the Wellcome Collection, London Metropolitan Archives, Royal College of Psychiatrists and the National Archives at Kew have helped sort endless requests for documents. The Wellcome Collection generously provided the funds to publish this book open access. Matt Smith and Cathy Coleborne, series editors, and Molly Beck, Joe Johnson and Meera Mithran at Palgrave, have been a supportive team to work with. Two anonymous peer reviewers, one who read the synopsis and another who read the entire manuscript offered valuable feedback and helped shape the final text. Rhodri Hayward read chunks of the work and his comments were much appreciated. Advice from Nicol Ferrier about post-mortems was most welcome and discussions with Louise Hide are always thought provoking and fruitful. Adrian James found time to write the foreword, and I am grateful for his continued interest in the history of psychiatry. Hugh and Gus Fowler-Wright and library staff at King's College London provided invaluable copyright information about illustrations. My husband Michael has allowed me to disappear into lengthy anti-social hibernation with my laptop, and he has continued to explore former asylums and asylum cemeteries with me. I am particularly indebted to David Jolley for his enthusiasm and encouragement and valuable comments after reading the entire manuscript, some parts more than once.

CONTENTS

ABBREVIATIONS

AR	Annual Report
BJPsych	*British Journal of Psychiatry*
BMJ	*British Medical Journal*
BoC	Board of Control
CiL	Commissioners in Lunacy
CMO	Chief Medical Officer
CRDI	England and Wales, Civil Registration Death Index, 1916–2007
d	'Old' penny. 1d = ½p
EC	Earth closet
GPI	General paralysis of the insane
HC	House of Commons
HL	House of Lords
HoP	*History of Psychiatry* (Journal)
JMS	*Journal of Mental Science*
LAB	Lancashire Asylums Board
lb	Pound weight. 1 lb = 0.45 kg
LCC	London County Council
LMA	London Metropolitan Archives, City of London
MACA	Mental After Care Association
MDA	Mental Deficiency Act 1913
MOH	Medical Officer of Health
MRC	Medical Research Committee/Council
MP	Member of Parliament
MPA	Medico-Psychological Association
MS	Medical superintendent
NAWU	National Asylum Workers' Union

oz	Ounce. 1 oz = 28 grams. 16 oz = 1 lb
PoW	Prisoner of War
Q	Question number (in Cobb Inquiry)
RBNA	Royal British Nursing Association
Proc RSM	*Proceedings of the Royal Society of Medicine*
s	Shilling. 1 s = 5 p
TNA	The National Archives, Kew
UK	United Kingdom
USA	United States of America
VC	Visiting committee
WC	Water closet
W/FM	Weekly or fortnightly meeting of Board of Control
WL	Wellcome Library

LIST OF FIGURES

LIST OF TABLES

CHAPTER 1

Introduction: Civilians, Lunacy and the First World War

Britain declared war against Germany on 4 August 1914. For the next four years military priorities overrode those of civilians. The entire population faced hardships, but for those people designated "pauper lunatics" in public asylums, life became very harsh. At the beginning of the war, the asylums were a story of good intentions gone awry, the failed dreams of social reformers and psychiatrists. They had become "vast warehouses for the chronically insane and demented."[1] Richard Hunter and Ida Macalpine, in their history of Colney Hatch Asylum, commented about the gloomy picture: "Custodial care was forced on asylums as a way of life....paralysed by sheer weight of numbers of patients" and financial constraints.[2] "Nothing", they said, showed "more blatantly how relentless pressure for more and more beds forced the asylum further and further away from the idea of a hospital."[3]

Public lunatic asylums in England and Wales changed in the decades before the war, arguably for the worse. Reflecting Hunter and Macalpine's dismay, earlier good intentions such as implementing "moral treatment", a social intervention involving trust, sympathy and group activities, alongside good food, fresh air, occupation and exercise, disappeared, even though the approach benefitted patients with reversible disorders of recent onset and those chronically unwell on long-stay wards.[4] Alongside moral treatment, principles of "non-restraint" were valued, but not uniformly implemented. Both these methods were effective and gained

© The Author(s) 2021
C. Hilton, *Civilian Lunatic Asylums During the First World War*,
Mental Health in Historical Perspective,
https://doi.org/10.1007/978-3-030-54871-1_1

prominence in smaller institutions through the work of enthusiastic lay leaders, such as the Tuke family at the Retreat in York, and medical leaders such as John Conolly at Hanwell and Robert Gardiner Hill at Lincoln. The methods worked less well in larger asylums, and never achieved widespread implementation, remaining as an ideal rather than reality.

Many other aspects of the asylum changed, influenced by stakeholders with different opinions, including doctors, lawyers, social reformers and the general public. Sometimes they agreed on priorities, but often not. The role of the medical profession became more dominant, in part due to legislation which stipulated that every institution of more than 100 lunatics must have a resident physician.[5] No other profession vied for the leadership.[6] New lunacy laws became more rigid and complex, tending to focus on the safety of the public rather than on the wellbeing of those suffering from mental disorders.

By 1870, public asylums had an average of 500 beds. Total annual admissions rose steeply after 1890, associated with the new Lunacy Act, but then stayed roughly in line with demographic trends (Fig. 1.1).[7] The death rate remained stable, but the discharge rate declined.[8] There is no evidence that the type or severity of mental disorders accounted for the changes. The increasing size of asylums, beyond that which could be accounted for by demographic changes, is likely to have been due to the decades-long mental disability caused by chronic psychotic disorders, such as schizophrenia,[9] accompanied by a changing balance of therapeutic interventions and custodial care. By the beginning of the war, in England and Wales, an average asylum had 1000 beds[10] and over 100,000 people were certified as pauper lunatics. Wartime shortages of staff and material goods, and overcrowding after the War Office requisitioned asylums to use as military hospitals, were associated with a calamitous fall in standards of care for mentally unwell civilian patients. The situation was a sad commentary on the low social priorities attached to people identified as suffering from mental disorders.[11]

A substantial historiography exists on "shell shock", the syndrome of mental disturbances suffered by war-traumatised soldiers during the First World War.[12] By contrast, the historiography of civilian asylums and their patients at the same time is meagre, featuring in a few academic journal articles and chapters in some general asylum histories.[13] No in-depth historical studies have specifically drawn together the various elements of the story to provide a contextualised and detailed analysis, as this book sets out to do. It tells the story of four asylums on the periphery of

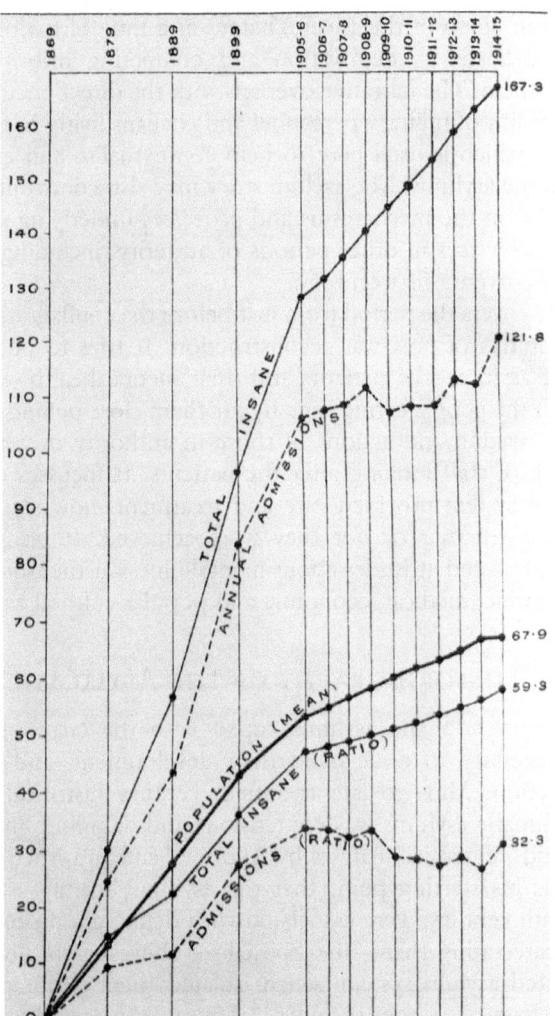

Fig. 1.1 Percentage change in "insane" patients relative to population of England and Wales (1869–1915). From top to bottom: Patients resident ("total insane"); Annual admissions; Population of England and Wales; Ratio of patients to population; Ratio of admissions to population. (*First Annual Report of the Board of Control, for the Year 1914* (London: HMSO, 1916), between pp. 8–9).

London to the north of the River Thames at a time of national turmoil, when intense austerity, deprivation and competing priorities affected those within them. The narrative overlaps with the direct effects of war on the mental health of military personnel and civilians living in the community, material which is used here to help contextualise and explain what happened in the asylums. The asylum story may also contribute to debate and shed light on the mechanisms and processes underlying standards of mental health services in other periods of austerity, including in the first decades of the twenty-first century.

This study covers the period from just before the conflagration through to the beginnings of post-war reconstruction. It tries to put the *raison d'être* of the asylum—the patients and their mental health—in the foreground, with the people caring directly for them close behind. It explores the decision making and actions of those in authority over the asylums and the work of staff looking after the patients. It focusses on how the public asylum system provided care and treatment, how standards were envisaged and whether or not they were achieved. It brings together knowledge, ideas and attitudes about mental illness at the time, including political, scientific, medical, economic and popular cultural aspects.

Historiography of the Asylums

To comprehend how the asylums coped with the crisis of the Great War, it is necessary to understand their development, and disentangle fact from fiction. Mid- to late twentieth century historical interpretation of the lunatic asylums was contentious and damning, including the persuasive and influential analyses by Andrew Scull and Michel Foucault. Scull took as his starting point that the asylums, mainly established in the nineteenth century, were associated with defining a problem population and incarcerating them "in a specialised, bureaucratically organised, state-supported asylum system which isolated them geographically and symbolically from the larger society."[14] Foucault also attributed asylums' rural locations to the public desire to segregate "mad" people from the majority of the population, drawing analogies between asylums and leper houses of the middle ages.[15] Even though, like leprosy, mental disorders were tainted by fear and stigma, in the nineteenth century there was also a public perception that people with disturbed minds required protection, care and compassion. These notions contributed constructively to new lunacy legislation, asylum building and asylum care in England.[16] Despite good intentions of the reformers, as sometimes revealed verbatim in their reports in *Hansard*,[17] Scull and Foucault identified the underlying ethos of the asylums as inherently and inevitably damaging to those within. Their conclusions linked to the theoretical and ideological standpoints which they held. Scull took a Marxist perspective in his analysis,[18] which fits with his description of asylums as "Warehouses of the Unwanted", "largely receptacles for the confinement of the impossible, the inconvenient and the inept",[19] the economically unproductive sector of the population. Foucault's analysis was cotemporaneous and convergent with that of the anti-psychiatry movement, which regarded mental illness as socially fabricated and those afflicted as wrongfully confined and medicated. Anti-psychiatry activists who wrote at the same time as Foucault included RD Laing and Thomas Szasz who expounded on social causes of insanity, and Erving Goffman, who scrutinized regimes of institutional living, with particular attention to their harmful effects.[20] David Cooper, the psychiatrist said to have coined the term "anti-psychiatry", wrote the introduction to Foucault's *Madness and Civilisation* when published in England, endorsing its link to anti-psychiatry ideology.[21]

So contentious were the writings of Scull, Foucault and others in the second half of the twentieth century, that historians since then have criticised their methodologies.[22] Joseph Melling and Bill Forsythe argued that Foucault displayed some "extravagant historical inaccuracies", such as in his analysis of confinement of the insane in early modern Europe.[23] Louise Hide described Foucault's study as "brilliant but flawed", such as his arguments about industrial society being increasingly intolerant of its non-productive members so beginning to lock them away in institutions.[24] Jonathan Andrews and Anne Digby regarded some twentieth-century historiography as too divorced from wider historical issues and "overly ideologised and unconvincingly theorised" in its approaches to asylums and psychiatry, lacking a firm and comprehensive grounding in archival sources.[25] Hugh Freeman found no evidence to support Scull's economic and social exclusion model of the asylums. Instead, he found severely ill patients whose relatives had done all they could to contain the situation before seeking admission.[26] Edward Shorter also criticised historians of the 1960s and 1970s, who

> constituted a kind of lost generation in that they have chosen to pursue puffs of smoke, displaying no interest in the question of just what happens historically to make mind and brain go awry. If we wish to tell the story

of psychiatry empathetically, we must deal with the story of illness rather than arguing that it is a nonstory or that it is unknowable.[27]

Paul Tobia also argued that understanding asylums in depth can only be done by uncovering detailed source material, although that risks creating studies overly detailed and too divorced from wider historical issues.[28]

Another sort of historiography, which has coloured our understanding of psychiatric history, comprises accounts written by medical professionals about their own institutions.[29] These authors also conveyed biased perspectives, often as culprits of "whiggish" research, according to Juliet Hurn, adopting a "style of history-writing in which it is assumed that scientific progress can be charted through the approach towards an objective scientific truth."[30] Their work tended to be founded on hindsight, comparing the past with scientific evidence and medical standards to which they had aspired during their clinical careers.[31] They were also judgmental, praising the work of those perceived to have aided "progress" and dismissing others.[32] They tended to focus on the leadership rather than the patients and on what happened, rather than on analysing processes of why and how things occurred in broader contexts. John Crammer, a psychiatrist who wrote the history of the Buckinghamshire Asylum summarised: "the history of psychiatry was left to medical men with a fondness for anecdote, a reverence for pioneers, and a belief in 'progress'."[33]

Aware of the many concerns about the nature of the evidence and analysis used in historical studies of mental disorder and institutional care, this study uses standard historical methodology,[34] and draws extensively on archival and published sources, aiming to achieve a balanced understanding of the asylums, contextualised in the circumstances of the day.

FROM BROAD THEORIES AND GENERALISATIONS TO SPECIFICS AND DIVERSITY

Despite some historical analyses suggesting that the segregation and exclusion of mentally disturbed people was a key rationale for building asylums in rural areas, there are alternative explanations. One was the belief, in line with moral treatment, that the location would provide a healthy environment to benefit recovery and recuperation. Similar principles applied to building rural sanatoria for treating tuberculosis in the pre-antibiotic era. Asylums were frequently located on the best sites—on a hillside and above urban pollution, and south-facing to maximise sunshine and give shelter from the prevailing winds—to allow employment and leisure in the fresh air. The building of many asylums in the early to mid-nineteenth century was also concurrent with the founding of specialist hospitals, each dedicated to a group of related diseases or a single bodily organ or organ system. In the London area, for example, specialist hospitals opened for eye and ear diseases, bowel problems, cancer and neurological conditions. They raised interest in the diseases on which they focussed, and the knowledge and expertise in treatment which developed in them were gradually adopted by general (physical illness) hospitals, thus becoming part of mainstream medicine and surgery.[35] There are parallels in the asylums, where the medical leadership sought to better understand the disorders they diagnosed and to find effective treatments, preferably cures.

The architecture of the asylums, the palatial façade of Colney Hatch (Fig. 1.2) or the prison-like central towers at Hanwell (Fig. 1.3) were emblematic of the diversity of the asylums in terms of practices and

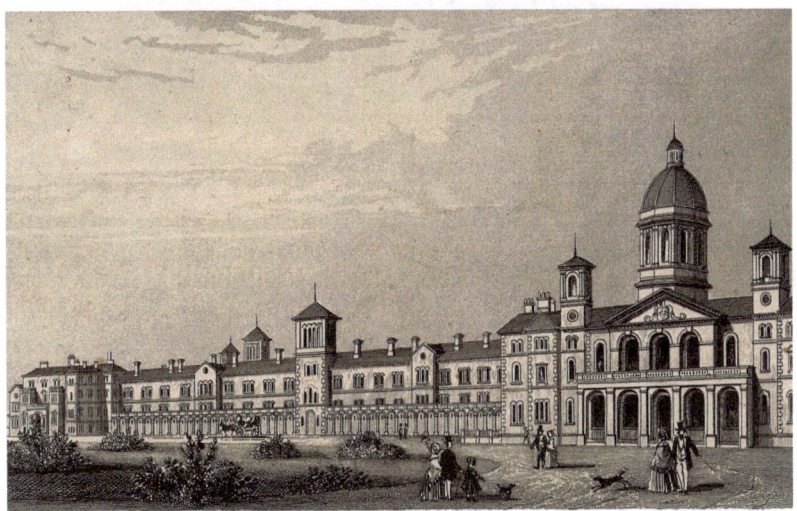

Fig. 1.2 Colney Hatch Lunatic Asylum, Southgate, Middlesex: panoramic view, undated (Wellcome Collection CC BY licence)

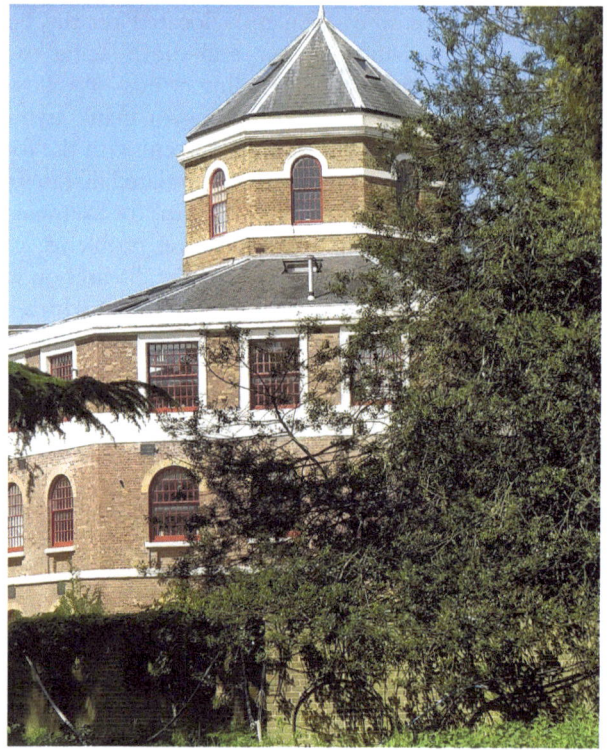

Fig. 1.3   Hanwell Asylum (Photograph by author, 2017)

standards within them. These varied despite the Lunacy Act 1890. The Act mandated legal, financial and organisational structures, and the hierarchy of authority, oversight and regulation stemming from the central government body, the Commissioners in Lunacy until 1914 and the Board of Control ("the Board") thereafter, which had responsibility for civilian asylums in England and Wales. The rigid, legalistic approach of the Lunacy Act also reflected increased societal and legal concerns about public safety, ensuring detention of "dangerous" lunatics while preventing wrongful incarceration of "sane" people. Beyond these requirements, the public generally distanced themselves from happenings inside the asylums, their perspectives reinforced by novels about lunacy which tended to emphasise the frightening and the macabre, and rarely encouraged sympathetic interest in the asylums or their occupants.[36]

Historian Roy Porter wrote in 1991 that many dimensions of recent psychiatric institutional history "remain a blank".[37] Since then, understanding of the philosophy, uniformities and diversity of the asylums, has been enhanced by in-depth "hospital biography" investigations into individual asylums, or small groups of them, including in Hampshire, Norfolk, Bristol, Essex, and on the London borders.[38] These institutional biographies give nuanced insights into asylum organisation, patients, staffing, care and treatment within the wider societal context. In exemplary asylums shortly before the First World War, many patients reportedly undertook manual work appropriate to their pre-admission employment, participated in leisure activities, sports and entertainments, and had leave off the premises, including trial leave before discharge with a meaningful monetary allowance to help cover their personal expenses. Some asylums endeavoured to model their clinical approaches on practices in general hospitals. They placed patients on different wards according to whether they were deemed curable or chronic, used the most up-to-date treatments to ameliorate symptoms, and educated and professionalised their staff.[39] Diane Carpenter, however, in her comparison of two Hampshire asylums, described the "postcode-lottery" of variability of care and treatment, from custodial to rehabilitative.[40]

Hospital biographies challenge many generalisations made by Scull and Foucault, but they also demonstrate troubling variation, conflicts and mismatches between ideals and reality, intention and implementation, and numerous facets which came together to influence the functions of the asylums and the outcomes for individuals inside them. Mathew Thomson highlighted how individual and collective factors inside and outside the asylum system influenced policy and provision.[41] Knowledge, understanding and value systems of the medical profession, lawyers, architects, reformers, national and local government, macro- and micro- political networks, and the broader public, all interacted. Together they affected asylum practices and contributed to maintaining the *status quo* or pacing the speed and mapping the route of any significant change. In histories of psychiatry dedicated to a particular aspect of science, philosophy, psychopathology or individual mode of therapy, "single-issue mythologies" have evolved to explain change or stagnation.[42] To avoid these mythologies, the multiplicity of threads indicate the need for a multi-faceted historiographical approach, digging deep into a range of archives and published sources, to reach an understanding about whether, how and when aspects of asylum care altered.

SHELL SHOCK: HISTORIOGRAPHY AND CHANGE

Regarding mental disorders and psychiatric services at the time of the First World War, historians of psychiatry have focussed on shell shock. Public sympathy for soldiers who became mentally disturbed while serving their country contrasted with fear and stigma concerning mental disorders of civilian pauper lunatics in asylums. The socially entrenched pattern of moral judgement of dividing needy people into "deserving" and "undeserving" was reshaped into provision for war-torn soldiers compared to civilians.

Commentators Anne Rogers and David Pilgrim inferred that shell shock plus industrial fatigue at home combined to "change irrevocably the face of twentieth-century psychiatric services". They proposed that shell shock encouraged environmental theories of aetiology and displaced bio-deterministic ideas: to describe soldiers—"England's finest blood"—as biologically "degenerate" and predisposed to mental disturbance "was logically impossible and tantamount to treason." They linked shell shock to the establishment of out-patient clinics and to neurosis becoming a focus of professional interest, although that was also associated with psychoanalytic theory developing pre-war.[43]

Shell shock may have contributed to re-conceptualising some mental disorders, but overall it stimulated little change in asylum treatment.[44] If anything, learning arising from the treatment of shell shock could be detrimental to patients with other severe, disabling mental disorders. Methods used to treat shell shock could be harsh, such as "bullying" electric shocks.[45] Psychological therapies for shell shock, such as cure by suggestion, promoted the idea that patients could control their symptoms, a view which would be inappropriate for people suffering from psychoses, such as schizophrenia, or from organic brain diseases such as general paralysis of the insane (GPI, brain syphilis).[46] Goals of treating shell shock, to send soldiers back to the front line, meant that medical ethics, humanity and measures of "success" were abstruse when compared to ideals of conventional aims of treatment to promote the health and wellbeing of individuals.

In contrast to Rogers and Pilgrim, Jose Harris and Peter Barham were cautious about attributing change in psychiatry primarily to shell shock. Harris raised the question of how far the war itself transformed British society, or merely channelled and accelerated germinating seeds of change sown pre-war when "Britain appeared to be on the cusp of radical change".[47] Social welfare and universal suffrage, for example, had roots pre-war, but wartime priorities diverted good intentions away from peacetime objectives, and direct implementation ground to a halt. The war, however, generated debate on many aspects of life, including roles and opportunities for women, priorities for reconstruction and the meaning of "civilisation",[48] which informed public attitudes and helped shape the course of post-war policy.

Regarding mental health policy and provision, shell shock was just one factor alongside others, including clinical and scientific research; the psychiatric clinics in Germany envied by psychiatrists in England; and the rise of trade unions and disenchantment with conditions of employment in the asylums. Arguably, *The Experiences of an Asylum Doctor* by Montagu Lomax, a retired doctor in his late 50s and temporary wartime asylum assistant medical officer at Bracebridge Asylum, Lincolnshire and Prestwich Asylum, Lancashire (1917–1919), had a profound effect on instigating change in the asylums.[49] For this reason, and as we shall refer to the author, his book and its aftermath several times in the course of the present study, they deserve introduction here. Tim Harding and John Hopton appraised Lomax's work and its outcome.[50] Lomax was particularly critical of the conditions which he observed at Prestwich, although in his book he did not reveal the identity of the asylum. He advocated more active therapeutic interventions to secure the return of patients to the community, he called for wide-reaching changes in asylum management, and a complete reform of existing mental health legislation. Published post-war, when the public had more emotional energy for considering such matters, it raised public awareness and spearheaded further thought. The psychiatric establishment, however, rejected his descriptions of inhuman, custodial, and antitherapeutic conditions.[51] Despite publication coinciding with competing economic struggles nationally, likely to deflate interest in asylum patients' welfare, the aftermath of Lomax's exposé was an inquiry into the "administration of public mental hospitals" chaired by Sir Cyril Cobb in 1922. This led to the appointment of the 1924–1926 Royal Commission on Lunacy and Mental Disorder and to the enactment of the more therapeutically orientated Mental Treatment Act 1930.[52]

PLACING THE PATIENTS CENTRE STAGE

Some historians of psychiatry, as Roy Porter advocated, have succeeded in placing patients centre stage in their narratives.[53] Louise Hide's study about gender and class in asylums between 1890 and 1914 and Paul Tobia's study of the Bristol Lunatic asylum were both bottom-up and top-down, valuing the lives and experiences of patients and those in direct contact with them, as well as those in authority in the asylum hierarchy up to national level.[54] Allan Beveridge analysed 1000 letters written by patients at the Royal Edinburgh Asylum (1873–1908) which were retained by the authorities rather than sent to the addressee. A complex picture emerged in their accounts, which included both humanity and coercion. Many patients spoke warmly of the asylum and its staff and frequently thanked the medical superintendent for his kindness and concern. Some patients, rejected by family and friends, made some sort of life for themselves within the asylum which was more tolerant of their behaviour than the society outside. Letters, like many other single classes of document from the asylum world, have limitations, but Beveridge concluded that the contents should militate against painting too crude a picture of the asylum with staff in the guise of oppressors and inmates as innocent victims.[55] His conclusions contrasted with studies which create an overwhelmingly negative image of the asylums, such as those by Scull.[56]

Peter Barham also wove individual life stories into his history of shell shock, *Forgotten Lunatics of the Great War*. He placed the sufferers' mental disturbances in the context of their lives and the lives of their families and community, giving voice to their personal experiences. In contrast to the *forgotten* soldier patients during the war, civilian patients in the lunatic asylums were almost *invisible* and usually without a voice. Barham described his research experience, that "fossicking in the archival undergrowth frequently yields scraps that, once juxtaposed, deliver startling insights into what was at stake" for individuals.[57] The same was true when researching this study of civilians, which, like Barham's and Beveridge's work, aims to tell the patients' stories and how their needs were, or were not, met.

A variety of bottom-up sources are available to historians of asylums in the early twentieth century. Within individual asylum records, material written by patients, their families and friends can be found pasted into clinical notes and committee minutes. Some documents are positive, including letters of thanks, but more relate to disputes about treatment, thefts, escapes, discharge and money, and other unfavourable aspects of asylum life. As in Beveridge's study, some accounts by patients derive from un-posted, asylum-censored letters. Regarding patients' letters to friends and family, staff had authority to read them. Staff justified their probing in this way as a means of finding out about their patients in order to help them, but this probably reflected, and caused, a lack of trust and face to face conversation between patients and staff. Patients who were aware of the censorship of their letters might also have adjusted their content and tone.

In contrast to personal letters, the Lunacy Act stipulated that letters from patients to the authorities who oversaw their certification and care should be forwarded unopened, but this correspondence was often destroyed after being dealt with.[58] A few patients wrote memoirs. Whereas letter writing is influenced according to who the recipient might be, memoirs can be shaped by time between the experience and the writing, affected by personal reflection, changing knowledge and social expectations giving new emphases. Diaries, generally written for the authors themselves, are the least likely to be tailored to an anticipated external readership. No diaries, however, were identified while researching the present study. Another source of patients' views was their evidence to the Cobb Inquiry as a result of Lomax's book.[59]

Some of the patient vignettes used in this study were identified serendipitously in clinical records or committee minutes. Others derived from a sample I gathered of 600 civilian patients from the national registers of asylum admission and discharge (1913–1918).[60] The sample consisted of every thirtieth patient (the last entry on each page) in the register. Each entry recorded the asylum's name, and patient's name, gender, dates of admission and outcome (recovered, relieved, not improved, died), but not age, date of birth, diagnosis or other clinical information. The method ensured that the sample was clinically, socially and demographically un-biased. In total, 58 of the 600 patients were admitted to Colney Hatch, Claybury, Napsbury and Hanwell. Detailed social and clinical data were sought for them, with the aim of analysing the reasons for their admission and their "journey" through the institution.

STANDARDS OF CARE AND HOW TO MEASURE THEM

Several historians have attempted to ascertain the standards of care achieved in asylums. Carpenter concluded that "basic determinants of the quality of life" for patients in the Hampshire asylums pre-war were "preferable to its alternatives": diet, cleanliness, personal hygiene and clothing, all compared reasonably with poorer private dwellings and the workhouse. Other living conditions were similar to many poorer homes, such as gas lighting, open fires, no electricity and lack of privacy.[61] Kathleen Jones, who investigated mainly social and legal aspects of mental health policy and practice, commented that for asylum patients who worked during the day and took part in social activities in evenings and weekends, "it was a full life – often much more so than their life outside."[62] She did not state a particular period to which this referred, or whether it was reality at times of greatest austerity.

Standards and quality of care, the parameters which underpinned them, and how and why they changed, often for the worse during the war, are explored thematically in this book. The Board had responsibility for setting and monitoring standards and determining the adequacy of the care provided. It benchmarked asylums against ideals and expectations which were often inferred from its annual reports and letters and circulars of guidance, rather than stated systematically. During the war, with pressure on resources and an assumption of compromise, the Board modified its ratings and accepted lower standards. Its methods of assessing asylum standards were also unconvincing: inspectors focussed on documentation and basic, easily observable physical matters, such as cleanliness. Less tangible and more complex human needs[63] were rarely assessed in a balanced way such as by talking frankly to patients. Patient-derived data is hard to identify and neither Carpenter nor Jones reflected directly on patients' perspectives of their treatment or quality of life.

Developments since the First World War in setting standards and parameters to evaluate healthcare quality can provide useful tools in structuring an historical analysis. Formal mechanisms for conceptualising and measuring healthcare standards originated in the United States of America in the 1930s, aligned to the insurance-based healthcare system.[64] Louis Reed and Dean Clark in 1941 defined healthcare quality according to the scope, quality, quantity and continuity of care, and coordination with social services.[65] In the 1950s, Mindel Sheps acknowledged the intangible nature of healthcare quality, and its assessors tendency to focus on correcting abuses and setting minimum standards, rather than achieving excellence,[66] much as the Board did. Ideas about standards obtained a wider organisational acceptance from the 1960s, based on the work of Avedis Donabedian. Donabedian[67] wrote about the need to define dimensions of quality before specifying what constitutes "goodness" or "badness". However, since stakeholders value quality according to their own interests, defining dimensions is complex. Value for money, system capacity and outcome of treatment, for example, hold different salience for patients, policy makers, financial providers and clinical staff,[68] resulting in conflicting priorities underpinning distribution and utilisation of resources.

Additional concepts derived from new organising categories about mental health services, such as costs, risks, needs and values, and their use in historical analysis were discussed by John Turner et al.[69] He recommended their incorporation into historical research about modern mental health services, but the concepts are also useful markers for studying services in the more distant past. The Care Quality Commission, today's independent regulator of all health and social care services in England, aims to judge whether services are safe, caring, effective, responsive and well led, based on criteria founded on a human rights agenda.[70] Reports of asylum inspectors a century ago reveal their concerns on similar human matters, such as dignity, meaningful life, sense of community, as much personal freedom as possible, and contact with family and the outside world. Achieving a consensus regarding standards of healthcare is challenging. Although there was no consensus for the asylums, awareness of the multiple components of standard setting can assist with focussing historical analysis on a range of issues concerning formulating, prioritising and evaluating earlier standards.

THE LANGUAGE OF THE ASYLUMS

There are many other methodological considerations when writing the history of psychiatry and its institutions, but the use of language looms large. The term "asylum" was itself was controversial. In 1841, a handful of psychiatrists proposed replacing it with "hospital".[71] In 1908, the Royal Commission on "the feeble-minded" also recommended the substitution. It reasoned that the word asylum was misleading as it "savours of the mere detention of extreme cases". Treatment was the goal, so they should be called hospitals.[72] The term was already permitted for privately-run and military psychiatric establishments. A name change alone would not change practice, but it had the potential to influence expectations about treatment and recovery from mental disorders.

Attitudes towards people suffering from mental disorders were expressed by the language of public and official discourse. The public referred to asylum staff as "keepers", more in line with prisons or zoos than hospitals.[73] An "escaped" patient might be described as "at large", a term generally used to refer to a criminal or dangerous animal, and a resident staff member might be "absent without leave", a military term.[74] Patients conflated their asylum experience with prison jargon, substituting seclusion in a side-room or "padded" room with solitary confinement in a "cell".[75] The Lunacy Act designated asylum patients "pauper lunatics", the "pauper" label adding an extra layer of stigma to their "lunacy". Much of the Act's vocabulary resembled that of prisons and workhouses, such as detention, parole, escape and recapture. Nevertheless, the Act used the word "patient" or "lunatic", reserving the more derogatory word "inmate" for occupants of workhouses, although "inmates" continued to appear in asylum committee minutes during the war years when referring to people under their care.[76] Overall, deprecatory language articulated apprehension and fear of asylums and mentally disturbed people, and lack of empathy and compassion, distancing those outside from the human needs of those within.

Another word, "control", commonly features in historiography of asylum practice. The Lunacy Act used the word "control" in several contexts: concerning the administrative control of asylums; when a person in the community was "not under proper care and control, or is cruelly treated"; and for defining the need for urgent admission to a workhouse when behaviour due to a mental disorder risked causing direct harm to the disturbed individual or to others.[77] Control can be an emotive word with multiple connotations which beg the question of who controlled whom, and how and why. The word itself gives no indication of the rationale (such as to protect the patient or others) or the means (humane or coercive) to achieve it, but critics interpret it to imply abuse. Scull described the asylum as "the new apparatus for the social control of the mad", with control the primary objective.[78] This contrasts with the stated aims of the Act for asylums to provide "care and treatment",[79] which inevitably included control of a patient's disturbed behaviour. The aims, means and outcomes of therapeutic and harmful control of asylum patients, are recurring themes in this book.

How to deal sensitively with stigmatising terminology is another conundrum for historians. This is particularly problematic in the history of psychiatry as language associated with mental disorders changes in attempts to discard associated stigmata and to dispel prejudice and discrimination. These attempts often fail: new names selected to replace them tend to acquire old humiliations, while the old language can linger colloquially and in official documents and debates, including in parliament.[80] Old technical terms which perpetuate may acquire broadly derogatory meanings, such as the words imbecile, idiot, spastic and mongol, and may indicate out-dated attitudes of the speakers.

Many historians, including Foucault, Porter and Scull loosely referred to "madness", a generic term for mental symptoms.[81] This may have been appropriate to earlier centuries but was outdated by Edwardian times when "insanity" or "lunacy" were the characteristic generic terms.[82] For historians of psychiatry, antiquated terms may best help understand highs and lows and obstacles and opportunities facing those who tried to cope with, survive in, or improve institutions and clinical practices. In this book antiquated term are therefore used, but with respect for patients and with the intention of illuminating how they fared at the hands of the asylum system.

Over the last century, the meaning of much psychiatric terminology shifted. "Mania", for example, as used in asylums a century ago, meant any mental disturbance characterised by overactivity. In contrast, today it refers specifically to a diagnosis of bipolar disorder. "Dementia", a chronic deterioration of intellectual and social function, was used to refer to GPI or chronic stages of schizophrenia. Dementia could also be categorised as primary, secondary or senile, but the word senile carried multiple meanings and assumptions relating to chronological age, ageing, old age or conditions assumed to be age-related.

Another pair of words, "illness" and "disease", have influenced the choice of language in this book. Eric Cassell, a public health physician, used the word "illness" to mean "what the patient feels when he goes to the doctor", and "disease", "what he has on the way home from the doctor's office."[83] From an anthropological viewpoint, a disease is an independent entity which has specific properties and a recurring identity in whichever setting it appears, and illness relates to the personal experience of it. A disease is assumed to comprise a universal "syndrome", with pathology, causation, symptoms and signs, natural history, treatment and prognosis similar in whatever individual, culture or ethnicity it occurs.[84] If, as in mental disorders, brain disease may be undetectable, the boundaries between illness and disease can be blurred. With lack of clarity and inconsistency in some source material, I have frequently used the deliberately vague terms "disorder", "disturbance" or "distress", meaning a disruption of the individual's usual mental and bodily function.

Some diseases and illnesses can be identified historically if adequate evidence is available. Evidence may be found by careful examination of patients' clinical notes, revealing history, symptoms and physical and mental state examinations. For psychiatric disorders, ascertaining the patterns of symptoms over time is invaluable for determining the type of disorder. Many First World War asylum records allow this sort of clinical analysis. However, since precise psychiatric diagnostic criteria and illness classifications continue to be disputed and to change, detailed "retrospective diagnosis" comparisons with twenty-first century terminology lack meaning. Nevertheless, there is room to construct a "working diagnosis" relating to a class of disorders. A working diagnosis can assist in clarifying other historical evidence, such as about detention, recovery or chronicity requiring long term support. "Translations" into current terminology are sometimes given to enhance understanding for a readership more familiar with twenty-first century mental health vocabulary.

Other less contentious areas of asylum terminology, which nevertheless still require clarification, are professional designations, such as "psychiatrist" and "attendant". The Royal Society of Medicine established a "Section of Psychiatry" in 1912 and "psychiatrist", referring to a medical doctor who specialised in mental illness, replaced the older term "alienist", meaning a doctor who treated "mental alienation".[85] The term psychiatrist gained acceptance in the early twentieth century and is used in this book. Concerning asylum ward staff, "attendants" were generally male and "nurses" female, but this could be inconsistent, such as in the title of the textbook for both, the *Handbook for the Instruction of Attendants on the Insane*, a general training manual for asylum ward staff.[86] Historians have adopted various ways to deal with this gendered language, such as using the generic term "asylum nurse".[87] In this study, as far as possible, I have kept the terminology as it appears in archival sources, but when referring to the combined male and female ward workforce, I have generally called them "ward staff".

Other Methodological Considerations

Four asylums provide the core, in depth source material for this study: Claybury, Colney Hatch, Hanwell and Napsbury. Claybury, Colney Hatch and Hanwell were London County Council (LCC) asylums, and Napsbury served the county of Middlesex, particularly the more urbanised part, coterminous with the LCC's northern administrative border. Despite the distance between any two of these asylums being under 25 miles by road, each had a different institutional wartime footprint. Part of Napsbury was taken over as a war hospital in 1915, the rest in 1916. Colney Hatch had a large proportion of patients from abroad, including Belgian refugees, prisoners of war, interned foreign nationals, and Jewish people from the East End of London.[88] Claybury lost its prestigious scientific research laboratories during the war and suffered extraordinarily high death rates in 1917–1918.[89] Hanwell steered a middle path, receiving hundreds of patients from other asylums vacated for military use, but it experienced neither the diverse ethnic mix of Colney Hatch nor the extreme death rates at Claybury.

Each asylum has an extensive, but not too unwieldy, range of archived records. They provide a flavour of the challenges, contrasts and commonalities of each in a context of prolonged austerity. Some have unique records which were not preserved by the others. Only Colney Hatch, for example, has records of staff salaries and wages,[90] and only Hanwell has note books of staff misdemeanours.[91] Management committee minutes vary in their detail, such as Claybury's which list issues raised by the medical superintendent without giving particulars, contrasting with the others which generally record associated discussions.[92] Reasons for degree of thoroughness of minute keeping were not revealed, but they may have included staff availability to take minutes and to type them, or the wishes of the medical superintendent and management committee, but some give an impression of concealing problems.

Colney Hatch archives include albums of photographs of patients taken for identification purposes shortly after admission.[93] Photographing patients was a common practice in many asylums in the early twentieth century, but the images have received relatively little attention by historians of medicine. Katherine Rawling argued that examining the visual patient record can enhance, and even challenge, established histories of mental illness and medico-psychiatric practice: they may give clues to the doctor–patient encounter, to diagnosis and treatment, and to the patient's experience.[94] In some asylums, photographs of patients resembled police mug-shots,[95] but those from Colney Hatch are varied. They demonstrate aspects of mental and physical health, and attitudes and attire, thus indicating something of the patient's experience. Ludmilla Jordanova recommends that images should be "integral parts of historical arguments" and that historians must be particularly aware of their ethical obligations to their sources, being reflective, accurate, compassionate and responsible.[96] Regarding ethics, all the images of patients conform to the 100-year rule for confidentiality of personal archives. In addition to this, to help preserve anonymity, surnames are not used when discussing them. First names are used to engender a sense of empathy and identification with them, to emphasise that each was a human being whose experience in the asylum we are attempting to understand. The images may also help reveal how the staff—doctors and others—would begin to understand their patients: "Much can be learned" staff were instructed, "from how a person looks, and the expression of the face, the attitude, the dress and other visible signs of a person's emotional and mental state."[97] The images also need to be interpreted in the context of the experience of having one's photograph taken. Some patients may never have been photographed before, so might have found the process unsettling or amusing, although in general, posing for a photograph was a formal event, with facial expressions usually emotionally neutral. Thus, patients in asylum photographs who are smiling may have had an abnormal state of mind, or the image reflected their interactions with the photographer or other staff. As with other sources, there are multiple layers of interpretation.

Another aspect of asylum archives concerns the historical usefulness of clinical notes. Tobia regarded them as bearing the "imprint and prejudices" of the asylum staff,[98] and Andrews suggested that clinical notes "convey more about the preoccupations of the asylum's medical regime than about the patients and their histories".[99] Although clinical notes need to be read critically using knowledge of prevailing medical theories and social views, Tobia and Andrews may have overestimated their subjectivity. Medical notes comprised two main components. First, demographic data plus biographical information, clinical history and examination which were largely objective and collected in a standard way. Second, the medical officer's interpretation of the findings to identify causes, formulate treatment plans and consider prognosis. The medical officer making the notes would have been aware that the Board might scrutinise them during an inspection or the medical superintendent might peruse them when reviewing the patient sometime later.[100] The doctor compiling them would therefore have had a vested interest in demonstrating his (rarely, her) expertise and clinical objectivity in order to enhance his professional reputation. The overall uniformity of clinical note keeping, at least within the asylums investigated in the present study, suggests little scope for personal views.

Archives relating specifically to the four asylums focussed on in this book complement national records but cannot be assumed to be representative of asylums elsewhere across England and Wales. Eight of the nine LCC lunatic asylums had over 2000 beds each, making them larger than most others nationally. In addition, in most lunatic asylums, a significant proportion of patients had a "mental deficiency" (later known as learning disability). This was less so in the London area where the Metropolitan Asylums Board managed many health and welfare institutions, including those for mental deficiency, separate from the lunatic asylums which were the direct responsibility of the LCC.[101] Regarding other effects of wartime contributing to making London's asylums unrepresentative, this is hard to ascertain: according to Stefan Goebel and Jerry White, except for air raids, revisited from the standpoint of the Second World War, First World War London has had relatively little historical analysis.[102] The German bombing raids on London, initially by Zeppelins and later by Gotha bombers, were more intense than in other parts of the country, and induced fear and panic in civilians, but how that affected asylum admissions and the patients and staff within them, is less clear.[103]

Despite the differences, the four asylums did have commonalities with those elsewhere. Their patients suffered the same range of mental and physical disorders. They were all subject to the Lunacy Act, regulation by the Board of Control, and pressures to release staff to serve in the war and to provide beds for physically and mentally injured soldiers. Scotland had separate legislation and some of their asylum practices were more liberal than those south of the border. Scottish records can shed light on happenings in English and Welsh public asylums, as can developments internationally and sources relating to private and military mental hospitals.

In addition to archives relating to each asylum, the Board's records include minutes, unpublished documents and published annual reports. The annual reports have extensive statistical tables about asylums, including disease and death, but they are far from fool-proof. Their focus and extent vary from year to year and administrative categories can be confusing: some tables, for example, include all patients detained under the Lunacy Act, others only those in public asylums. Data were collected according to information priorities, and during the war many details were abandoned due to lack of staff to gather, sort, collate and transcribe them.

Investigating the period 1914–1918 has pros and cons. One con is that much record keeping was abandoned due to staff shortages. A major pro is that archive sources are now beyond the 100-year rule for personal information. Many records, however, have been destroyed. The Board discarded records they considered obsolete, such as letters of complaint, registers of seclusion and restraint, and notices of discharge and death.[104] Survival of other Board records was partly governed by rules about disposing of papers for which preservation for the public record could not be justified.[105] In addition, with space for storing notes at a premium, and wartime paper shortages, some Board and LCC records were pulped.[106] Further destruction took place later. Three-hundred metres of files stored below King Charles Street, Westminster, became unusable by the 1930s: the air "was foul and stagnant" and periodically the vaults flooded necessitating using duck boards to avoid having "to wade in water to get to the shelving".[107] Later, the archiving of records from individual asylums was hardly systematic: Dawn Galer, archivist at the Redbridge Heritage Centre, recalled that most records from Claybury were incinerated when the hospital closed in 1997.

Overall, archives and published sources are available which relate to many aspects of the asylums, including the lives of patients and staff. To best understand what happened to the people, and to attempt to decipher how the asylums functioned during the war years, this book takes a thematic approach. The narrative and argument are clearest when beginning with the context of the relatively fixed infrastructure of the asylums (Chapter 2). The *raison d'être* of the asylums, and the central theme of this book, the people who suffered from mental disorders, their routes into the asylums, their difficulties, care and treatments, are discussed after that (Chapter 3). This is followed by exploring the challenges of staffing the asylums (Chapter 4) and obtaining goods and consumables to satisfy daily living needs during the war (Chapter 5). These themes come together to create an understanding of the patients' daily lives (Chapter 6) and to contextualise and inform the narrative of how physical illness, particularly potentially avoidable infectious diseases (Chapter 7), and "accidents" and suicides and other undesirable outcomes (Chapter 8), affected the lives of those in the institutions.

NOTES

1. Edward Shorter, *A History of Psychiatry* (New York: John Wiley and Sons Ltd, 1997), 33.
2. Richard Hunter and Ida Macalpine, *Psychiatry for the Poor: 1851 Colney Hatch Asylum-Friern Hospital 1973: A Medical and Social History* (London: Dawsons of Pall Mall, 1974), 158.
3. Hunter and Macalpine, *Psychiatry for the Poor*, 50.
4. Hugh Freeman, "Psychiatry in Britain c.1900," *History of Psychiatry* 21 (2010): 312–24, 313.
5. Lunacy Act 1845 section 57.
6. Lord Ashley, Earl of Shaftesbury, in: Treatment of Insane Persons in England and Wales. *Hansard* HC Deb 06 June 1845 vol 81 cc180-202.
7. *First Annual Report of the Board of Control, for the Year 1914* (London: HMSO, 1916) (*BoC AR 1914*), Part 1, 4.
8. *BoC AR 1914*, Part 2, 29–30, 32–33.
9. Freeman, "Psychiatry in Britain": 313.
10. *BoC AR 1914*, Part 1, 8.
11. Steven Cherry, *Mental Healthcare in Modern England: The Norfolk Asylum/St. Andrews Hospital 1810–1998* (Woodbridge, Suffolk: Boydell Press, 2003), 144–45, 170.
12. Peter Barham, *Forgotten Lunatics of the Great War* (New Haven and London: Yale University Press, 2004); Suzie Grogan, *Shell Shocked Britain: The First World War's Legacy for Britain's Mental Health* (Yorkshire: Pen and Sword Books, 2014).
13. E.g. John Crammer, "Extraordinary Deaths of Asylum Inpatients During the 1914–1918 War," *Medical History* 36 (1992): 430–41; Cherry, *Mental Healthcare*; Diana Gittins, *Madness in Its Place: Narratives of Severalls Hospital, 1913–1997* (London: Routledge, 1998).
14. Andrew Scull, *The Most Solitary of Afflictions: Madness and Society in Britain, 1700–1900* (New Haven: Yale University Press, 1993), 1.
15. Michel Foucault, *Madness and Civilization: A History of Insanity in the Age of Reason* (tr. Richard Howard) (London: Routledge, 1989), 4.
16. Lunatic Asylums and Pauper Lunatics Bill. *Hansard* HL Deb 29 July 1845 vol 82 cc1186-93.
17. The official report of all parliamentary debates.
18. Andrew Scull, *Decarceration: Community Treatment and the Deviant: A Radical View* (New Jersey: Prentice Hall, 1977), 25–27.
19. Scull, *Solitary*, 370.

20. Michel Foucault, *Folie et Déraison: Histoire de la Folie à l'Âge Classique* (Paris: Union Générale d'Éditions, 1961); Ronald "RD" Laing, *The Divided Self: An Existential Study in Sanity and Madness* (Harmondsworth: Penguin, 1960); Thomas Szasz, *The Myth of Mental Illness: Foundations of a Theory of Personal Conduct* (London: Paladin, 1961); Erving Goffman, *Asylums: Essays on the Social Situation of Mental Patients and Other Inmates* (1961; Harmondsworth: Penguin, 1980).

21. David Cooper, "Introduction," vii–ix, in Foucault, *Madness and Civilisation* (1989).

22. Paul Tobia, "The Patients of the Bristol Lunatic Asylum in the Nineteenth Century" (PhD thesis, University of the West of England, 2017), https://eprints.uwe.ac.uk/29359, 11.

23. Joseph Melling and Bill Forsythe, *The Politics of Madness: The State, Insanity and Society in England, 1845–1914* (London and New York: Routledge, 2006), 3.

24. Louise Hide, *Gender and Class in English Asylums, 1890–1914* (London: Palgrave Macmillan 2014), 5.

25. Jonathan Andrews and Anne Digby, "Gender and Class in the Historiography of British and Irish Psychiatry," 7–44, in *Sex and Seclusion, Class and Custody: Perspectives on Gender and Class in the History of British and Irish Psychiatry*, ed. Jonathan Andrews and Anne Digby (New York: Rodopi, 2005), 13.

26. Hugh Freeman, "Psychiatry and the State in Britain," 116–40, in *Psychiatric Cultures Compared: Psychiatry and Mental Health Care in the Twentieth Century: Comparisons and Approaches*, ed. Marijke Gijswijt-Hofstra, Harry Oosterhuis, Joost Vijselaar and Hugh Freeman (Amsterdam: Amsterdam University Press, 2005), 119.

27. Shorter, *A History of Psychiatry*, 49.

28. Tobia, "Bristol Lunatic Asylum": 20; Andrews and Digby, "Gender and Class": 13.

29. E.g. Hunter and Macalpine, *Psychiatry for the Poor*.

30. Juliet Hurn, "The History of General Paralysis of the Insane in Britain, 1830 to 1950" (PhD thesis, University of London, 1998), https://discovery.ucl.ac.uk/1349281/1/339949.pdf, 7–8.

31. Claire Hilton, "Psychiatry Past and Present: Do We Need History?" *BJPsych Bulletin* 43 (2019): 126–30.

32. Hurn, "History of General Paralysis": 7–8.

33. John Crammer, *Asylum History: Buckinghamshire County Pauper Lunatic Asylum—St John's* (London: Gaskell, 1990), ix.

34. E.g. Simon Gunn and Lucy Faire (eds), *Research Methods for History* (Edinburgh: Edinburgh University Press, 2016).

35. George Rosen, *The Specialization of Medicine with Particular Reference to Ophthalmology* (New York: Froben Press, 1944).

36. Valerie Pedlar, *The Most Dreadful Visitation: Male Madness in Victorian Fiction* (Liverpool: Liverpool University Press, 2006); Fiona Subotsky, *Dracula for Doctors: Medical Facts and Gothic Fantasies* (Cambridge: Cambridge University Press, 2019).
37. Roy Porter, "History of Psychiatry in Britain," *History of Psychiatry* 2 (1991): 271–79, 277.
38. Diane Carpenter, "'Above All a Patient Should Never Be Terrified': An Examination of Mental Health Care and Treatment in Hampshire 1845–1914" (PhD thesis, University of Portsmouth, 2010), https://researchportal.port.ac.uk/portal/files/5877161/Diane_Carpenter_PhD_Thesis_2010.pdf, 120; Cherry, *Mental Healthcare*; Tobia, "Bristol Lunatic Asylum"; Gittins, *Madness*; Hide, *Gender and Class*.
39. Hide, *Gender and Class*, 171.
40. Carpenter, "'Above All'": 230–31.
41. Mathew Thomson, *The Problem of Mental Deficiency: Eugenics, Democracy, and Social Policy in Britain c.1870–1959* (Oxford: Clarendon Press, 1998): 3–4, 6.
42. German Berrios, *The History of Mental Symptoms: Descriptive Psychopathology since the Nineteenth Century* (Cambridge: Cambridge University Press, 1996); FE James, "Insulin Treatment in Psychiatry," *History of Psychiatry* 3 (1992): 221–35; Edward Shorter and David Healy, *Shock Therapy: A History of Electroconvulsive Treatment in Mental Illness* (London: Rutgers University Press, 2007); John Turner, Rhodri Hayward, Katherine Angel, Bill Fulford, John Hall, Christopher Millard, et al., "The History of Mental Health Services in Modern England: Practitioner Memories and the Direction of Future Research," *Medical History* 59 (2015): 599–624.
43. Anne Rogers and David Pilgrim, *Mental Health Policy in Britain* (London: Macmillan Press Ltd, 1996), 57–58.
44. Freeman, "Psychiatry and the State": 120.
45. Harold Merskey, "Shell Shock," 245–67, in *150 Years of British Psychiatry 1841–1991*, ed. German Berrios and Hugh Freeman (London: Gaskell, 1991), 264.
46. Charles Myers, "A Contribution to the Study of Shell Shock," *Lancet* 13 February 1915: 316–20; Merskey, "Shell Shock": 246–47, 264.
47. Jose Harris, *Private Lives, Public Spirit: Britain 1870–1914* (New York: Oxford University Press, 1993), 1, 251–52; Barham, *Forgotten Lunatics*, 3.
48. Tracy Loughran, *Shell Shock and Medical Culture in First World War Britain* (Cambridge: Cambridge University Press, 2017), 26–27.
49. Anon. "Montagu Lomax MRCS Eng, LRCP Edin," *Lancet* 25 March 1933, 668.

50. Tim Harding, "'Not Worth Powder and Shot': A Reappraisal of Montagu Lomax's Contribution to Mental Health Reform," *BJPsych* 156 (1990): 180–87; John Hopton, "Prestwich Hospital in the 20th Century: A Case Study of Slow and Uneven Progress in the Development of Psychiatric Care," *History of Psychiatry* 10 (1999): 349–69.

51. Montagu Lomax, *The Experiences of an Asylum Doctor* (London: Allen and Unwin, 1921); Harding, "'Not Worth Powder and Shot'": 180.

52. Ministry of Health (MoH), *Report of the Committee on Administration of Public Mental Hospitals* Cmd. 1730 (Chairman: Sir Cyril Cobb) (London: HMSO, 1922); *Report of the Royal Commission on Lunacy and Mental Disorder* (Macmillan Commission) (London: HMSO, 1926); Hopton, "Prestwich Hospital in the 20th Century": 356.

53. Alice Brumby, "'A Painful and Disagreeable Position': Rediscovering Patient Narratives and Evaluating the Difference Between Policy and Experience for Institutionalized Veterans with Mental Disabilities, 1924–1931," *First World War Studies* 6 (2015): 37–55; Roy Porter, "The Patient's View: Doing Medical History from Below," *Theory and Society* 14 (1985): 175–98.

54. Hide, *Gender and Class*; Tobia, "Bristol Lunatic Asylum."

55. Allan Beveridge, "Life in the Asylum: Patients' Letters from Morningside, 1873–1908," *History of Psychiatry* 9 (1998): 431–69, 465.

56. Scull, *Solitary*.

57. Barham, *Forgotten Lunatics*, 7.

58. Lunacy Act 1890, section 41; BoC, "Orders for Destruction of Documents," 31 March 1909 MH 51/723 TNA.

59. MoH, *Committee on Administration*.

60. BoC, Patients admission registers: Rate aided admissions 1913–1918 MH 94/48–53 TNA.

61. Carpenter, "'Above All'": 67, 166.

62. Kathleen Jones, "The Culture of the Mental Hospital," 17–27, in *150 Years of British Psychiatry* ed. Berrios and Freeman, 24.

63. E.g. Abraham Maslow, "A Theory of Human Motivation," *Psychological Review* 50 (1943): 370–96.

64. Roger Lee and Lewis Jones, *The Fundamentals of Good Medical Care* (Chicago: Chicago University Press, 1933).

65. Louis Reed and Dean Clark, "Appraising Public Medical Services," *American Journal of Public Health and the Nation's Health* 31 (1941): 421–30.

66. Mindel Sheps, "Approaches to the Quality of Hospital Care," *Public Health Reports* 70 (1955): 877–86, 883–84.

67. Avedis Donabedian, "Evaluating the Quality of Medical Care," *Milbank Memorial Fund Quarterly* 44 (suppl) (1966): 166–206.

68. Veena Raleigh and Catherine Foot, *Getting the Measure of Quality: Opportunities and Challenges* (London: King's Fund, 2010), 5; World Health Organisation, *Mental Health Policy and Service Guidance Package: Quality Improvement for Mental Health* (Geneva: WHO, 2003), 2.
69. Turner et al. "History of Mental Health Services."
70. Care Quality Commission, "The Five Key Questions We Ask," https://www.cqc.org.uk/what-we-do/how-we-do-our-job/five-key-questions-we-ask.
71. Thomas Bewley, *Madness to Mental Illness: A History of the Royal College of Psychiatrists* (London: RCPsych Publications, 2008), 11.
72. LCC LCC/MIN/00583 Meeting, 18 December 1917, 234, citing *Royal Commission on the Care and Control of the Feeble-Minded* Cd. 4202 (Radnor Report) (London: HMSO, 1908) LMA.
73. William Stoddart, *Mental Nursing* (London: Scientific Press, 1916), 9.
74. BoC, Representative case papers of patients: Eliza Garratt, *Daily Sketch* 21 May 1923 MH 85/62 TNA; Hanwell LCC/MIN/01096 Meeting, 28 August 1916, 156 LMA; "absent without leave," *Oxford English Dictionary Online* (Oxford University Press, 2020) https://www.oed.com/view/Entry/647?rskey=bxHyz2&result=1&isAdvanced=false#eid 5286197.
75. D Davidson, *Remembrances of a Religio-Maniac* (Stratford-on-Avon: Shakespeare Press, 1912), 50–51.
76. Lunacy Act 1890 section 24 (1); e.g. LCC LCC/MIN/00583 Meeting, 30 October 1917, 143 LMA.
77. Lunacy Act 1890 section 169 (3); 13 (1); 21 (1).
78. Scull, *Solitary*, 1–2.
79. Lunacy Act 1890 Form 8.
80. Lunatic Asylum, Worplesdon. *Hansard* HC Deb 24 June 1937 vol 325 cc1369-70.
81. Roy Porter, *A Social History of Madness: Stories of the Insane* (London: Weidenfeld and Nicolson, 1989); Foucault, *Madness and Civilisation*; Roy Porter, *Madness: A Brief History* (Oxford: Oxford University Press, 2003); Andrew Scull, *Madness in Civilization: A Cultural History of Insanity, from the Bible to Freud, from the Madhouse to Modern Medicine* (London: Thames and Hudson, 2015).
82. Crammer, *St John's*, 4.
83. Eric Cassell, *The Healer's Art: A New Approach to the Doctor-Patient Relationship* (Harmondsworth: Penguin Books, 1978), 42.
84. Cecil Helman, "Disease Versus Illness in General Practice," *Journal of the Royal College of General Practitioners* 31 (1981): 548–52, 548.
85. George Savage, "The Presidential Address, Delivered at the Opening Meeting of the Section of Psychiatry of the Royal Society of Medicine,

on October 22nd, 1912," *Journal of Mental Science* 59 (1913) 14–27, 14.

86. Medico-Psychological Association (MPA), *Handbook for the Instruction of Attendants on the Insane* (London: Baillière, Tindall, & Cox, 1885).

87. Neil Brimblecombe, "Asylum Nursing as a Career in the United Kingdom, 1890–1910," *Journal of Advanced Nursing* 55 (2006): 770–77, 771.

88. David Berguer, *The Friern Hospital Story: The History of a Victorian Lunatic Asylum* (London: Chaville Press, 2012), 106.

89. Eric Pryor, *Claybury 1893–1993: A Century of Caring* (London: Forest Healthcare, Mental Health Care Group, 1993), 64.

90. Colney Hatch H12/CH/C/04/004 Male attendants' wages book 1917–1918 LMA; H12/CH/C/03/004 Officers' salaries book 1910–1917 LMA.

91. Hanwell H11/HLL/C/05/008 Female attendants' fine book 1911–1916 LMA.

92. Claybury LCC/MIN/00947 Meetings, 2 March 1916, 56; 30 March 1916, 73 LMA.

93. Colney Hatch H12/CH/B/18/004 Photographs of female patients 1918–1920; H12/CH/B/19/003 Photographs of male patients 1908–1920 LMA.

94. Katherine Rawling, "The Annexed Photos Were Taken Today: Photographing Patients in the Nineteenth-Century Lunatic Asylum," *Social History of Medicine* (2019): https://doi.org/10.1093/shm/hkz060.

95. Rawling, "The Annexed Photos": 10.

96. Ludmilla Jordanova, "Approaching Visual Materials," 30–47, in *Research Methods for History*, ed. Simon Gunn and Lucy Faire (Edinburgh: Edinburgh University Press, 2016): 31.

97. MPA, *Handbook for Attendants on the Insane* (6th Edition) (London: Baillière, Tindall and Cox, 1911), 216.

98. Tobia, "Bristol Lunatic Asylum": 7.

99. Jonathan Andrews, "Case Notes, Case Histories, and the Patient's Experience of Insanity at Gartnavel Royal Asylum, Glasgow, in the Nineteenth Century," *Social History of Medicine* 11 (1998): 255–81, 265.

100. Colney Hatch LCC/MIN/01005 Meeting, 24 March 1916, 103–4 LMA; Lunacy Act 1890 section 38 (4).

101. Ayers Gwendoline, *England's First State Hospitals and the Metropolitan Asylums Board, 1867–1930* (London: Wellcome Institute of the History of Medicine, 1971); Frederick Mott, "Tuberculosis in London County Asylums," *Archives of Neurology and Psychiatry from the Pathological Laboratory of the London County Asylums, Claybury, Essex* 4 (1909): 70–116, 74.

102. Stefan Goebel and Jerry White, "London and the First World War," *London Journal* 41 (2016): 199–218, 200.
103. Joanna Bourke, *Fear: A Cultural History* (London: Virago, 2005) 225.
104. BoC, "Orders for Destruction of Documents," 31 March 1909 MH 51/723 TNA.
105. Public Record Office Act 1877 and 1898. "Rules for the Disposal of Documents which are not of Sufficient Value to Justify their Preservation in the Public Record Office," MH 51/723 TNA.
106. Claybury LCC/MIN/00945 Meeting, 1 October 1914, 185–86 LMA; Public Record Office circular, "Destruction of Papers, Records and Documents," April 1918 MH 51/723 TNA; LCC LCC/MIN/00581 Meeting, 21 March 1916, 476 LMA.
107. BoC, unsigned note, 26 July 1932; Charles Raithby, 2 January 1933, MH 51/723 TNA.

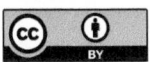

CHAPTER 2

Infrastructure: Rules, Walls, Obstacles and Opportunities

INTRODUCTION

Lunatic asylum practice shifted, arguably for the worse, in the first decade of the twentieth century. Sir George Savage informed his fellow psychiatrists in 1912:

> Fifty years ago we were proud in thinking that we English were the great protectors of the insane. We introduced humane treatments and were content that the patients should be protected, while also society was safeguarded from injury.[1]

In early 1914, the *Lancet* published a letter from psychiatrist Dr. Lionel Weatherly, concerned about declining rates of recovery in the asylums, and the problem of "large asylums for the insane, wherein individualism is so much lost and where, to a very large extent, patients are herded in large numbers together."[2] The asylums were submerged under countless pressures, partly stemming from the Lunacy Act 1890, and associated with long-term detention, overcrowding, and larger institutions having a diminished sense of community.[3] The Board of Control ("the Board"), the central government authority responsible for supervising and regulating the asylums, praised those which managed to preserve patients' individuality and make their lives meaningful,[4] but their praise suggests that high standards were noteworthy rather than universal. The Medico-Psychological Association (MPA, the asylum doctors' professional body,

© The Author(s) 2021

C. Hilton, *Civilian Lunatic Asylums During the First World War*,
Mental Health in Historical Perspective,
https://doi.org/10.1007/978-3-030-54871-1_2

forerunner of the Royal College of Psychiatrists) discussed how to over-come the "grave defects" in British psychiatry. Its recommendations, made in July 1914,[5] vanished amid the turmoil when war broke out a few weeks later.

Outside the asylums, a shifting landscape of national political, social and economic change preceded the war.[6] The Labour Party was formed in 1900. Some movement towards social reform emerged under the Liberal government which came to power in 1905. A state old age pension was first paid in 1909, and the National Insurance Act 1911 created health and unemployment benefits for the workforce, although not for their dependents. The poverty of working-class people more generally, however, received little practical attention. Society was still largely divided by class and functioned in a duty bound, paternalistic, conservative, gender segregated and moralising way. New knowledge and ideas, such as about science, belief in God, the unconscious, the global village and gender, affected outlooks, social interactions and behaviours.[7] However, regarding the asylums, well entrenched older attitudes persisted. In the view of psychiatrist Bernard Hollander in 1912:

It is difficult to get rid of antiquated notions on the subject of lunatics. The popular impression would seem to be that the insane are generally raving and desperate people, whose actions resemble those of beasts and whose language is that of Billingsgate; that consequently they ought to be deprived of their liberty and kept in specially built places of safety where they are protected from doing harm either to themselves or others.[8]

Limited information passed between institution and community, creating a restricted and often unbalanced view of life inside, open to speculation by the general public and contributing to Hollander's "popular impression". The separate world of the asylums fitted with Erving Goffman's model of a "total institution", a place of residence and work where a large number of like-situated individuals, cut off from wider society for an appreciable period of time, together lead an enclosed and formally administered round of life.[9]

The London County Council (LCC) managed nine lunatic asylums of the total institution pattern, altogether comprising about 19,000 patents and 3500 staff.[10] The LCC aimed to achieve a ratio of about 1 staff member to 10 patients during the day and 1–70 at night, in accor-dance with the Board's advice. Montagu Lomax, however, based on his wartime work as an asylum medical officer, regarded these ratios as insufficient to manage patients humanely[11]: they were scarcely enough to allow staff to know all the patients' names, let alone to develop therapeutic relationships.

The staffing situation deteriorated dramatically within weeks of the outbreak of war due to many male asylum workers volunteering or being called up as army reserves.[12] Whether any, let alone suitable, other staff could be obtained partly depended on competition with local industries which might pay better wages and have more desirable hours and conditions of employment.[13] Medical staff levels, already low because of a "shortage of qualified practitioners willing to enter this branch of their profession" worsened.[14] Reduced staffing, accompanied by financial constraints and problems obtaining supplies, risked prejudicing patient care.[15]

The LCC had oversight of staffing and other aspects of its asylums, although it generally delegated implementation to each asylum's lay management, or "visiting", committee (VC). One of the LCC's proposals in 1914 to improve the lives of asylum patients was to provide cinematograph lantern appliances to screen films for them.[16] The course of events goes someway to demonstrating the bureaucracy and complexity of making constructive changes in the asylums. Pre-war, noting that public audiences were reported to panic more frequently at "picture theatres" than in other places of entertainment, the LCC pondered over the likelihood that low levels of lighting required to watch the films might make patients panic.[17] However, the asylum engineers and medical superintendents agreed that lights "sufficiently bright for attendants to see their patients" with the hall having as many exits as public picture theatres, would suffice.[18] The war halted implementation, but the plan re-emerged post-war. A few VCs regarded film-shows as a therapeutic form of recreation and supported their introduction, but others opposed the idea, reiterating the pre-war rhetoric that patients would panic in the dark.[19] Their argument disregarded the fact that, during the war, asylums were bound by the same rules for low-level indoor lighting as domestic households, and they ignored the evidence that patients did not panic more than the general public in the dark, during air raids or if fires broke out at night.[20] Post-war, Herbert Ellis, a VC member who was also a magistrate, declared that he did not want patients "more mad than they are. I hope they won't have cinemas. I think that is what drives many patients in."[21] As well as VC discussions influenced by personal opinions rather than evidence, other factors thwarted implementation, including the poor state of the economy and the Board's preoccupations about licences and legalities of film-shows more than their contribution to normalising patients' lives.[22] Rules, regulations and personal opinions influenced decision making, contributing to a mismatch between evidence, ideals of care and experiences of asylum patients who remained virtually voiceless.[23] Sometimes, the Board admitted, rules were too rigid,[24] and, inequitably, the patients and lowest tiers of staff, comprising the largest groups in the institution, had the least say in decisions and bore the brunt of the mismatch.

The introduction to this chapter sketches out some of the organisational challenges faced by the asylums in 1914, including: staffing difficulties; falling standards of care; bureaucratic and uninformed decision making; and the public keeping the asylums at arm's length. The rest of this chapter will explore in more depth aspects of asylum management which maintained the total institutions, exerted control over them and shaped the lives of patients and staff within them. The Lunacy Act was a *fait accompli*. Heavily legalistic and created with the needs of the general public rather than the patients in mind, it stipulated asylum rules which constrained practice in ways which some said made it unfit for purpose. In Kathleen Jones' view it was "out of date before it was passed."[25] The Act shaped the asylum organisational hierarchy, with the Board at the top and local tiers of lay management which coordinated the asylums day-to-day in association with senior asylum employees, particularly the medical superintendent. National and local government and professional organisations interacted with and influenced this hierarchy. As the war progressed, the asylums made compromises to meet military requirements, providing accommodation for both mentally and physically injured soldiers. These compromises revealed, and added to, the poor standards of care provided to civilian patients. Moving forward into the plans for post-war reconstruction, the government prioritised physical health over mental health.

The Lunacy Act 1890: "Red Tapism", Admissions, Finance, Reform and Change

James W, a 57-year-old middle class man from Sussex, was certified under the Lunacy Act and detained in Hanwell Asylum. Two weeks later he was "discharged not insane".[26] We know from court records that his wife Mary petitioned for a judicial separation, raising suspicion that perhaps, vindictively, she tried to have him "put away".[27] Although wrongful confinement appeared rare, and as with James W, the decision could be overturned, when it occurred it frightened the public and jolted the authorities into considering ever more legalistic measures to avoid repetition.[28] Thus lawyers had played a major part in creating the Lunacy Act 1890, whereas asylum physicians with practical experience of treating insane people had little influence.[29] The outcome was an Act which prescribed everything in great detail with nothing left to chance or to professional discretion and provided little scope for future development.[30] It undermined the flexibility required for rehabilitation and compromised therapeutic interventions for patients.[31] It set penalties for infringements,[32] which fostered a risk-averse culture and created fears of punishment for staff and loss of reputation for the leadership. Mary Riggall, a patient, provided an example of the defensive, risk-averse stance in her memoir. She described how one woman was discharged then readmitted a week later after she hurled a knife at her family doctor. The medical superintendent told Riggall: "If people have to come back again as quickly as this, the doctors outside will say I don't know my job."[33]

Some psychiatrists openly criticised the Act. Daniel Hack Tuke, a psychiatrist at the time it became law, commented that "the great evil of the Act was that it was red tapism from the beginning to the end".[34] Some red tape was undoubtedly necessary, but administrative minutiae and bureaucratic form filling could detract from caring for patients and inhibit innovation. Sir Frederick Needham, a senior member of the Board, also reflected on the Act which may have suited the public but hardly worked in the patient's best interest:

> let the public feel the inconvenience of this Act which *they demanded* and has been passed in obedience to this demand, and as soon as the public have sufficiently felt the inconvenience of the Act, which we always objected to, I think they will demand a public remedy.[35]

Lionel Weatherly (Fig. 2.1), one of the most outspoken psychiatrists of his generation, regarded the Act as "obnoxious" and "To tinker with [it] is no use. It should be burnt on the rubbish fire of pernicious Acts."[36] Weatherly's book on lunacy law reform, *A Plea for the Insane*, was welcomed by his colleagues.[37] Tuke, Needham, Weatherly, Hollander and Lomax all challenged the value of the Act and its consequences for asylum practices and patient wellbeing.

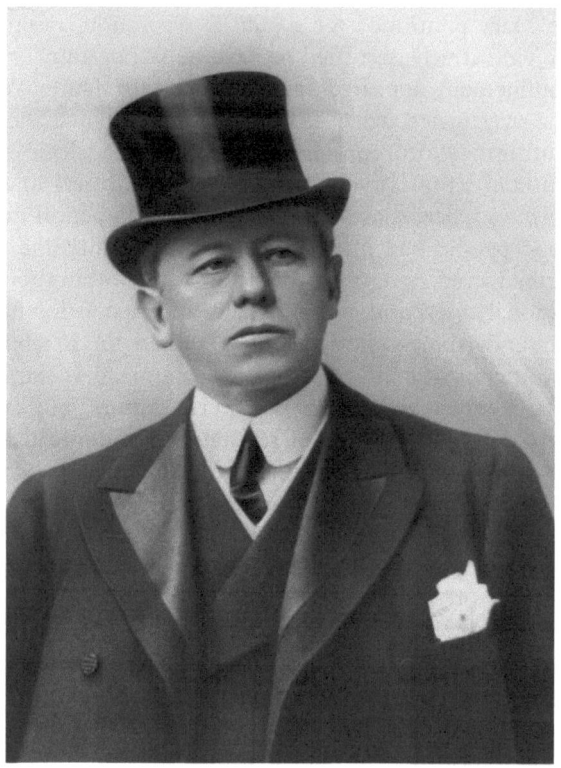

Fig. 2.1   Dr. Lionel Weatherly (Copyright: Bradford upon Avon Museum)

The Act prohibited public expenditure on out-patient clinics or on using asylums as hospitals for voluntary patients who required treatment for their early, mild, or "borderland" (uncertain) mental disturbance.[38] Thus, only people who had the means to pay privately could consult a psychiatrist in the early stages of their mental disorder, a clinically unreasonable situation.[39] Psychiatrists regarded the private-public divide as invidious. They wanted more flexible access to their services. They alleged that mentally disturbed people sought help from alternative, ill-trained and inexperienced practitioners, such as "psycho-therapeutists", hypnotists, faith healers, occult magnetic healers, quacks who made money from selling cheap medication, and physicians "who not infrequently recommend a sea voyage for an early suicidal melancholic, who returns to trouble them no more."[40] Hollander viewed delays caused by the Act's restrictions on early treatment as scandalous: "In no other form of disease is 'appropriate' treatment so tardily initiated and so difficult of attainment."[41] Drawing on his experience of continental clinics and private practice in London, he wrote that delaying treatment worsened outcomes, patients "becoming confirmed lunatics by neglect".[42] He wanted facilities for advice and early treatment for lower classes as well as the more well-to-do "which would do away with half of the difficulty we experience in treating the insane to-day."[43] Dr. Wolsely-Lewis of the Kent County Asylum, Barming Heath, argued that a less restrictive Act could prevent much suffering

> a wife who has a husband subject to attacks of recurrent insanity, with intervals of mental health, is obliged when the attacks are coming on and before the law can intervene to endure the misery of living with him as his wife, of seeing daily the evil influence he exercises on the home, and of watching his reason tottering to its fall – perhaps in constant dread for the safety of her children and herself; or, again, a husband whose wife suffers from recurrent attacks – finds his home and children neglected while he is away at work, well knowing from past experience what harm can be done before his wife again becomes certifiable.[44]

The Board agreed with Wolsely-Lewis, commenting that "the medical side of insanity was to some extent sacrificed to the legal".[45]

A certificate for admission was binding on an asylum to accept a patient, and without it, the asylum would turn a patient away. At one asylum: "A former patient came back in pouring rain and asked to be admitted, but had to be refused".[46] At another, the porter recognised a former patient when she arrived by taxi in a distressed state. He told the driver to take her to the police station and informed the medical superintendent about his action.[47] Under the Lunacy Act, "certifying" patients for admission usually fell to doctors who were general practitioners or workhouse medical officers who lacked specific expertise or post-graduate training in psychiatry, and to magistrates, more often associated with making judgments in criminal cases. Concurring with public concerns, the magistrate's role was to ensure that no one was unjustly deprived of their liberty. Delegating certification to non-psychiatrists aimed to prevent asylum doctors from admitting patients into their own institution which might provide them with personal or pecuniary advantage.

As a result, asylum doctors who had the specialist knowledge and experience of treating mental disorders were excluded from deciding who might be best placed in an asylum. The asylum admission process was closer to prison detention than an admission to a general hospital for a physical ailment, which was under the control of the patient and hospital doctor. Since asylum certification could be prolonged indefinitely, it could create more fear than a prison sentence of finite duration. Discharge from an asylum was also cumbersome. A medical officer and two VC members had to approve it for each patient. Coordinating this often delayed discharge, inadvertently increasing bed occupancy and overcrowding.

People certified under the Act and admitted to public asylums were designated by the doubly stigmatising term "pauper lunatic". The word "pauper" was associated with poverty and destitution and the demeaning epithet of "undeserving". It came to signify any financial dependence on the Board of Guardians ("the Guardians"), the locally elected body which oversaw welfare in its neighbourhood, payed for by local taxation. The Guardians had direct responsibility for social welfare, public health and the workhouse infirmaries which functioned as local general hospitals. For the asylums, the Lunacy Act delineated the Guardians' obligations: to fund the treatment of patients usually resident in their locality, and to delegate the asylum's management to the VC.[48] Typically, when an asylum sought funding from the Guardians to support a patient, the Guardians would assess the patient's finances to determine if they were able to make means-tested contributions to their care. Despite the contributions, the patient was still designated a pauper lunatic. This was raised by Labour Member of Parliament (MP) John Clynes in the House of Commons in 1910, on the grounds that the term pauper lunatic was misleading and offensive to their relatives. The Home Secretary disregarded the emotional distress, blamed the Lunacy Act,[49] and stated that relatives' contributions did not cover the full cost of the patient's stay, so patients were still dependent on the Guardians.[50] The combination of lunatic and pauper designations with "undeserving" implications, plus the need for a magistrate to oversee admission to an asylum, created a multiple whammy of indignity. It also contributed to deterring people from seeking psychiatric help until they, or their family, could cope no longer.[51]

In the context of overcrowded asylums during the war, some leniency appeared in the way the Lunacy Act was interpreted, such as responding to requests from relatives of patients for the patient to be discharged into their care. Some of these requests, refused shortly before the war on the grounds that the patient remained too unwell, were suddenly agreed when the war began, despite no clinical improvement. Other patients, less helpfully, were discharged from asylums, still unwell, into the care of relatives who had previously been unable to manage them.[52] By interpreting some sections of the Lunacy Act more flexibly, asylum admissions could be limited to the most disturbed civilian patients, while those considered, dependent, harmless or senile were placed in workhouses.[53] Marriott Cooke, who may have had some conflict of interest as a Board member delegated to work with the War Office, stated that long-term workhouse placements suited many asylum patients: they worked well, became attached to the Master and Matron, and had social networks in the local community which would not have been feasible had they stayed in the asylum. An additional motivation was that placements in workhouse were cheaper than in asylums. Conveniently for the Board and the budgets, as Cooke reassured the social welfare reformer Beatrice Webb, former patients "need never be returned to the more expensive asylum accommodation".[54] Occasionally, contingency plans necessitated ignoring the Lunacy Act altogether, such as when considering how to manage the worst scenario, that of a German invasion into Essex: for Severalls asylum near Colchester, the Board and medical superintendent agreed that helpless and violent patients would remain in the asylum under the Red Cross flag and the remainder would "take their chance with other inhabitants" of the area, free to leave without formality.[55]

The Lunacy Act stipulated the maximum amount that a VC could charge the Guardians for each patient: 14s (shillings; 70p) a week. This covered staff salaries and related expenses, some maintainance of the buildings and estate, and allowed for expenditure on consumables, such as food and clothing, at around the level of the poorest of urban households.[56] Asylum fees could only be raised above 14s if the proposal was first published in a local newspaper.[57] In the context of negative pubic perspectives and fear about mental disorder and its treatment which discouraged expenditure on anything other than the cheapest containment in asylums, the Guardians were reluctant to take steps which might make them unpopular with their electorate.[58] In Lomax' words, the "welfare of patients is pitted against the cost to the ratepayers".[59]

With almost no inflation between 1890 until 1914, the 14s maximum was tolerable, but fear of exceeding it ensured that many VCs strived to minimise their expenditure. With wartime inflation, the asylums tried to remain within the 14s stipulated, despite having to increase staff salaries to cover the higher cost of living.[60] In mid-1915, the LCC was relieved to find that costs of care had risen slower than expected mainly due to economies in the asylums. It did not refer to the possibility that economies might be detrimental to patients, but warned that war time inflation would continue to rise and that asylums must comply with public retrenchment directives,[61] a tall-order for an already cash-strapped system. Financial constraints contributed to friction between VC members and medical superintendents who objected to being told to reduce standards which were "the result of many years of thought and experience" with the warning that "a lowering of standard does not necessarily lead to a saving".[62] Psychiatrist and pathologist Richard Gundry Rows berated the asylum authorities for their financial preoccupations. He expected that if mental disturbance was treated in the early stages (in line with provision for private patients) and that treatment was founded on science, the public would grumble less about expense, in the same way as they accepted rising costs of treating physical disorders.[63] Another psychiatrist, John Keay, then president of the MPA, put asylum expenditure into perspective: the war cost £6.8 million a day compared to £4.6 million annually for the entire UK asylum system. Keay argued that the country could afford better if it wished: prevention was preferable, for both mental disorder and war, but otherwise, like the war, care and treatment for mentally unwell people was a necessity.[64]

As well as minimising expenditure, the asylums tried many ways to subsidise their budgets, with practices established pre-war including recycling, selling or otherwise putting surplus asylum material to good use. These practices continued during the war, but with austerity and material shortages, lower standards were permitted when considering what should be repaired, condemned or recreated.[65] The LCC enquired of their asylums how they economised, such as whether they cooked potatoes in their jackets, and how many garments nurses were allowed to send to the laundry.[66] Some measures showed ingenuity and skill: Colney Hatch, for example, installed tanks in the sculleries to collect grease for making soap, and Hanwell sold hundreds of empty jam tins for 2d (old pence; 1p) each.[67] Colney Hatch also advertised tar, a by-product from the asylum gas-works, at 6d (2½p) a gallon and invited tenders for tons of unwanted lead which had accumulated.[68] Lead was used in munitions manufacture, so was in demand, but it was also a constituent of paint.

Asylums required permission to use their own stocks of paint, but only for essential maintenance, such as repainting rust-prone, out-door iron emergency staircases (Fig. 2.2).[69]

Lunacy law in England and Wales contrasted with that in Scotland which permitted less legalistic approaches to treating mental disorders in publicly funded institutions, ideas which the Board and other psychiatrists were keen to follow.[70] One manifestation of Scottish innovation was the "psychiatric observation unit" established in 1887 at Glasgow's Barnhill Hospital, the local "poorhouse", by John Carswell, a psychiatrist committed to improving public health.[71] Similar units followed in Edinburgh and Dundee. Their wards ran under psychiatric leadership, in contrast to similarly named "observation wards" in England which were led by non-psychiatrically trained workhouse infirmary physicians, and although they aimed to provide initial assessment of mental disturbance, this was often cursory. Standards varied and at times were "disquieting."[72]

Fig. 2.2 Emergency staircase at Hanwell (Photograph by author, 2017)

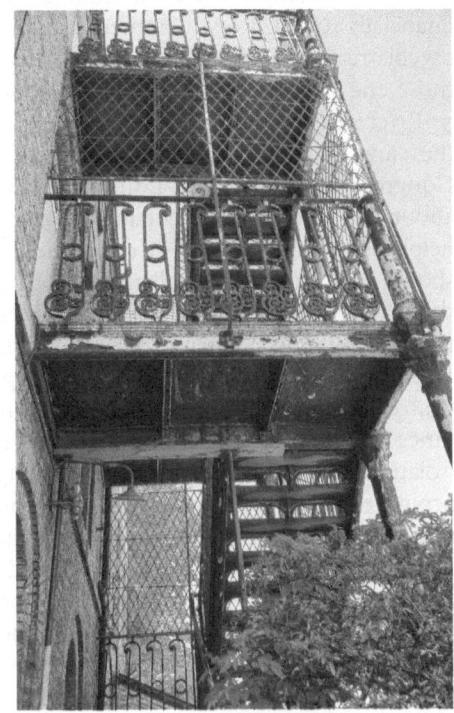

The model of having psychiatrist-led units outside the asylums and associated with universities was also part of the scene in Germany and Austria and much admired by psychiatrists in England. Emil Kraepelin, a physician, led one of these, a university-funded, research and teaching focussed, psychiatric "clinic" in Munich which allowed admission of patients with early stages of mental disorders on their own volition without legal procedures.[73] Kraepelin's clinic admitted over 1500 patients a year for early treatment.[74] It comprised 120 in-patient beds and out-patient facilities. Wards were quiet and un-crowded with no more than 10 beds in each, contrasting with wards of 50 or more beds in many English asylums. It was well-staffed, with 16 doctors and 53 ward staff plus out-patient physicians, compared to an English asylum, typically with 4 doctors and around 120 ward staff for 1000 patients.[75] High staffing levels were inevitably costly, but with thorough medical assessment and active treatment many patients were discharged, although local long-stay asylums backed up clinics when that was not feasible. Overall, avoiding long-term admissions meant that the clinics were financially sound. Rows commented that Kraepelin's model would enable psychiatrists in England "to take a more honourable position amongst those engaged in the conflict with disease." [76]

Psychiatrist Adolph Meyer in Baltimore was also an advocate of the clinic model. When Meyer addressed the seventeenth International Congress of Medicine in London in 1913,[77] he expressed hopefulness about the treatment of mental disorders, compared to the "pessimism and helplessness" of his English colleagues.[78] He recommended that clinics should be in hospitals familiar to local people, not in asylums. He noted the clinics' goals of "service to the patient rather than to an administrative system" and compared them to "wholesale handling" in asylums.[79] Placing psychiatrists in clinics alongside physicians and surgeons in major centres of clinical practice, teaching and research, could provide opportunities for better psychiatric training, help alleviate some of the professional isolation and acquired stigma of working in a typical rural asylum, and promote exchange of ideas across disciplines. Meyer attributed the slow rate of up-take of the clinic model in Britain to the moralising attitude of Anglo-Saxon communities, which aimed to regulate and remove, rather than to understand psychiatric conditions.[80] Although the observation wards in Scotland were superior to those in England, none of them provided the intensive assessment or treatment of their German counterparts.[81] A few German-style psychiatric clinics emerged in the USA, founded on the understanding that they were as necessary to psychiatry as to any other medical discipline.[82] In England, Hollander criticised the inhumanity associated with the lack of similar facilities:

> The want of such an establishment in every great urban centre in the country is an expression of passive cruelty and indifference which can only be described as a blot upon our much vaunted civilisation.[83]

University teaching hospital psychiatric facilities were not alien to England,[84] but their value was debated, with particular concern that they might encourage neglect of incurable patients in asylums.[85] Teaching hospital facilities would be permitted under the Lunacy Act because these hospitals were funded from voluntary or charitable sources, rather than drawing on local authority public funds. By 1913, several London teaching hospitals had some sort of out-patient department, but still no in-patient facilities.[86]

Frederick Mott, a dedicated physician and researcher in psychiatry who directed the LCC's Central Pathological Laboratory, proposed the first publicly run German-style psychiatric clinic in England after visiting Kraepelin's clinic in Munich. A gift of £30,000 to the LCC in 1907 by another psychiatrist, Henry Maudsley, kick-started the project, with Mott facilitating the protracted negotiations behind it.[87] Negotiating and building this new "Maudsley Hospital" took eight years.[88] Planned for civilian patients, it became a military mental hospital in which Mott took a significant lead, and only when no longer required for that purpose, in 1923, were its doors opened to its original target population.

THE BOARD OF CONTROL, ASYLUM LEADERSHIP AND THEIR CHALLENGES

The Lunacy Act delegated oversight and regulation of the asylums to the Commissioners in Lunacy. This body was reformulated as the Board of Control by the Mental Deficiency Act 1913, but the leadership remained largely unchanged, maintaining stability and expertise, but hardly introducing new blood. The Mental Deficiency Act stipulated Board membership: salaried lawyers and doctors; unpaid lay-commissioners; at least two women, one paid and one unpaid; and at least one member able to undertake inquiries in Welsh.[89] The Board had no direct health-related ministerial-level oversight but was accountable to the Lord Chancellor for some legal matters, and to the Home Office for many other duties under the rubric of protecting the public and safeguarding rights and liberties of individuals. Within the asylums it worked with the medical superintendents, other senior asylum officers, and the VCs. The VCs were appointed annually[90] and consisted of well-meaning lay people of relatively high social standing in the local community but with little expertise in subjects on which they were expected to make decisions.

In addition to monitoring and regulating public lunacy and mental deficiency institutions, the Board directly managed the criminal lunatic asylums and oversaw many small private establishments which consumed a disproportionate amount of its time. Its lunacy, mental deficiency and criminal asylum roles developed separately, reflecting public understanding. The public regarded mentally deficient people as unfortunate and generally harmless, thus worthy of compassion and philanthropic co-operation with the statutory services. By contrast, according Kathleen Jones, "emotions aroused by the thought of mental illness were so painful that the whole subject tended to be blocked". The public offered little support for mentally disturbed people, for whom care was largely provided by statutory organisations and salaried workers.[91] One small charity, the Mental After Care Association (MACA), functioned mainly in the London area and aimed to assist people regain their confidence and independence after discharge from lunatic asylums.[92] As a further indication of the pecking order of sympathy, philanthropic support was more readily available to criminals on release from prison than pauper lunatic patients on discharge from asylums.[93]

A time-consuming and prolonged dispute about a single patient greeted the Board at its first committee meeting in April 1914, just four months before the war: which institution, a workhouse infirmary or a lunatic asylum, should provide care for 80-year-old Ellen Q? The stalemate was attributed to an invalid Lunacy Act certificate.[94] Since a certificate was normally binding on an asylum to accept a patient, questioning its legality was a convenient way to allow the asylum to refuse to do so, but the deadlock allowed other more fundamental concerns to surface.

The Barnet Guardians approached the Board to intervene in the dispute between them and Napsbury's VC who refused to admit Ellen Q from their workhouse infirmary. Ellen's disturbed behaviour had necessitated the Guardians employing two nurses specifically to look after her over several months "at a cost of Two Guineas a week for salaries besides rations and other expenses."[95] From Napsbury's perspective, a shortage of female beds meant that "senile" women should not be admitted for care; vacant beds "were to be reserved for patients obviously requiring Asylum care and treatment," a recurrent theme in the twentieth century, of excluding older people on the assumption that they would not benefit from care and that younger people were automatically more deserving of expert attention.[96] The Board objected to this discriminatory stance, stating that Ellen's on-going disturbed behaviours meant that she required admission and should not be "deprived of such care merely on the score of age."[97] Napsbury's VC did not budge.[98] The Board expressed "grave dissatisfaction"[99] stating that the VC showed "a callousness and indifference to the welfare of the insane, which the Board cannot consider creditable to any lunacy authority."[100] Eventually Dr. Rotherham from the Board, and Dr. Rolleston, medical superintendent at Napsbury, jointly assessed Ellen, but we are not privileged to know their opinions: minutes at Napsbury and from the Board fell silent on the matter as the country moved into war.[101] Bed shortages, monetary concerns, rejection of older people from hospitals and asylums, and rigid but opposing perspectives of different players in the fragmented healthcare system were among the tension-creating issues looming large when war broke out.

Visiting committee minutes chiefly recorded practical problems of asylum management and attempts to solve them. Minutes at Colney Hatch demonstrated a range of wartime challenges, such as: providing for refugees, enemy aliens and military patients; managing staff sickness, vacancies, salaries and "war bonuses"; and dealing with infestations of rats, mice and beetles and an outbreak of typhoid fever.[102] Minutes which reported more problems and the actions taken to remedy them could be interpreted in several ways, including that those asylums had higher, rather than lower, standards. The VC's minutes rarely mentioned individual patients, except in the context of discharge or untoward incidents, although occasionally they recorded gifts from former patients, their relatives and staff, grateful for care and support given. Overall, however, since the management hierarchy assumed that asylum care was humane, good practice and kindnesses received little direct comment. Minutes also give insight into activities arranged for patients, and asylum practices such as arranging trial leave before discharge and providing a monetary allowance to assist the patient during it. The Lunacy Act recommended this leave plus the allowance, but VCs often overlooked it, even if the patient had no other means of support, reinforcing the impression that VCs cut corners on short-term expenditure, even if that might hamper recovery in the longer term.[103]

The Board desired to solve problems in asylums and to ensure good standards, to promote innovation, staff education, research into mental disorders and more liberal lunacy legislation, but it only had authority to advise and lacked power to mandate change.[104] It relied on naming and shaming, suggestion, cajoling and using "informal tactics of persuasion".[105] It did not shy away from criticising medical superintendents and VCs. The Board, for example, pointed out that the medical superintendent at Colney Hatch needed to keep a close eye on ward safety and "impress upon the nurses the absolute necessity of refraining from anything in the nature of rough treatment", with the implication that rough treatment had occurred under his leadership.[106] The Board described another superintendent as "able and energetic in the discharge of his duties" but he needed to develop his asylum "on enlightened modern lines",[107] implying that he was behind the times. The Board could be precise and targeted, verging on harsh, with their criticism sometimes rejected hostilely by the recipient.[108]

To help monitor asylums the Board undertook annual inspections of all the institutions in its charge. However, without formally defined or agreed concepts and criteria for standards of care, Board members judged quality against ideals and expectations inferred from the annual reports, and letters and circulars giving guidance, and from their own experience, including from previous inspections and discussions in their regular team meetings. The effect of subjective, non-standardised values for determining standards could be moderated when two inspectors worked together, but it was problematic when an inspector worked alone. Aware of this, pre-war, the Board delegated two people, usually a doctor and a lawyer to undertake inspections together, but, by 1915 staff shortages reduced this to one.[109] That a lawyer could undertake an inspection alone indicated the emphasis placed on law, rules and regulations, rather than the care and treatment provided and the patients' mental and physical wellbeing. Lawyers were confident that they could undertake the task, although it is hard to believe that they could advise on clinical matters, make judgements on patterns of illness or death statistics or judge conclusively that a patients' complaints were "evidently based on a delusional condition of mind"[110] so that they could justify ignoring them.

Asylum inspections were meant to be unannounced, to give a true understanding of practices within. However, a "mysterious telepathy" between asylums could provide a couple of hours warning during which time staff were stirred into action, getting patients up, sorting out bed covers, cleaning side rooms, tidying, and improving the visual impression to which the inspectors paid particular attention. A message from the porter's lodge, or a warning along a corridor of approaching senior people, or even an unexpected turn of the key in a locked ward door, could alert staff to their approach.[111] Inspections often lasted one or two days, providing ample time for further window-dressing.[112] Many Board members had previously worked as medical superintendents, so were likely to be aware of the mechanisms by which an asylum could demonstrate high standards during an inspection. If the Board challenged those practices it risked exposing past practices of its own elite membership. By not doing so, the Board contributed to perpetuating the inspection culture and its drawbacks which could undermine rather than enhance patients' wellbeing. Ultimately, a good rating mainly reassured the leadership and the public that all was well, fitting with Goffman's assertion that total institutions present themselves to the public as rational organisations designed "as effective machines for producing a few officially avowed and officially approved ends."[113] Beyond those endpoints, few questions were asked about asylum processes and outcomes.

Preoccupied with asylum safety and disasters which could generate adverse public opinion, the Board scrutinised management of dangerousness and risks of all sorts.[114] Inspectors might initiate a fire drill,[115] aware of the high fire risk with asylums typically having coal fires and gas lighting in wards with wooden floorboards shined with inflammable floor polish and where patients smoked.[116] In 1914, the Board was encouraging installation of central heating, electric lighting and electric fire alarms.[117] Later that year it added telephones and chemical fire extinguishers, both necessary in the event of bombing, with extinguishers essential in the event of a bomb destroying the water mains supplying the fire hydrants.[118] Asylums which lacked the new technologies devised their own fire and air raid warning systems: at Colney Hatch in the event of an air raid warning, the police informed the gate porter or the attendant manning the switchboard who informed the medical superintendent[119]; at Hanwell, if the boiler house engine driver heard a local explosion, he sounded the hooter to summon attendants and workmen who were off duty.[120]

Lomax described inspectors as hurried and blasé, ward staff as constrained and anxious, medical superintendents bored and indifferent, and lunatics composed and critical, realising that it was all staged.[121] Inspectors focussed largely on the fabric and facilities and what could be observed directly, and senior asylum staff generally accompanied them around the site.[122] This gave patients little chance to speak to inspectors in confidence. Officials who spoke with patients tended to accept their compliments but discount their criticisms, which they attributed to distorted judgement due to their mental disorder. This selectivity was illogical. It also meant that formal inspections were unlikely to detect abusive practices which left no visible bodily or documentary trace. In addition, quiet patients were interpreted as being well cared for, rather than intimidated into submissiveness. Although Lomax referred to the eminent psychiatrist Henry Maudsley using the term "asylum-made lunatics",[123] there was little acknowledgement of the effects of institutionalisation on the behaviour and mental state of patients. That understanding developed several decades later, particularly from the work by Russell Barton in the UK and Erving Goffman in the USA.[124]

As well as ignoring most criticisms by patients, the Board was intolerant of other negative comments, particularly from people of lower social or employment ranks. The Board received a report written by some temporary attendants during the war which mentioned harsh treatment of patients. In response, the Board justified cold-hearted practices and low standards as inevitable due to wartime constraints.[125] Attributing poor care to the war, passed the buck and alleviated pressure on the Board to attempt to advocate for the patients and remedy the situation. Abdicating responsibility was more comfortable psychologically than the uncertainty of having to deal creatively and effectively with substandard care. However, their responses were questionable ethically: physician-members of the Board would have been familiar with the medical ethics principle *primum non nocere*, first do no harm. Denying or hiding problems gave the outside world the impression that all was well. The leadership feared adverse publicity which might undermine the reputation of the asylums and their own status. When the press reported that food at Colney Hatch was "abominably cooked", and when Graylingwell Asylum appeared in the *Times* as "Graylingwell Hell", they responded with rebuttal rather than planning to investigate.[126] After the war, at the Cobb Inquiry, deeper probing into the standards of care and treatment provided in asylums revealed both evasiveness and ignorance of some of the leadership about the poor care they provided for patients.[127]

As with other criticisms of the asylums by those of lower rank, when faced with Lomax's critique of wartime Prestwich Asylum, the Board maintained its usual tactic of downplaying the allegations.[128] This contrasted with the stance taken by Chief Medical Officer Sir George Newman, who acknowledged the variable asylum standards. Newman wrote that Prestwich was one of the least satisfactory asylums:

> buildings are antiquated, and the Medical Superintendent is not conspic-
> uously efficient....Dr Lomax saw the English asylum system at its worst,
> the normal defects of Prestwich being aggravated by shortage of staff and
> strict rationing of food....Broadly speaking it is true that our asylums are
> barracks rather than hospitals and the insane are treated more like prisoners
> than patients.

Newman attributed the difficulties to broader organisational factors pre-war, including: the Lunacy Act; local funding without central government funding; penny-pinching VCs; and the Board being expected to undertake "police duties." He asserted that the issues Lomax raised were well known, an indictment of a government which failed to remedy them. He was pleased that Lomax's book "directed public attention to the defects of a system which has hitherto been taken on trust."[129]

Another aspect of the Board's work concerned collating data, aimed to detect trends to help guide the asylums. Pre-war, asylum staff filled numerous registers and forms which the Board then examined, including about infectious diseases, suspicious deaths, suicides, disciplinary matters, finances, facilities and numbers of "escapes".[130] The Board's first annual report, for 1914, made information available concerning benchmarks, pitfalls to avoid and goals to emulate. The report included quantitative statistical tables and rich narratives of each asylum's inspection: strengths and weaknesses, innovation and stagnation, praise and criticism. Some asylums were good, others far from ideal, but overall, the Board described them as "creditable", even though, by the end of the year, the war had "affected the Asylums to a serious extent".[131] Unfortunately, the asylum narratives were omitted from the annual reports from 1915 until after the war due to staff and paper shortages. The Board also recognised the time-consuming nature of data collection and suspended much of it during the war. As with inspections undertaken by a lone non-medical inspector, amid many other changes occurring simultaneously, it is unclear whether, or how much, these data and publishing cutbacks affected patients' wellbeing.

General histories of psychiatric services express divergent views about the Board, from Kathleen Jones' praise for their good work, to criticism, such as by Charles Webster, that under its "jealous eye...the system ossified."[132] Marriott Cooke, a member of the Board (and its chairman 1916–1918),[133] was cited as saying that it regarded itself as "the particular friends of the lunatics".[134] Sir Robert Armstrong-Jones, medical superintendent at Claybury until 1916 (knighted in 1917), concurred:

> It may be said without fear of contradiction or exaggeration, that the Board of Control are the best friends of the Insane, and it is to this Board that is due the credit for the high place that the treatment of the Insane is known to occupy in the mind of the informed public in this country.[135]

Armstrong-Jones wrote this just after the Cobb Inquiry. He may have written it to counteract negative public opinion at that time, but it is difficult to justify his sentiments.

Special Care? Service Patients and Other Groups

In contrast to lack of public interest in the welfare of mentally disturbed civilian patients in the asylums, public concern and sympathy was aroused by distressing mental symptoms presenting in soldiers fighting in the front line early in the war. In February 1915, Captain Charles Myers of the Royal Army Medical Corps described three soldiers suffering from mental and physical disturbances but without physical injury. Their symptoms were attributed to shells bursting close to them, but curiously, despite the noise of the blast, their hearing was not disturbed. This observation contributed to Myers concluding that the condition resembled hysteria. The term "shell shock" was already used by the soldiers, and Myers adopted it in his report.[136] The War Office intended to treat men with this condition in the "mental section" of Netley Military Hospital near Southampton and, when faced with growing numbers, in the 2000 beds allocated for the purpose within the war hospitals.[137]

The challenges of providing care and treatment for shell shocked soldiers also inform us about patients and practices in civilian asylums and public perceptions of them. The public, and some members of the medical profession, opposed mentally disturbed soldiers being treated as, or alongside, pauper lunatics whose care could be demeaning: it would be disrespectful to men whose mental distress was caused by fighting for king and country. Dr. White, "a lady member of the profession", protested in 1917 against nerve-stricken soldiers being sent to lunatic asylums, "worse prisons", she said, than Germany provided for prisoners of war. An anonymous report in the *Journal of Mental Science* expressed outrage at her criticisms, describing them as "unjustified...likely to make a very unfavourable impression on the minds of the public, and [they] are not creditable to any person who makes them."[138] Dr. White's colleagues dismissed her comments, appearing more concerned about adverse publicity. Shooting the messenger for exaggerating or making unjustifiable comparisons allowed the message to be rebutted, the public to be reassured by those with greater authority, and the reputation of the institutions to remain intact.

Many others wanted to prevent traumatised soldiers from entering the asylum system. Robert Cecil MP argued that soldiers with "nerve strain" should "not be placed under asylum administration or in charge of officials connected with lunacy",[139] indicating his lack of confidence in a system regarded as tainted with stigma. Cecil Harmsworth MP proposed a Mental Treatment Bill, to facilitate treatment of mentally disturbed soldiers outside the authority of the Lunacy Act,[140] but it was dropped when it became clear that the Army Act 1881 covered these contingencies.[141] The Army Act gave soldier lunatics the special status of "service" patients, unencumbered by certification or the pauper lunatic label. Some medical superintendents argued that all patients should have the same status, and some VCs responded with objections to *any* patient having the opprobrious label of pauper.[142] According to Marriott Cooke and Hubert Bond, members of the Board who wrote a government endorsed report on the war hospitals, the Board approved avoiding Lunacy Act certification for soldiers as it was "a boon and a solace to the men and their relatives". Alongside this, they promoted the cause of civilian asylum patients, noting long-term problems of negative public attitudes "to be recognised and reckoned with," and that the standards for soldiers should "be extended at the earliest practicable moment to the civilian population."[143]

Military hospitals and dedicated shell shock beds in the war hospital were insufficient to treat large numbers of soldiers so some were transferred to civilian asylums. In these cases, the Ministry of Pensions (created to handle war pensions for former members of the armed forces and their dependants) would pay the asylum charge, rather than the Guardians.[144] It also paid 3s9d (18½p) a week over and above the usual asylum charge—a third more than the average for a pauper lunatic—plus half-a-crown (12½p) to the individual patient for extra comforts, plus financial support when on trial leave and a war disability pension. These benefits emphasised the meagre provision for civilian patients. On the wards, the special privileges could create jealousy and resentment.[145] For the Treasury, the care package was seen as too lavish and it proposed that the service patient status should expire after one year, to which the Board responded: "Do they then become "paupers" through no fault of their own, indicating the short lived nature of the country's gratitude to them?"[146] An assumed hopeless outlook for lunatics, and qualms about asylums syphoning off public resources which could be spent more constructively on non-psychiatric health and welfare needs, coloured the decisions of those in power.

Within the asylums, particularly Colney Hatch, refugees, prisoners of war (PoWs), "undesirable" aliens under the Aliens Act 1905, and enemy aliens were treated alongside service and pauper patients. For the authorities, the different groups created administrative work as each had a different legal standing with time-consuming bureaucratic technicalities and financial implications. Financing refugees in asylums was relatively simple as they were directly chargeable to Whitehall's Local Government Board, thus imposing no additional expenditure on local authorities.[147] Regarding PoWs, Swiss officials inspected to check their well-being[148] and Colney Hatch's medical superintendent resented the amount of Home Office paperwork associated with monitoring them, the need to liaise with the police who inspected their belongings and interviewed them, and the time spent making plans to ensure their safe departure.[149] Sometimes staff were required to escort them to the port of embarkation or to another destination, creating further demands on the asylum.[150]

A different set of rules regarding residency and finance applied to patients who fell under the Aliens Act 1905. Prompted by concern over mainly Jewish immigration from Eastern Europe, this Act was the first attempt to establish a system of immigration control.[151] Under it, if an immigrant became dependent on poor law relief, which included asylum admission, within 12 months of arriving in England, they could be deported as an "undesirable" alien.[152] This aimed to avoid cost to ratepayers.[153] Mayer L, a patient at Colney Hatch, was Jewish and from

Jerusalem, then under rule by the Ottoman Empire. Just before war broke out, the Home Office decided not to deport him[154]; the VC appealed, but the Home Office stuck to its decision stating that it would be inhumane to do so as he was unlikely to receive adequate treatment in Jerusalem.[155] Mayer L remained in Colney Hatch for two years, and was discharged to the Jews Temporary Shelter, funded by the Jewish community, to avoid him becoming dependent upon poor law relief.[156] After war broke out, as well as being undesirable aliens, people from Germany, Austria-Hungary or Turkey were also designated enemy aliens.

Creating Military Hospitals from Asylums

The War Office requisitioned asylums for billeting soldiers and treating military casualties, creating challenges for the whole asylum system.[157] In 1914, 300 men, 400 horses and "a park of guns" arrived at one Kent asylum and Severalls billeted 4000 troops.[158] The Board transferred newly built but unoccupied asylums, including Moss Side State Institution, Liverpool, and the Maudsley Hospital, to the War Office for treating mentally traumatised soldiers.[159] With the intention of freeing initially 2000 asylum beds for military use,[160] the 97 county and borough asylums were divided geographically into groups, to facilitate the transfer of patients to alternative asylums as locally as possible. Eventually 24 asylums were vacated, comprising over 23,000 beds, almost one quarter of the asylum total.[161] The Board complied with War Office requests half-heartedly, with occasional rhetoric but little more forceful advocacy on behalf of their civilian patients.[162]

Many asylums had to make space for patients transferred from others which were vacated when the War Office requisitioned them. The Board authoritatively stated that 20 per cent overcrowding (i.e. 120 beds in the space usually allocated to 100) would not incur "serious detriment" to the health of civilian asylum patients.[163] Their reassurance was speculative, if not fraudulent, but with their foremost priority being to support the country during the crisis.[164] In mid-1916 Sir William Byles MP asked in the Commons about the degree of asylum overcrowding, receiving the official response that no further reduction in accommodation was proceeding or contemplated.[165] That plan did not hold.

The War Office was particularly keen to take over asylums which had their own railway sidings, useful for transporting wounded men, coal, stores and other essentials. Of the LCC asylums, the "Epsom cluster" of four, south-west of London, was linked by the Horton Light Railway to Ewell West main line station. It was an obvious location for a war hospital. The LCC negotiated with the Board about providing beds for injured soldiers, contingent upon the Board "giving definite assurance that they will not raise objection to the infraction of rules and regulations" particularly concerning overcrowding and omissions in routine paper-work.[166] Thus Horton Asylum became "The County of London War Hospital Epsom", mainly for soldiers with physical injuries, and the LCC was reassured that compromises were acceptable when providing for civilian patients in its other asylums.

The peace-time arrangement whereby asylums receiving out-of-county patients could demand a higher fee from the requesting authority,[167] ceased for transfers made when creating war hospitals. In theory, within the Epsom cluster, it should have been straight forward to empty one asylum by transferring patients to the others. In practice, many were transferred further afield, in open-top "motor char-a-bancs and by omnibuses."[168] Hanwell accepted 173 patients, using basements, halls and whatever other space could be found.[169] Colney Hatch took 300 patients who all arrived on one afternoon.[170] The influx of patients added to the worsening staff-to-patient ratios.[171] Decisions to transfer patients long distances, over 150 miles in some cases, were taken locally, a difficult task for the VCs, disapproved of by the Board, and resented by patients and their families.[172] However, where possible, asylums took account of people's personal circumstances before moving them: when James R was transferred from Cane Hill, a LCC asylum in Surrey, to Gateshead in County Durham, his brother requested his return so that he could visit him: the VC refused, on the grounds that no one had visited him since his admission 14 years previously.[173]

Patients moved from their asylum lost their "home" and many familiar faces associated with it. The VC and medical superintendent usually remained at the vacated asylum, to equip the hospital, engage more staff and manage it under the direction of the War Office which also defrayed additional costs and provided "fully trained nurses".[174] Most asylum doctors and ward staff remained at their asylum, rather than accompany their mentally unwell patients elsewhere.[175] Ward staff retained their salaries, but were demoted: experienced nurses to probationer grade, and attendants to orderlies, reflecting the standards of their physical-disorder nursing skills. The War Office also agreed to make available additional surgical support for "serious operations", although routine surgical procedures and anaesthesia, as when pauper lunatics required comparable interventions, continued to be undertaken by the asylum medical officers based on their medical student training.[176]

Many modifications, of various sorts, were made to convert asylums into war hospitals. Work undertaken improved the ward lighting and heating; introduced electricity (ostensibly for X-ray equipment); and provided more toilets and bathrooms and better internal décor.[177] This upgrading had the implication that mentally unwell civilian patients, and their staff, could cope with antiquated facilities but wounded soldiers and those tending them deserved better. Regarding asylum paraphernalia, "everything in the buildings which might be objectionably reminiscent of their normal purposes" had to go, such as padded rooms, blocks on windows to prevent escape, and the excessive number of doors locked with a key. Lunacy stigma might also taint soldiers in death: if they died in a war hospital they were to be buried with military funerals and "In no case should a soldier be buried in that part of a local cemetery which has been specially set apart for insane patients dying in the Asylum".[178] A rare glimpse of equality between asylums and war hospitals was indicated in the decision that labour-saving devices installed in war hospital kitchens and laundries would remain on site when the building reverted to civilian use.[179]

Horton received mainly physically injured soldiers. Additional beds were required for those with mental disturbances. Napsbury Asylum, like Horton, had a dedicated railway siding so was favourable to the War Office. Napsbury also had 1500 civilian patients, with 1200 in its main building and 300 in a separate admissions unit. Initially, the War Office acquired the smaller building for mentally traumatised soldiers, its civilian occupants being transferred to the main asylum.[180] A high fence separated the new 300-bed Middlesex County War Hospital from the main asylum a few metres away,[181] protecting the sensibilities of the soldiers and their visitors from association with the pauper lunatics. The war hospital also provided a superior level of leisure facilities for the soldiers compared to the civilian patients: new purchases included 2 billiard tables with all accessories at a cost of £73, more than the annual salary of many asylum staff.[182]

The rest of Napsbury was vacated to become a war hospital for physically injured soldiers in May 1916.[183] In line with the Board's guidance, Napsbury aimed to transfer its asylum patients as short a distance as possible.[184] However, many were transported 70 miles away to Severalls, with others scattered across at least 18 asylums, mainly in south east England.[185] Eighty civilian patients remained at Napsbury to work the 426 acre farm and gardens.[186] The Edgware Guardians queried this: surely if these patients were working, the Guardians need not pay for them? There was no flexibility when it came to these costs: the VC informed the Guardians that the standard fees covered all patients, whether usefully employed or not.[187]

Almost half a million men received treatment in asylum war hospitals, more than one-sixth of the total number of those sick and wounded from all fronts,[188] including 38,000 with mental disturbances.[189] In April 1919, Napsbury still had over 1000 military patients, and VC minutes gave no clue as to when civilian patients might return. Staff were restless, still working wartime shifts, longer than their pre-war hours.[190] Contrary to promises earlier in the war,[191] the authorities planned to remove the kitchen and laundry labour-saving devices before the civilian patients returned, on the grounds that patients would otherwise be unable to take up their former roles, and because machinery would "reduce the useful work upon which patients can now be employed."[192] With a high turnover of civilian patients—admissions, discharges and deaths—in the intervening years, how many would actually return was unclear. Unrealistically, the authorities wanted to pick up where they had left off, bizarrely seeming to regard patients as a group whose insanity was so all-encompassing that it made them oblivious to the war and unaffected by the changes imposed on their lives.

RECONSTRUCTION

The Cabinet established a Reconstruction Committee in 1916 to plan for after the war. Demoralisation at home and devastation abroad made planning essential, for economic and social welfare recovery, and to convince people that things could get better.[193] The Committee sought advice from numerous statutory bodies, including the Board, but the Board was disturbed by its emphasis on physical health without mental health. The Committee's stress was probably due to competing priorities, with deep concern about maternal ill-health, high infant mortality and a declining birth-rate, and because between 40 and 60 per cent of recruits for the British Army were turned down as physically unfit for service.[194] Failing to mention mental health, however, suggested that the

Committee did not appreciate the incapacitating nature of severe mental disorders, whether suffered by soldiers or civilians. The Board did not reply to the circular until prompted by the Committee to do so.[195] The Board's reply respectfully stated that it hoped the Committee's expression "health of the population" included both mental and physical health and that the Committee agreed that they were equally important. It informed the Committee of the benefits of admitting mentally disturbed soldiers without certification to allow early treatment which could facilitate recovery and it reiterated the need for similar admission procedures for civilian patients, which had so far only been achieved to facilitate admission to the Maudsley Hospital when it could eventually open its doors to them.[196]

Alongside seeking advice for post-war health priorities, the Reconstruction Committee was interested in plans to create a Ministry of Health, to improve and coordinate health care and public health more generally, which, according Walter Holland and Susie Stewart, were "something of a patchwork of ramshackle and uncoordinated services".[197] Public opinion also favoured the creation of the Ministry, which came into being post-war after "much political machination".[198] The Board feared that the new Ministry might remove its independence, but it also envisaged advantages of mental health being part of a comprehensive national health scheme, giving opportunities for prevention and treatment, and reducing stigma.[199] The Board had insightful ideas to improve services and to counteract damaging public opinion, but its ability to implement them was questionable.

For public opinion to benefit patients, the authorities had to take it seriously. Occasionally this happened. In 1917, the LCC noted that patients, their relatives and the wider public preferred the designation "hospital" over "asylum" and acknowledged their backing as "an important factor in the success or failure" of planning. LCC asylums thus became "mental hospitals".[200] A year later, other asylums followed.[201] For economy's sake, the Board insisted that supplies of old headed paper would have to be used before ordering new, and legal documents would retain the old designation until altered by law.[202] The law, by then almost 30 years old, was a stumbling block to fully implementing this change, as it was to allowing a more flexible system of admission.

Also linked to public opinion, the MPA was optimistic about the speed at which legal reform might materialise:

public attention has been awakened by the mental cases resulting from the war, and that during the era of reconstruction that must inevitably follow when peace is finally declared....a more enlightened opinion may prevail which may lead to better provision being made for the treatment of certain types of mental disorder.[203]

In 1920, however, the Board acknowledged its failure to achieve prompt amendment to the Lunacy Act to enable early and voluntary treatment and to establish psychiatric wards and out-patient clinics in general hospitals. The Board suggested other ways for VCs to fulfil their duty to ensure that patients received "treatment on modern lines". These included encouraging VCs to make postgraduate psychiatric training with paid study leave mandatory (a financial issue), and setting a maximum of 50 new patients to be under the care of a single medical officer (with both recruitment and financial implications).[204] These recommendations hardly reached the standard of Kraepelin's clinic established 15 years earlier, and the competing pressures meant that the reality of implementing them was far from certain.

In October 1918, with the expectation that the war was nearly over, the Board met with VCs from across the country. Much of their discussion consisted of reiterated, unimplemented ideas, such as: the need for more research; better public and staff education on mental disorders; administrative support for medical superintendents, as in general hospitals; standardised wages, terms of employment and hours of duty; and abolishing the stigmatising labels of pauper, lunatic and asylum.[205] Novel recommendations derived from wartime experiences were lacking. The Cabinet Committee on Post War Priority, and its successors, would help shape if, how and when the ideas could be taken forward.[206] Mental health had never been at the top of the national priority ladder and it seemed unlikely to reach that position soon, despite MPA optimism.

Lack of priority for asylum change was likely to have been associated with the fall in number of civilian patients during the war. Admissions fell from over 23,000 a year in 1914 to around 20–21,000 annually during the war. Lower admission rates were attributed to better population mental health linked to greater social cohesion and high employment rates, a notion which has some support from the international decline in suicide rates in countries directly involved in the conflict.[207] Alcohol related admissions also declined, associated with restricted licencing hours and reduced liquor consumption.[208] High asylum death rates also

contributed (see Chapter 7), and doctors and magistrates may have interpreted the Lunacy Act more liberally, being reluctant to certify patients
into overcrowded, understaffed and sub-standard facilities. Also, men who
became mentally unwell while on military service were initially admitted
to war hospitals, beyond the Board's statistical radar.[209] Optimistically, or
perhaps naïvely, the Board did not envisage an more patients post-war,
with the consequences that it took a *laissez faire* approach to seeking
more resources in the reconstruction period.[210]

Bedford Pierce, medical superintendent at the York Retreat and president of the MPA in 1919 wrote optimistically in the *Journal of Mental
Science*:

> I cannot but think that the old days of autocratic management are over,
> and though some who think a beneficent autocracy is the best form of
> government may lament the change, we can nevertheless look forward
> without dismay to the new era of democratic control if the proletariat
> recognises its responsibility.[211]

His political insights aligned with other social and political changes.
From abroad came news of the Russian Revolution.[212] At home changes
included the Representation of the People Act 1918, the Education
Act 1918, the Ministry of Health Act 1919 and the Sex Disqualifica-
tion (Removal) Act 1919. These changes had potential to expand social
opportunities and wellbeing for people with the least voice, both inside
and outside the asylums. On the other side of the coin, post-war, the
government had to pay off an enormous national debt. Local authorities
curbed spending in every direction and the Board only authorised capital
expenditure for essential maintenance of the fabric of asylums or for "promoting the health of the patients and the staff."[213] "Geddes Axe", the
outcome of Sir Eric Geddes' Committee on National Expenditure in
1922, further restricted public spending. Without public demand, despite
being chronically underfunded, the asylums were "low-hanging fruit"
whose fortunes were unlikely to improve. [214] Public support for mentally
disturbed soldiers during the war dwindled, and provision for them gradually merged into the existing asylum system rather than leading to asylum
reform. By 1922, 5000 soldiers resided in public asylums in England
and Wales alongside the pauper lunatics.[215] The same year, the report of
the War Office committee of enquiry into shell shock, made no recommendations about reform of civilian asylum law or practice.[216] A further

eight years would elapse before the Mental Treatment Act 1930 which created a less legalistic approach to admission and discharge. Overall, the shell shock legacy added little to debate on post-war improvements for patients in civilian asylums and mental hospitals. Lomax's critique, the voice of a low status temporary member of staff whose views were typically discounted by the asylum leadership, ultimately proved more effective.[217]

Conclusions

The process of creating the war hospitals and the military, political and public responses to shell shock indicated inadequacies of the asylums and the lunacy system, but did not directly trigger reform of asylum culture and practices.[218] The Board lacked authority to prevent low standards or enforce the best practices for which it and a few psychiatrist-reformers advocated. The tactics of persuasion allowed to the Board were insufficient to change a complex conservative culture where multiple stakeholders had divergent concerns, lay VCs were insufficiently trained to make the decisions expected of them, patients' voices were barely audible or credible and a moralising public was largely unsympathetic, including as ratepayers. The top-down hierarchical management structure meant that the Board obeyed, almost without question, the obligations placed on it by its task masters in central government and by the Lunacy Act, passed a quarter of a century earlier and criticised at the time by psychiatrists as unfit for purpose. The Board policed compliance with the Lunacy Act by its bureaucratic monitoring of all aspects of asylum practices. The importance of this legal role was demonstrated when lawyer Board members inspected asylums alone. Policing and legal compliance helped transmit an authoritarian culture into the asylums, which neither inspired nor encouraged lateral-thinking, creativity or innovation. A few chinks of flexibility appeared in the Lunacy Act, apparently without adverse consequences.

Occasionally the Board challenged its superiors, but it is debatable how much it could do this without threatening its own reputation as a compliant and effective body. Its position was particularly difficult when higher-ranked authorities, such as the Reconstruction Committee, lacked understanding of mental disorders and asylums. The hierarchical assumption within the asylum system that the most senior knew best, meant that criticism, especially from people lower in the hierarchy was explained away rather than evaluated. Despite rhetoric about tackling asylum problems, the top-down approach inhibited the leadership from engaging with lower ranks to understand what needed to be done.

In Peter Barham's view the Board was "squeezed between conflicting interests and visions of its objectives".[219] The Board and other leaders in the asylum hierarchy appeared satisfied to stick with what they knew best, which maintained the organisational *status quo* as far as possible. But as circumstances changed, the *status quo* was not necessarily fit for purpose.

NOTES

1. George Savage, "The Presidential Address, Delivered at the Opening Meeting of the Section of Psychiatry of the Royal Society of Medicine, on October 22nd, 1912," *Journal of Mental Science* (*JMS*) 59 (1913): 14–27, 14.
2. Lionel Weatherly, "The Treatment of Incipient and Unconfirmed Insanity," *Lancet* 14 February 1914, 497.
3. Kathleen Jones, *Mental Health and Social Policy, 1845–1959* (London: Routledge and Kegan Paul, 1960), 94.
4. *First Annual Report of the Board of Control, for the Year 1914* (London: HMSO, 1916) (*BoC AR 1914*), Part 2 Upton Asylum 16 March 1914, 206.
5. "Report of the Committee on the Status of British Psychiatry and of Medical Officers," *JMS* 60 (1914): 667–68.
6. Louise Hide, *Gender and Class in English Asylums, 1890–1914* (London: Palgrave Macmillan, 2014).
7. Mike Jay and Michael Neve (eds), *1900: A Fin-de-siècle Reader* (Harmondsworth: Penguin, 1999).
8. Bernard Hollander, *The First Signs of Insanity: Their Prevention and Treatment* (London: Stanley Paul and Co, 1912), 15; Anon. "Dr. Bernard Hollander," *BMJ* 17 February 1934, 316.
9. Erving Goffman, *Asylums: Essays on the Social Situation of Mental Patients and Other Inmates* (1961; Harmondsworth: Penguin, 1980).
10. *BoC AR 1914*, Part 2, 154; Anon. *The LCC Hospitals: A Retrospect* (London: LCC, 1949), 108; LCC LCC/MIN/00754 Minutes of miscellaneous sub-committees 1915–1919: Summary of staff numbers required for 48-hour week, LMA.
11. *BoC AR 1914*, Part 2, Glamorgan Asylum 4 November 1914, 230; Montagu Lomax, *The Experiences of an Asylum Doctor* (London: Allen and Unwin, 1921), 73.
12. LCC LCC/MIN/00579 Meeting, 29 September 1914, 645 LMA.

13. Richard van Emden and Steve Humphries, *All Quiet on the Home Front: An Oral History of Life in Britain during the First World War* (London: Headline, 2003), 302.
14. *BoC AR 1914*, Part 1, 15–16.
15. *BoC AR 1914*, Part 1, 14.
16. LCC LCC/MIN/00579 Meeting, 16 December 1913, 117 LMA.
17. Hanwell LCC/MIN/01093 Meeting, 22 December 1913, 24 LMA.
18. LCC LCC/MIN/00579 Meeting, 16 December 1913, 117–18 LMA.
19. Pamela Michael, *Care and Treatment of the Mentally Ill in North Wales 1800–2000* (Cardiff: University of Wales Press, 2003), 112.
20. Hanwell LCC/MIN/01096 Meeting, 9 October 1916, 200 LMA; R Percy Smith, "Mental Disorders in Civilians Arising in Connexion with the War," *Proceedings of the Royal Society of Medicine* 10 (1917): Section of Psychiatry, 1–20, 19; Hanwell LCC/MIN/01095 Meeting, 7 June 1915, 99 LMA; Claybury LCC/MIN/00946 Meeting, 4 February 1915, 10–11 LMA.
21. Committee on the Administration of Public Mental Hospitals (Chairman: Sir Cyril Cobb) (Cobb Inquiry), 16 March 1922 Herbert Ellis Q:890, MH 58/219 TNA.
22. Colney Hatch LCC/MIN/01007 Meeting, 16 May 1919, 311 LMA; LCC LCC/MIN/00584 Meeting, 24 June 1919, 550 LMA; Cobb Inquiry, 16 February 1922 Dr. Rotherham Q:306, MH 58/219 TNA; BoC, letter to MSs "Cinematograph Installation," 9 March 1923 MH 51/240 TNA.
23. Joseph Melling and Bill Forsythe, *The Politics of Madness: The State, Insanity and Society in England, 1845–1914* (London and New York: Routledge, 2006), 206.
24. *BoC AR 1914*, Part 2, Wells Asylum 15 October 1914, 301.
25. Jones, *Mental Health and Social Policy*, 93.
26. *Medical Directory* (London: John Churchill and Sons, 1917); Hanwell H11/HLL/B/09/031 Discharge book 1912–1916 LMA.
27. Divorce Court File 2441. Wife's petition for judicial separation J77/1069/2441 TNA; Cobb Inquiry, 15 March 1922 Mr. Sale Q:742, MH 58/219 TNA.
28. Lunacy Law (Committal of Sane Persons). *Hansard* HC Deb 28 February 1910 vol 14 c562.
29. Lionel Weatherly, *A Plea for the Insane: The Case for Reform in the Care and Treatment of Mental Diseases* (London: Grant Richards Ltd, 1918) 23.
30. Kathleen Jones, "Law and Mental Health: Sticks or Carrots," 89–102, in *150 Years of British Psychiatry 1841–1991*, ed. German Berrios and Hugh Freeman (London: Gaskell, 1991), 96.

31. Jones, *Mental Health and Social Policy*, 35; Jones, "Law and Mental Health," 95; Hugh Freeman, "Psychiatry in Britain c.1900," *History of Psychiatry* 21 (2010): 312–24, 312.
32. Lunacy Act 1890, sections 31, 64, 255, 258.
33. Mary Riggall, *Reminiscences of a Stay in a Mental Hospital* (London: Arthur Stockwell, 1929), 12.
34. Weatherly, *Plea*, 34.
35. Weatherly, *Plea*, 13. Unclear from the text whether Weatherly or Needham added the emphasis.
36. Weatherly, *Plea*, 36, 47.
37. Henry Devine, "*A Plea for the Insane* by LA Weatherly," *JMS* 65 (1919): 208–9.
38. Voluntary Mental Treatment Bill. *Hansard* HL Deb 22 July 1914 vol. 17 cc89-92.
39. Melling and Forsythe, *Politics of Madness*, 208.
40. A Helen Boyle, "Observations on Early Nervous and Mental Cases, with Suggestions as to Possible Improvement in Our Methods of Dealing with Them," *JMS* 60 (1914): 381–99 (including discussion) 382–83.
41. Hollander, *First Signs*, 17.
42. Hollander, *First Signs*, 16; Anon. "Voluntary Mental Treatment Bill. Presented by The Earl Russell. Ordered to be Printed July 22nd, 1914," *JMS* 61 (1915): 481–82.
43. Hollander, *First Signs*, 195.
44. Anon. "Asylum Reports," *JMS* 59 (1913): 371–92, 379.
45. BoC, memo to Lionel Shadwell for comment. c. November 1918 MH 51/521 TNA.
46. Anon. "Asylum Reports," *JMS* 59 (1913): 130–44, 132.
47. Colney Hatch LCC/MIN/01003, Meeting, 6 November 1914, 150 LMA.
48. Lunacy Act 1890 sections 241–46.
49. Lunacy Act 1890 section 341.
50. Deaths in County Asylums (Form of Notice). *Hansard* HC Deb 6 April 1910 vol. 16 cc422-3.
51. Weatherly, *Plea*, 23.
52. Steven Cherry, *Mental Healthcare in Modern England: The Norfolk Asylum/St. Andrews Hospital 1810–1998* (Woodbridge, Suffolk: Boydell Press, 2003), 157.
53. LCC LCC/MIN/00580 Meeting, 18 May 1915, 479–80 LMA.
54. BoC, Marriott Cooke letter to Mrs. Webb, 11 May 1917 MH 51/688 TNA.
55. BoC W/FM, 16 December 1914, 279 MH 50/43 TNA.

56. Central government provided grants for capital expenditure: Sir George Newman CMO memo to Sir Aubrey Symonds, c. August 1921, 4 MH 52/222 TNA; Benjamin Seebohm Rowntree, *Poverty: A Study of Town Life* (London: Macmillan and Co, 1902).
57. Lunacy Act 1890 section 283 (1) (2).
58. Lunatic Asylums Regulation Bill. *Hansard* HL Deb 29 April 1828 vol. 19 cc196-9; Richard Rows, "Clinics and Centres for Teaching," *JMS* 60 (1914): 674–81, 677; Jane Hamlett and Lesley Hoskins, "Comfort in Small Things? Clothing, Control and Agency in County Lunatic Asylums in Nineteenth- and Early Twentieth-Century England," *Journal of Victorian Culture* 18 (2013): 93–114, 103.
59. Lomax, *Experiences*, 48.
60. JM Winter, "The Impact of the First World War on Civilian Health in Britain," *Economic History Review* 30 (1977): 487–507, 499.
61. LCC LCC/MIN/00581 Meetings, 30 November 1915, 145; 14 March 1916, 431–32; LCC LCC/MIN/00583 Meeting, 30 April 1918, 534 LMA.
62. LCC LCC/MIN/00580 Meeting, 27 July 1915, 699 LMA.
63. Rows, "Clinics": 679.
64. John Keay, "Presidential Address on the War and the Burden of Insanity," *JMS* 64 (1918): 325–44, 326, 331–32.
65. Claybury LCC/MIN/00949 Meeting, 23 May 1918, 68–69 LMA.
66. LCC LCC/MIN/00759 Presented papers of sub-committee 1909–1923: letter LCC to superintendents 5 November 1915 LMA.
67. Colney Hatch LCC/MIN/01007 Meeting, 22 February 1918, 42; LCC LCC/MIN/00583 Meetings, 30 April 1918, 500; 26 March 1918, 442 LMA; Hanwell LCC/MIN/01096 Meeting, 25 September 1916, 183; LCC/MIN/01094 Meeting, 29 March 1915, 309 LMA.
68. Colney Hatch LCC/MIN/01006 Meeting, 4 May 1917, 173; LCC/MIN/01001 Meeting, 25 April 1913, 50; LCC/MIN/01003 Meeting, 25 September 1914, 106 LMA.
69. Hanwell LCC/MIN/01097 Meetings, 18 June 1917, 109; 2 July 1917, 125 LMA.
70. Weatherly, *Plea*, 53.
71. Meyer, "Aims": 2; Matt Egan, "The 'Manufacture' of Mental Defectives in Late Nineteenth and Early Twentieth Century Scotland" (PhD thesis, University of Glasgow, 2001) 57–58. http://theses.gla.ac.uk/1040/1/2001eganphd.pdf.
72. Richard Mayou, "The History of General Hospital Psychiatry," *BJPsych* 155 (1989): 764–76, 767–68.
73. Ronald Chase, *The Making of Modern Psychiatry* (Berlin: Logos Verlag Berlin, 2018), 108.
74. Hollander, *First Signs*, 194.

75. *BoC AR 1914*, Part 2, Northumberland Asylum 4 May 1914, 293; Salop Asylum 8 July 1914, 298.
76. Rows, "Clinics": 675.
77. Adolph Meyer, "The Aims of a Psychiatric Clinic," 1–11, in *XVIIth International Congress of Medicine, London 1913. Section XII Psychiatry. Part 1* (London: Henry Fowde, Hodder and Stoughton, 1913).
78. Rows, "Clinics": 676.
79. Meyer, "Aims": 3–7.
80. Meyer, "Aims": 1–2.
81. "Report of the Committee on the Status of British Psychiatry": 669.
82. Meyer, "Aims": 1–2; Rows, "Clinics": 675.
83. Hollander, *First Signs of Insanity*, 195.
84. Mayou, "General Hospital Psychiatry: 765.
85. Patricia Allderidge, "The Foundation of the Maudsley Hospital," 79–88, in *150 Years of British Psychiatry*, ed. Berrios and Freeman, 80.
86. WR Merrington, *University College Hospital and Its Medical School: A History* (London: Heinemann, 1976), 227–28.
87. Edgar Jones, "'An Atmosphere of Cure': Frederick Mott, Shell Shock and the Maudsley," *History of Psychiatry* 25 (2014): 412–21.
88. Allderidge, "The Foundation of the Maudsley Hospital": 84, 86.
89. Mental Deficiency Act 1913 section 22 (1) (2).
90. Lunacy Act 1890 section 169 (1).
91. Jones, *Mental Health and Social Policy*, 73.
92. Mental After-Care Association, https://wellcomelibrary.org/collec tions/digital-collections/mental-healthcare/mental-after-care-associ ation/, WL.
93. W Norwood East, "On Attempted Suicide, with an Analysis of 1000 Consecutive Cases," *JMS* 59 (1913): 428–78.
94. Napsbury H50/A/01/021 Meeting, 3 April 1914, 264–65; H50/A/01/022 Meeting,1 May 1914, 32 LMA.
95. Napsbury H50/A/01/022 Meeting, 1 May 1914, 33 LMA.
96. Napsbury H50/A/01/021 Meeting, 12 March 1914, 224 LMA; Claire Hilton, "The Development of Psychogeriatric Services in England c.1940 to 1989" (PhD thesis, King's College London, 2014), 104–5.
97. Napsbury H50/A/01/021 Meeting, 3 April 1914, 264 LMA.
98. Napsbury H50/A/01/022 Meetings, 16 May 1914, 63; 20 June 1914, 117 LMA.
99. BoC W/FM 1 April 1914, 6; 1 July 1914, 113; 22 July 1914, 144, MH 50/43 TNA.
100. Napsbury H50/A/01/022 Meeting, 18 July 1914, 147 LMA.
101. Napsbury H50/B/02/003 Civil Register of Admissions: Female Patients, 1912–1915 LMA.
102. Colney Hatch LCC/MIN/01006 Meeting, 4 May 1917, 160–65 LMA.

103. Lunacy Act 1890 section 55; *BoC AR 1914*, Part 2, Berks Asylum 6 May 1914, 197; Cornwall Asylum 25 May 1914, 209.

104. Jones, *Mental Health and Social Policy*, 8.

105. Stephen Soanes, "Rest and Restitution: Convalescence and the Public Mental Hospital in England, 1919–39" (PhD thesis, University of Warwick, 2011) http://wrap.warwick.ac.uk/54604/1/WRAP_T HESIS_Soanes_2011.pdf, 120.

106. *BoC AR 1914*, Part 2, Colney Hatch 28 February 1914, 271–72.

107. *BoC AR 1914*, Part 2, Upton Asylum 16 March 1914, 207.

108. *BoC AR 1914*, Part 2, Cumberland and Westmorland Asylum 23 July 1914, 212.

109. BoC W/FM, 15 December 1915, 12 MH 50/44 TNA.

110. *BoC AR 1914*, Part 2, City of London Asylum 8 June 1914, 362.

111. Ministry of Health (MoH), analysis of BoC's response to Lomax, 11 October 1921 MH 58/221 TNA; Cobb Inquiry, 16 March 1922 Herbert Ellis Q:874, MH 58/219 TNA.

112. *BoC AR 1914*, Part 2, Barming Heath Asylum 12 November 1914, 237.

113. Goffman, *Asylums*, 73.

114. Wilfrid Llewelyn Jones, *Ministering to Minds Diseased: A History of Psychiatric Treatment* (London: Heinemann, 1983), 113.

115. *BoC AR 1914*, Part 2, Hanwell Asylum 25 July 1914, 273.

116. *BoC AR 1914*, Part 2, Lancaster Asylum 22 July 1914, 247; Canterbury Asylum 21 March 1914, 348; Yorkshire (East Riding) Asylum 13 October 1914, 326.

117. *BoC AR 1914*, Part 2, Gateshead Asylum 5 May 1914, 355; Parkside Asylum 2 July 1914, 208; Rainhill Asylum 21 February 1914, 250.

118. *BoC AR 1914*, Part 2, Cane Hill Asylum 6 October 2014, 267; Hanwell LCC/MIN/01097 Meeting, 14 January 1918, 288 LMA.

119. Colney Hatch LCC/MIN/01004 Meeting, 18 June 1915, 124 LMA.

120. Hanwell LCC/MIN/01095 Meeting, 7 June 1915, 99 LMA.

121. Lomax, *Experiences*, 79.

122. *BoC AR 1914*, Part 2, Leicestershire and Rutland Asylum 3 February 1914, 258; Bracebridge Asylum 26 January 1914, 260; Oxford Asylum 4 August 1914, 295.

123. Lomax, *Experiences*, 39.

124. Russell Barton, *Institutional Neurosis* (Bristol: John Wright and Sons, 1959); Goffman, *Asylums*.

125. *Seventh Annual Report of the Board of Control, for the Year 1920* (London: HMSO, 1921) *(BoC AR 1920)* 17–18, citing *The Friend* (Society of Friends) 28 May 1920; National Council for Lunacy Reform, minute books, 1920–1921, 30 September 1920; report of Mr. Parley SA/MIN/A/1 WL.

126. Colney Hatch LCC/MIN/01005 Meeting, 20 October 1916, 297–98 citing *Islington Daily Gazette* 15 October 1916, LMA; Anon. "Lunacy Law Reform: Criticisms at the Inquiry," *Times* 17 March 1922.
127. Cobb Inquiry, 11 April 1922 Rev WD Yoward (VC chairman) Q:3092–98, 3048–50, MH 58/220 TNA; MoH, *Report of the Committee on Administration of Public Mental Hospitals* Cmd. 1730 (Chairman: Sir Cyril Cobb) (London: HMSO, 1922).
128. MoH, GN to "Secretary," memo, 14 October 1921 MH 52/222 TNA.
129. Sir George Newman CMO memo to Sir Aubrey Symonds, c. August 1921, 3–4 MH 52/222 TNA.
130. BoC W/FM 30 September 1914, 202 MH 50/43 TNA.
131. *BoC AR 1914*, Part 1, 11, 14.
132. Jones, *Mental Health and Social Policy*, 135; Charles Webster, *The Health Services Since the War. Vol 1: Problems of Health Care: The National Health Service Before 1957* (London: HMSO, 1988), 10.
133. HB. "Sir Marriott Cooke KBE MB," *BMJ* 31 October 1931, 829–30.
134. Peter Barham, *Forgotten Lunatics of the Great War* (New Haven and London: Yale University Press, 2004), 123.
135. Robert Armstrong-Jones, "The Eighth Annual Report of the Board of Control for the Year 1921," *Eugenics Review* 15 (1923): 426–32, 432.
136. Charles Myers, "A Contribution to the Study of Shell Shock" *Lancet* 13 February 1915, 316–20, 320; Edgar Jones, "Shell Shocked," *Monitor on Psychology* 43, June 2012. http://www.apa.org/monitor/2012/06/shell-shocked.
137. E Marriott Cooke and C Hubert Bond, *History of the Asylum War Hospitals in England and Wales* (London: HMSO, 1920), 29; *Third Annual Report of the Board of Control, for the Year 1916* (*BoC AR 1916*) (London: HMSO, 1917), 2.
138. Anon. "Hostels for Heroes," *JMS* 63 (1917): 450–52.
139. Nerve Strain. *Hansard* HC Deb 11 March 1915 vol. 70 cc1563-4W.
140. Mental Treatment Bill. *Hansard* HC Deb 20 April 1915 vol 71 223.
141. Army Act 1881 section 91.
142. Napsbury H50/A/01/025 Meeting, 22 January 1916, 99 LMA.
143. Cooke and Bond, *War Hospitals*, 29.
144. BoC, letter Marriott Cooke to Sir Edward Troup, 1 November 1917 MH 51/693 TNA.
145. LCC LCC/MIN/00583 Meeting, 30 April 1918, 501–2 LMA.
146. BoC, letter and recommendations to War Pensions etc. Statutory Committee, 4 June 1917, MH 51/692 TNA.
147. Colney Hatch H12/CH/B/47/016 Reception orders, medical certificates, notices of death, discharge or removal and correspondence for female patients who died or were discharged or removed 1918 LMA.
148. Colney Hatch LCC/MIN/01006 Meeting, 10 August 1917, 223 LMA.

149. Colney Hatch LCC/MIN/01004 Meeting, 26 March 1915, 27 LMA; H12/CH/A/08/001 Meeting, 22 February 1918, 20 LMA.
150. LCC LCC/MIN/00584 Meeting, 27 May 1919, 477 LMA.
151. Helena Wray, "The Aliens Act 1905 and the Immigration Dilemma," *Journal of Law and Society* 33 (2006): 302–23, 302, 308.
152. Aliens Act 1905 section 3 (b).
153. Napsbury H50/A/01/024 22 May 1915, 26–27 LMA.
154. Colney Hatch LCC/MIN/01002 Meetings, 21 November 1913, 4; 5 December 1913, 30 LMA.
155. LCC LCC/MIN/00579 Meeting, 27 January 1914, 131–32 LMA.
156. Colney Hatch LCC/MIN/01005 Meetings, 30 June 1916, 202; 14 July 1916, 216 LMA.
157. BoC W/FM 25 November 1914, 256 MH 50/43 TNA.
158. *BoC AR 1914*, Part 2, Chartham Asylum 10 November 1914, 240; Severalls Asylum 27 October 1914, 226.
159. BoC W/FM, 4 November 1914, 229 MH 50/43 TNA; LCC LCC/MIN/00580 Meetings, 27 April 1915, 409; 18 May 1915, 486–87 LMA.
160. D Thomson, "A Descriptive Record of the Conversion of a County Asylum into a War Hospital for Sick and Wounded Soldiers in 1915," *JMS* 62 (1916): 109–35, 112.
161. Cooke and Bond, *War Hospitals*, 1; *BoC AR 1916*, 2.
162. David Pearce, "Evacuation and Deprivation: The War Time Experience of the Devon and Exeter City Mental Hospitals," *History of Psychiatry* 22 (2011): 332–43, 334.
163. Cooke and Bond, *War Hospitals*, 3.
164. BoC W/FM 3 November 1915, 577 MH 50/43 TNA.
165. Anon. "Asylum Accommodation," *JMS* 62 (1916): 827–28, 827; Asylum Accommodation. *Hansard* HC Deb 21 August 1916 vol 85 cc2260-1.
166. LCC LCC/MIN/00580 Meeting, 10 November 1914, 6 LMA.
167. Lunacy Act section 283 (3).
168. LCC LCC/MIN/00580 Meeting, 23 March 1915, 302 LMA.
169. Hanwell 11/HLL/A/14/003/012/001 Letter book, including in-letters and copies of out-letters, statistics and other information 1915–1927, 88 LMA.
170. Colney Hatch LCC/MIN/01004 Meeting, 2 March 1915, 9 LMA.
171. LCC LCC/MIN/00580 Meeting, 23 February 1915, 111–13 LMA; Colney Hatch H12/CH/C/04/003-4 Male attendants' wages books 1915–1918 LMA.
172. BoC W/FM 9 December 1914, 272 MH 50/43; 19 January 1916, 42 MH 50/44 TNA.
173. LCC LCC/MIN/00579 Meeting, 19 September 1914, S681 LMA.

174. James Chambers, "The Presidential Address, on the Prevention of the Insanities," *JMS* 59 (1913): 549–82.
175. Thomson, "Descriptive Record": 113.
176. Chambers, "Presidential Address"; Phyllis Bottome, *Private Worlds* (Harmondsworth: Penguin, 1934).
177. Cooke and Bond, *War Hospitals*, 14–15; *BoC AR 1914*, Part 2, Cambridge and Isle of Ely Asylum 21 October 1914, 201.
178. Napsbury H50/A/01/024 BoC letter 18 June 1915 to VC, 65–69 LMA.
179. Cooke and Bond, *War Hospitals*, 15.
180. Napsbury H50/A/01/024 Meetings, 22 May 1915, 2, 23; 4 June 1915, 42 LMA.
181. Napsbury H50/A/01/026 Meeting, 7 July 1916, 29 LMA.
182. Colney Hatch H12/CH/C/04/003 Male attendants' wages book 1915–1916 LMA.
183. Cooke and Bond, *War Hospitals*, 31.
184. Cooke and Bond, *War Hospitals*, 3.
185. Cooke and Bond, *War Hospitals*, 31.
186. Napsbury H50/A/01/025 Meeting, 19 February 1916. Between pp. 143–44 LMA.
187. Napsbury H50/A/01/026 Meeting, 1 December 1916, 186–87 LMA.
188. Cooke and Bond, *War Hospitals*, 2.
189. Cooke and Bond, *War Hospitals*, 29.
190. Napsbury H50/A/01/029 Meetings, 1 March 1919, 252; 5 April 1919, 275 LMA.
191. Cooke and Bond, *War Hospitals*, 15.
192. LCC LCC/MIN/00584 Meeting, 28 January 1919, 224 LMA.
193. Pat Thane, *Divided Kingdom: A History of Britain, 1900 to the Present* (Cambridge: Cambridge University Press, 2018), 56.
194. Thane, *Divided Kingdom*, 56–57; JM Winter, "Military Fitness and Civilian Health in Britain During the First World War," *Journal of Contemporary History* 15 (1980): 211–44, 211.
195. Reconstruction Committee, letters to BoC 14 August 1916 and 2 January 1917 MH 51/687 TNA.
196. Lunacy Act Amendment Bill 1905; BoC, letter to Reconstruction Committee, 9 February 1917 MH 51/687 TNA; London County Council (Parks etc) Act 1915.
197. Walter Holland and Susie Stewart, *Public Health: The Vision and the Challenge* (London: Nuffield Trust, 1998), 30.
198. Holland and Stewart, *Public Health*, 31, 33.
199. BoC, letter to Home Office, 16 July 1918, and memo "Transfer of Lunacy Work to a Ministry of Health" 15 July 1918 MH 51/631 TNA.
200. LCC LCC/MIN/00583 Meeting, 18 December 1917, 234–36 LMA.

201. Napsbury H50/A/01/029 Meeting, 4 January 1919. Between pp. 205–6, "Report of the Committee Appointed at the Conference of Visiting Committees of the Asylums of England and Wales," 29 October 1918 LMA.

202. LCC LCC/MIN/00583 Meeting, 18 December 1917, 234 LMA.

203. Anon. "Reform in Lunacy Law," *JMS* 63 (1918): 66–67.

204. *Sixth Annual Report of the Board of Control, for the Year 1919 (BoC AR 1919)* (London: HMSO, 1920), 19–20.

205. Napsbury H50/A/01/029 Meeting, 4 January 1919. Between pp. 205–6, "Report of the Committee Appointed at the Conference of Visiting Committees of the Asylums of England and Wales," 29 October 1918 LMA.

206. BoC W/FM 4 December 1918, 313 MH 50/46 TNA.

207. Maurice Halbwachs, *The Causes of Suicide* (tr. Harold Goldblatt) (London: Routledge and Kegan Paul, 1978), 209, 212.

208. *BoC AR 1919*, 11–12; Reginald Smart, "The Effect of Licencing Restrictions During 1914–1918 on Drunkenness and Liver Cirrhosis Deaths in Britain," *British Journal of Addiction* 69 (1974): 109–21.

209. Jones, *Mental Health and Social Policy*, 96–97.

210. *BoC AR 1914*, Part 1, 10; *BoC AR 1916* 10; *BoC AR 1919* 10, 23; *BoC AR 1920* Appendix A, 87.

211. Bedford Pierce, "Some Present Day Problems Connected with the Administration of Asylums," *JMS* 65 (1919): 198–201, 201.

212. Thane, *Divided Kingdom*, 62.

213. *Eighth Annual Report of the Board of Control, for the Year 1921* (London: HMSO, 1922), 5.

214. Christopher Hood and Rozana Himaz, *A Century of Fiscal Squeeze Politics: 100 Years of Austerity, Politics, and Bureaucracy in Britain* (Oxford: Oxford University Press, 2017).

215. Barham, *Forgotten Lunatics*, 371–73.

216. War Office, *Report of the War Office Committee of Enquiry into "Shell-Shock"* Cmd. 1734 (London: HMSO, 1922).

217. Tim Harding, "'Not Worth Powder and Shot': A Reappraisal of Montagu Lomax's Contribution to Mental Health Reform," *BJPsych* 156 (1990): 180–87.

218. Freeman, "Psychiatry in Britain": 319.

219. Barham, *Forgotten Lunatics*, 104.

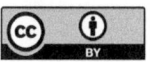

CHAPTER 3

Certified Insane: Concepts and Practices

INTRODUCTION: LILY'S STORY

Henry R was concerned about his wife Lily, a 43-year-old mother-of-two. She had been nursing his stepmother "which was very trying" and it had "unhinged her mind". Mindful of the stressful domestic environment, the family sought no treatment until the situation was desperate. The stigma of certification, the pauper lunatic label, and the belief that the war was nearly over so the stress would diminish, were likely to have contributed to their decision to wait. Lily was admitted to the mental observation ward at St. John's Road workhouse infirmary in Islington in July 1918, and from there to Colney Hatch Asylum.[1] Mentally disturbed people were frequently admitted first to an observation ward, likely to be relatively close to their home compared to an asylum beyond the suburbs. However, these wards were often ill-equipped and "without means of classification of maniacal, suicidal, or mildly affected patients".[2] Interactions between staff and patients could be unhelpful: a former asylum patient who had been certified while in an observation ward recalled that the workhouse medical officer was "a gentleman and very kind", but the head attendant was "a complete savage in every way".[3]

From observation ward to certification under the Lunacy Act 1890 was a small medico-legal step with profound implications for the patient. Once a person was certified under the Act an asylum was obliged to accept them, regardless of any underlying physical disorder causing their mental

© The Author(s) 2021   73
C. Hilton, *Civilian Lunatic Asylums During the First World War*,
Mental Health in Historical Perspective,
https://doi.org/10.1007/978-3-030-54871-1_3

disturbance. The most experienced psychiatrists, those working in the asylum, had no part in deciding who would be admitted under their care. This was inequitable with the authority given to general hospital doctors treating physical conditions, who decided which patients to admit to their wards. The system favoured the opinions of general hospital doctors who did not want to treat disturbed patients, especially if perceived as elderly or likely to have an unfavourable prognosis. As John Keay, president of the Medico-Psychological Association (MPA), commented in 1918: "the most trifling mental abnormality is used as the pretext for sending to the asylum".[4] One neurologist proposed that every general hospital should provide wards to treat mentally disturbed patients who had underlying physical disorders, including isolation wards where quiet was not essential, to ensure that they received the most appropriate treatment.[5] The existence of such wards is elusive.

Attitudes of senior doctors in general hospitals contributed to increasing the proportion of older people in asylums who were regarded as senile and untreatable. By the time war broke out, over 15 per cent of asylum patients were over 60 years old, drawn from five per cent of the population of the same age group.[6] Some, such as Emma Matilda L (Fig. 3.1), were admitted "in a dying condition and all [were] in a very reduced bodily condition."[7] Asylum staff were perplexed why such physically ill people were sent to their institutions rather than treated in the local general hospital.[8]

Returning to Lily, the obligatory doctor's certificate required for asylum admission recorded her disturbed behaviour:

> highly amused with herself; when asked questions she starts quoting some simple rhyme and keeps time to the metre by shaking her head from side to side and ends with an emphatic nod and then glares at you. She is sometimes very noisy and destructive, smashing the mug she is drinking from.

On arrival at Colney Hatch the medical officer examined her and summarised:

> She is suffering from mania. Is very noisy, restless and agitated – wanders about the room talking incessantly to herself, and is at times resistive to attention. She has obvious hallucinations, both visual and auditory – hears and answers the voices of imaginary persons, and describes the wonderful

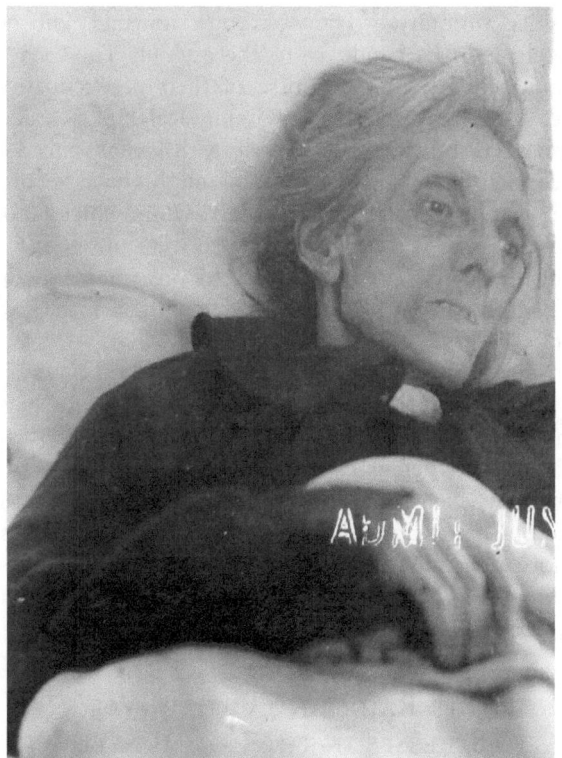

Fig. 3.1 Emma Matilda L, just after admission to an asylum (Photographs of female patients at Colney Hatch 1918–1920 H12/CH/B/18/004 LMA)

coloured lights which appear in the padded room at night and by their movements convey messages to her. She mistakes identities recognising strangers as old friends and is faulty in her personal habits. She is in great impaired health suffering from advanced Pulmonary Tuberculosis and is regarded as not likely to live long.[9]

The term mania indicated a general state of mental and physical over-activity, rather than the specific diagnosis of manic-depression (bipolar disorder).[10] Lily's mania was probably "acute delirious mania" or "acute delirium", both terms used at the time.[11] It was often rapidly fatal because it was associated with underlying severe physical illness, a relationship recognised since antiquity.[12] The workhouse infirmary did not mention Lily's tuberculosis in its handover to the asylum. They may have over-looked it or ignored it in the course of their preoccupation with her mental state. It is doubtful that Lily's physical illness trajectory could have been reversed, but for other people with less advanced or different illnesses, treatment in a general hospital might have secured a better outcome. Lily's transfer to an overcrowded asylum which lacked isolation facilities also jeopardised other patients who were put at risk of catching her infection. Lily died a few weeks later. Her post-mortem confirmed the diagnosis: "Both lungs riddled with tubercle with cavities of varying sizes in both lobes."[13]

Lily's journey from community, via the observation ward and into the asylum raises many issues about the mental disorders suffered by people admitted as pauper lunatics. This chapter seeks to explore some of them. The chapter begins by touching on the stresses of wartime life in the community, even though the Lunacy Act did not permit asylums to undertake out-patient or community work. It then focusses on mental disorders more generally, but with special reference to the patients in the public lunatic asylums: classification; research; nature and nurture hypotheses; treatment and convalescence.

Air Raids and Other War Stresses in the Community

During air raids early in the war, while some people ran for their cellars, others flocked onto the streets to watch the airships illuminated by search lights and to see their shells exploding. Anticipation of further raids caused some people anxiety, nightmares, insomnia and exhaustion. There was real danger, but Freudian interpretations also circulated, relating to the airships' phallic shape.[14]

Medical historians interested in the First World War have tended to focus on shell shock or the population's physical health, as reflected in national agendas at that time.[15] Concerning civilian mental health, there is little historical research about it, in contrast to much appertaining to it during the Second World War. Historical analysis about the latter provides some clues about issues likely to have been present in the earlier war, such as civilian morale, responses to threats of air raids and the presentation of symptoms. Edgar Jones and colleagues in their Second World War study, found that predictions of mass air raid neurosis failed to materialize: civilians proved more resilient than planners had predicted, largely because they had underestimated public adaptability and resourcefulness.[16] Hazel Croft, in a study of civilian neuroses also in the Second World War noted that wartime camaraderie, full employment, active roles in civil defence and war work may have assisted wellbeing. Reluctance to admit to mental symptoms which could be seen as personal failings, the incentive to be an ideal, stoical citizen, and that many people would not have taken their worries as a health matter to their family doctor, may have both concealed the true amount of mental disturbance and kept the sufferer away from mental institutions.[17] Croft's and Jones' analyses cannot be directly extrapolated backwards to the First World War, but they provide some possible explanations in support of the data which point to relatively few civilians being admitted to asylums due to unmanageable mental stress.

Of a random sample of 49 First World War civilian admissions to Colney Hatch, Claybury, Hanwell and Napsbury,[18] stress, worry, fright and fear relating to daily life in London were identified as presumed causes in five. On the one hand, this may be an under-estimate because attributing causes was an in-exact science and asylum records were incomplete. On the other hand, of these five, possibly three whose conditions were initially attributed to stress had other disorders to explain their symptoms. Lily was one. James N was another who was subsequently diagnosed with general paralysis of the insane (GPI, brain syphilis). He is discussed later in this chapter. Arabella M (Fig. 3.2), a 53-year-old house-

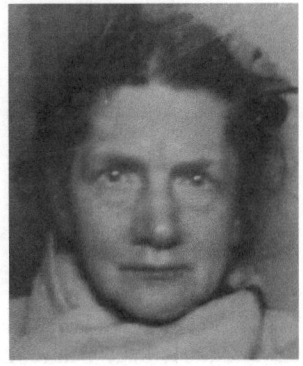

Fig. 3.2 Arabella M, admitted with "Worry and Zeppelin fright" (Photographs of female patients at Colney Hatch 1908–1918 H12/CH/B/18/003 LMA)

wife, was admitted to Colney Hatch, with mental distress attributed to "Worry and Zeppelin fright", but her case records also suggest overlap with physical illness.[19]

The figures do not suggest that the asylum population in the London area was overwhelmed with psychologically distressed patients. In contrast, in a study of the Denbigh Asylum serving north Wales, Pamela Michael identified 19 per cent of admissions in 1918 associated with "war worry".[20] Fear of raids in Wales may have caused more mental disturbance than for Londoners who developed strategies to deal with them. Similarly, as Harry Bernstein, born in 1910 and growing up almost 200 miles from London in Stockport, Cheshire, wrote: "The German zeppelins were bombing London and fear hung over us constantly."[21]

Threats other than bombs also created stress. Some people developed anxiety and depression fearful of the consequences for their loved ones fighting in the trenches or devastated by their deaths. For some women, keeping intensely busy was another way of coping, including making the most of new opportunities to work outside the home.[22] For others changes in roles and employment, and consequent financial difficulties, were traumatic. For Louise F (Fig. 3.3), a single 34-year-old Turkish "enemy alien", a financial crisis precipitated her admission to Claybury.

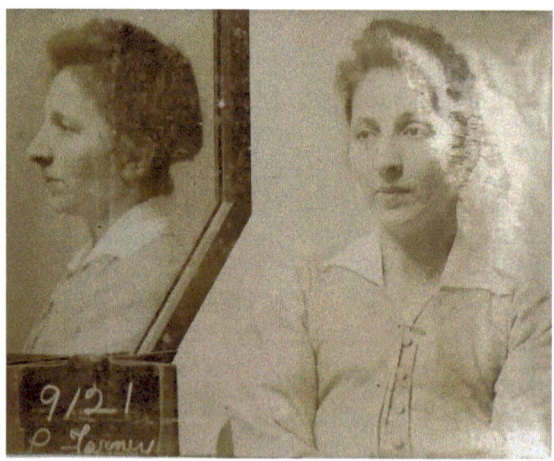

Fig. 3.3   Louise F, an enemy alien (Claybury: Female Patient Case Notes 1917; Redbridge Heritage Centre, 2020)

Louise had worked in England for 12 years, but in 1917 she was unemployed, her status making work hard to find. She sold her belongings to support herself. Almost destitute, when the coal merchant failed to deliver her coal, she smashed his shop window in despair and anger. The magistrate sentenced her to a week in Brixton Prison from where she was released to the workhouse. There, she was distressed and refused to eat, and was certified for asylum admission. Six months later, she was discharged fully recovered via a Mental After Care Association convalescent house.[23] The asylum had provided care and time for her to recover from her ordeal. She returned to work as a nurse and dress designer.[24]

Undoubtedly some people were admitted to asylums suffering directly from the effects of war time stress, but given the limited data collected during the war by the asylums' Board of Control ("the Board"), the patchiness of case notes, plus inaccuracies in specifying the causes of mental symptom and other factors affecting bed occupancy, it would be imprudent to estimate the number of asylum patients admitted directly and solely due to the stresses of war. Overall, asylum case notes suggest that they were admitted infrequently, and, as for Louise F, those whose symptoms were really due to stresses in civilian life, they improved and were discharged. This contrasts with the many admitted with life threatening or incurable mental and physical disorders.

UNDERSTANDING MENTAL DISORDERS: CLASSIFICATION

Concerning the healthcare of sick people in England, psychiatrist Adolph Meyer, looking on from the USA, commented:

> One comes closest to the truth about English medicine in saying that it's conceived as the art of healing, to which science is subordinated. Practical matters receive priority everywhere.[25]

Doctors were trained as apprentices to treat patients to the best of their ability guided by their professional ethics, with hypotheses less important. In asylum practice, the Lunacy Act undermined the tradition of medical empiricism, of helping people when they needed help. It introduced conflict for doctors between providing timely treatment when the sufferer sought it or needed it or might benefit from it, and delays because certification was only possible with more severe symptoms. Clinical records reveal patients' disabling psychiatric symptoms and the suffering of those admitted to the asylums. Sarah F's tortured expression indicated her anguish (Fig. 3.4).[26] She, and others unwell due to mental disorders, required compassion and help in the broadest sense, regardless of theories and legalities.

Meyer's observation fits with Tracy Loughran's argument that "British doctors were self-consciously proud of the empiricism of their medical tradition", in contrast to the "French and German taste for abstract theorisation."[27] Nevertheless, British psychiatrists were active in debates on some philosophical questions, such as the nature of insanity. There was no accepted single definition; all were unsatisfactory, vague and subjective with their value debated and with unclear dividing lines between normal, abnormal and eccentricity.[28] The Lunacy Act was unhelpful, stating that "'Lunatic' means an idiot or person of unsound mind".[29] Psychiatrist Charles Mercier wrote on the difficulties of defining insanity:

> No doubt we all have a certain vague notion in our minds, but the fact that we cannot put the notion into words shows that the notion is but vague and cloudy, sadly lacking in precision and definiteness.

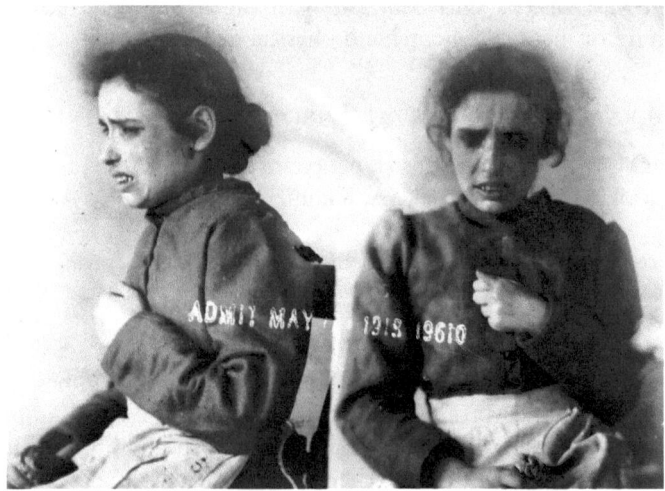

Fig. 3.4 Sarah F, in need of help (Photographs of female patients at Colney Hatch 1918–1920 H12/CH/B/18/004 LMA)

With his own characteristic eccentricity and boldness, lack of clarity did not stop him declaring that his own equally vague definition of insanity, an all-encompassing disorder of mind and conduct, was the best.[30] John Turner, medical superintendent of the Essex County Asylum at Brentwood, aimed for more precision and defined a "certifiable lunatic" as "one whose conduct (owing to disease) is persistently out of harmony with his environment, and who is, or may become, a source of harm to himself or a danger or annoyance to the community."[31] It too was inadequate, raising questions about the meaning of psychiatric "disease" and introducing social factors which could vary across place and time. Another physician, Edward Younger, advised that a doctor giving evidence in a law court should refuse to define insanity.[32] The difficulty of defining it was also a concern outside the medical profession. Earl Russell, perhaps influenced by personal experience, his own behaviours from time to time being on the fringes of public acceptability, commented in the House of Lords in 1914 that "whether a person is sane or insane is one of the most difficult matters that doctors have to decide, the dividing line being so fine".[33]

Not only was the overall definition of insanity inadequate, but classifying the array of different disorders within it was likewise problematic. Disease classification was founded on the system of the biological sciences. Meaningful categories depended upon whether symptoms were consistent across time and culture: if they had a biological basis they would exist in the same form in different places and times. This bore out the need to identify the *form* of symptoms, rather than their culture-bound *content* which varied across time and place, influenced by contemporary cultural issues and belief systems.[34] Classification was challenging for psychiatric symptoms which often lacked a clear underlying physical pathology, but identifying the type of disorder was important as each type would be expected to behave in a characteristic way with regard to causes, prognoses and treatments. Without clear physical pathology, psychiatric classification was (and is) based on clinicans' expertise in psychopathology, influenced by social and cultural expectations of disease and normality.[35] A degree of subjectivity was inevitable. Recognising these uncertainties could also contribute to public fear of wrongful confinement due to inaccurate medical assessments.[36]

Classification of psychiatric disorders was not just of interest in England, but was under consideration in Germany. Many psychiatrists outside Germany desired to emulate Emil Kraepelin's "clinic", but responses to his psychiatric classification varied.[37] Meyer initially welcomed Kraepelin's diagnostic classification, particularly concerning manic-depression and dementia praecox (later known as schizophrenia), as the break-through which psychiatry was waiting for, but he later criticised it for being too neurological and failing to take into account the context of the patient's life story.[38] Mercier accused his colleagues of following "Continental fashion"[39] and Havelock Ellis, a physician, better known for his studies on sexuality, acknowledged the snags of psychiatric classification generally and Kraepelin's classification in particular:

> It is impossible to consider the miscellaneous cases brought together by Kraepelin under the heading of manic-depressive insanity as a single disease....We learn nothing by placing a case in a "natural classification" which has no existence, and can have no existence, in the sense understood by Kraepelin.[40]

The war may have influenced negativity towards German psychiatric research. Near the end of the war, president of the American Medico-Psychological Association, James Anglin, described his colleagues as "infatuated with German pseudo-discoveries". Subjectivity associated with personal anguish may have clouded his views, mentioning in that lecture, the death of his eldest son at Vimy Ridge, his second a "permanent cripple", a third still fighting, and another preparing to travel to war.[41]

During the First World War and through to today, uncertainties in knowledge and understanding reflect different and evolving psychiatric classification systems and a thirst to find meaning, order and clinical guidance. In the context of many divergent views, the Board classified mental disorders based on their presumed causes, in the hope that it could reveal information useful for prevention and treatment.[42] Regarding causation, psychiatrist Bernard Hollander drew attention to the importance of environmental and social factors, Mercier emphasised concepts drawn from understandings about physical illness, while others favoured inherited risks.[43] A search for causes fitted with the belief that mental disease originated beyond skull and brain, in line with recent discoveries of invisible causes of physical disease identified through studies of physiology, pathology and bacteriology.[44] This was also compatible with observations that physical and mental disturbances overlapped, as in Lily's case, and that they had common causes, despite mechanisms remaining obscure.[45]

These overlaps encouraged the practice of carrying out post-mortems on almost all asylum patients (discussed further in Chapter 7): if causes could not be determined during life, it was appropriate to search for them after death. Biological explanations also had other advantages, such as the potential to avoid blaming patients for their own mental problems and reducing punitive responses to their otherwise inexplicable behaviours. The colloquialism "pull yourself together" was known by the mid-nineteenth century,[46] indicating that the speaker believed that a mentally disturbed person could immediately revert to normal. That was no truer for severe mental than physical illness: as Dr. Montagu Lomax advised in his critique of war time psychiatric practice: "it is as rational to punish a mental patient for refractory behaviour as it would be to punish a typhoid fever case for a rise in temperature."[47]

For each patient admitted, the Board pragmatically sought to record "predisposing" and "exciting" factors which could occur alone or in combination. These fitted with the need to disentangle multiple theories of causation, but as indicated for Lily R, Arabella M and James N, attributing causation was prone to inaccuracies. Before the war, from 1907 to 1911, the Board identified the main causes of admission to be alcohol, prolonged mental stress, "insane heredity", senility, GPI and epilepsy, with some gender variation for each (Table 3.1).[48] Pre-war data is the best available because the Board discontinued its multi-page tabular compilations of causation as part of reducing the administrative workload

Table 3.1 Yearly average of the total incidence of each cause (for first admissions) assigned without any correlated cause or factor, 1907–1911

	Males		Females	
	n	%	n	%
Alcohol	707	20.5	311	8.5
Prolonged mental stress	567	16.5	642	17.6
Insane heredity	399	11.5	538	14.7
Senility	328	9.5	416	11.4
Acquired syphilis (GPI)	311	9.0	40	1.1
Epilepsy	220	6.4	165	4.5
Total	3443		3649	

Source Commissioners in Lunacy, Tables xvii (male), xviii (female): causes of first admissions, excluding to idiot establishments, 1907–1911, MH51/687 TNA.

during the war. Of note, very few people were admitted with so-called "moral insanity", a subject which has entered recent public discourse through early twenty-first century novels depicting women incarcerated for no other reason than having given birth to an illegitimate child.[49] There is little evidence that unmarried mothers were admitted to asylums in the war years unless they also had mental symptoms, or they fell under the rules of the Mental Deficiency Act (MDA) 1913. The MDA, but not the Lunacy Act, obliged authorities to admit to an institution a woman known to be mentally defective "who is in receipt of poor law relief at the time of giving birth to an illegitimate child, or when pregnant of such child".[50] Objectives of this rule included preventing further pregnancies and preserving the woman's health and the ratepayers' pockets. Punishment was not integral to the plan, on the assumption that the pregnancies resulted from vulnerable women being exploited by men. The women tended to be admitted to mental deficiency institutions, lunatic asylums being considered inappropriate for their long-term detention.

Despite treatment implications derived from classifications based on symptoms or causation, they had little part in informing the organisation of asylums. Asylums adopted patient classifications based on "conduct, habits and bodily states" to place patients into "infirmary", "quiet", or "troublesome" wards.[51] These categories often had little to do with the individual's treatment or prognosis, but were convenient for the asylum. Some new patients were placed on wards appropriate to their needs, but others, such as some who were very disturbed, could be placed on wards with the most difficult to manage long-stay patients who had different disorders and therapeutic needs.[52] If the acutely disturbed new patient settled while on a ward of mainly long-stay patients suffering persistent behavioural symptoms, he could be overlooked relative to those who demanded more attention. Alternatively, if a new patient saw that difficult behaviours attracted staff attention, this could accentuate his disturbances, which could bring about the assumption that he had a similar chronic disorder. Either way, the new patient would be disadvantaged. The outspoken psychiatrist Lionel Weatherly criticised the combination of inadequate classification together with overcrowding.[53] The worst scenario, according to Nurse Jane Dagg who gave evidence to the postwar Cobb Inquiry, was overcrowding with no classification, as in the asylum where she had worked.[54] Little attention was paid to the merits of clinically focussed classifications or the understanding that acute disorders were more likely to improve than chronic. According to Weatherly, and to

Herbert Ellis, a magistrate and asylum management "visiting" committee member, the way patients were classified in asylums was influenced by short term financial considerations.[55]

RESEARCHING MENTAL CONDITIONS

"Scientific" classification of mental disorders was an aid to undertaking meaningful research, and its haphazard utilisation may have been one factor contributing to Hugh Freeman's analysis that British psychiatrists produced relatively little of importance from their research.[56] Despite this, the *Journal of Mental Science* (*JMS*),[57] published by the Medico-Psychological Association (MPA), brought together much research from home and abroad, pointing to diverse concerns and priorities, including a tendency for researchers to grapple with somatic, bodily processes thought to be associated with mental disorders, rather than the mental disorders themselves. Reports in the *JMS* on "vaccine therapeutics", dysentery, enteric fever (typhoid) and inflammation, read more like a journal of microbiology, rather than psychiatry.[58] Alongside the *JMS*, the *Lancet*, published for a broad medical readership, indicated other psychiatric preoccupations, including shell shock, lunacy legislation,[59] sedative medication[60] and "sexual perversion".[61] Weighing up the multiplicity of often contradictory research findings was far from straight forward, itself a demonstration of the lack of a secure scientific knowledge-base for clinical, policy and administrative decision making. Randomised controlled trials were not yet established in medical research, and together with embryonic statistical methodology, these factors often made conclusions hard to draw. George Savage commented that new discoveries challenged earlier certainties: "we must 'wait and see'; that we are prepared to follow truth where it leads, and that a dim light is better than none in such darkness as the realms of life and consciousness."[62]

Another factor contributing to the paucity of psychiatric research in England was the lack of an academic backbone for psychiatry, in contrast to the world-leaders in the field in German speaking countries.[63] Also, in contrast to the trend in much of western Europe, English-speaking countries separated the medical specialties of psychiatry (brain: mainly mental and behavioural manifestations) and neurology (brain: mainly bodily manifestations), despite much clinical overlap. British neurology became a discipline with high prestige and impressive clinical and scientific standards, in contrast to psychiatry. Many neurologists worked in private practice and had time for research. Most lacked experience of, or clinical responsibility for, patients in asylums although their research was pertinent to them. Neurologist John Hughlings Jackson, for example, researched epilepsy, yet he was unlikely to look after people with the severest forms of the disorder who frequently resided in asylums. In contrast to neurological research, little took place in asylums which were cut off, geographically and intellectually, at a distance from teaching hospitals and universities, and with their staff submerged by heavy workloads.

Despite lack of participation in research, as the content of the *JMS* indicated, psychiatrists sought answers to many of the problems faced in their clinical work. In 1912, almost every asylum authority in England and Wales sent delegates to a conference in London to discuss improving research into mental diseases. The conference stressed the importance of government funding for research (as provided in Germany) and informed the Prime Minister and Chancellor of the Exchequer of that.[64] Just before war broke out, the Board and MPA planned further discussions on taking research forward.[65] Later in 1914, the Treasury granted the Board £1500 to spend on research.[66] This was a pitiful proportion of the overall government medical research budget of £58,000.[67] The many applications for funding suggested interest in undertaking psychiatric research but limited expertise to carry it out.[68] Around the beginning of the war, the *JMS* and the Board reported on progress made in research from the asylums, including on the perennial enigmas of asylum dysentery, biological markers of insanities, and the relationship between insanity and mental deficiency.[69] Research on mental disorders was challenging, but financial priorities may have contributed to John Keay's frustration: "Why should insanity be left behind when so much forward endeavour is made in general medicine?".[70]

Most psychiatric research ceased during the war but a fresh clinical challenge loomed at its end: to unravel the new, disabling condition of encephalitis lethargica, later immortalised in Oliver Sacks' *Awakenings*[71] and Harold Pinter's *A Kind of Alaska*.[72] Despite an early consensus that the disorder resulted from the 1918–1919 influenza pandemic, evaluating the evidence was tricky and the hypothesis was gradually replaced by scepticism.[73]

GPI: CLINICAL CHALLENGE, RESEARCH AND CAUTIOUS RESPONSES TO INNOVATION

Research guided by the desire to identify physical causes of mental disorders had direct relevance to the welfare of patients in the asylums. General paralysis of the insane (GPI) provides an illustration of this. GPI could be difficult to diagnose from the patient's history and mental state examination, hardly surprising given that its symptoms were multiple and variable. The Wassermann blood test introduced in 1907 helped, but could give false positives. In 1913, Noguchi identified the spirochaete treponema pallidum, a bacterium, in the cerebro-spinal fluid surrounding the brain, thus verifying that syphilis caused GPI. Cautious psychiatrists in England, however, remained wary of both the Wassermann test, which moved slowly and erratically into asylum use,[74] and of Noguchi's evidence, acknowledging in 1918 that the spirochaete "probably" caused GPI.[75]

Some patients with GPI were women but most were men, often described as "powerful, hearty men, who had lived hard and never ailed...had 'burnt the candle at both ends,' and had led irregular if not debauched lives".[76] Syphilis was acquired sexually, but the spirochaete could spread to many body organs. When in the brain, its array of symptoms often included delusions of grandeur, which could result in financial ruin for a family.[77] Salvarsan, an arsenic-based drug, could cure bodily syphilis[78] but had no effect on the spirochaetes once they had entered the brain.[79] Some men so feared developing GPI that, after an "indiscretion with a woman", they developed another psychiatric disorder—syphilophobia—which could "drift into insanity" or lead to suicide.[80]

GPI was inevitably fatal: disinhibited behaviour, restlessness, seizures and difficulty swallowing food were associated with an undignified asylum death, such for Emma Sarah M who gave birth at Claybury in November 1914 while suffering from seizures caused by the disorder. Her baby survived, and, aware of the stigma derived from insanity, the asylum arranged a birth certificate which did not state the place of birth.[81] James N, a more typical patient with GPI, was a single, 34-year-old clothing factory machinist,[82] admitted to Colney Hatch. He was described as suffering from stress, and was sullen, melancholic, and restless. He refused food, likely associated with his "delusions that he is 'full up' to the neck and that he cannot pass his water or faeces." He developed seizures and died shortly after admission.[83]

Given the progressive and fatal nature of GPI, finding effective treatment was essential, even if the treatment itself had risks. During the war, Julius Wagner-Jauregg in Vienna, inoculated patients with malaria parasites to induce high fevers to kill the heat-sensitive spirochetes. He published his findings in 1919.[84] Malaria treatment was dangerous, but until penicillin became available nearly three decades later, it was the only hope. Malaria treatment, alongside other clinical innovations, received a characteristically cautious reception from psychiatrists in England. Drastic treatments in psychiatry were appearing around the same time as risky interventions for other fatal disorders. William Halstead, for example, introduced the "radical" mastectomy for breast cancer, in the belief that cure was more likely with ever wider surgical resection.[85]

Caution and scepticism about innovative clinical methods was a double-edged sword. On the one hand it could prevent harm by avoiding insufficiently proven new methods, and on the other, it could cause harm by rejecting new and effective procedures. In contrast to the conservative approach of psychiatrists in England, and in the context of multiple hypotheses about infections combined with ideas about the benefits of radical treatments, less conformist colleagues risked generating over-zealous and unregulated treatments. This happened in the USA. Henry Cotton at Trenton State Asylum instigated a programme of radical surgery for psychiatric patients, to remove various organs harbouring suspected "focal infection" which supposedly produced or perpetuated their mental disorder.[86] Some of Cotton's patients, probably coincidentally, recovered mentally after his interventions, but evaluation of the treatment neglected the overall balance between healing and harm, including death. Surgery for focal infection, however, was not confined to psychiatry. It was also used for preventing physical disorders, such as "routine" tonsillectomy in children, once commonplace but later discredited as a prophylactic public health measure.[87] Despite some admiration for Cotton's work in the UK, his regime was not replicated on this side of the Atlantic where psychiatrists were arguably less innovative and more restrained in their treatments.[88]

English psychiatrists weighed up risks in a generally risk-averse asylum culture. They took clinical risks from time to time, usually in desperation. Tube feeding, is one example, undertaken on patients usually gravely ill, likely to have severe mental illness, stupor, food refusal and dehydration, all compounding the risks of the feeding.[89] English psychiatrists also adopted some fashions or fads used for treating physical illness. The Royal

Society of Medicine (RSM), alongside its more traditional medical and surgical sections, had a "Section of Electrotherapeutics", which advocated the use of X-rays and therapeutic electricity, the latter compatible with the understanding of electrical impulses in the nervous system. It also had a "Section of Balneology and Climatology" which included therapeutic bathing considered beneficial for many physical and mental disorders. Accepted but unproven, balneological therapeutic measures in asylums included prolonged warm baths for "motor excitement", Turkish baths for "simple melancholia" and brief cold showers or baths "to overcome certain resistances in the nervous system" in stupor.[90]

Use of electricity became an attractive therapeutic tool, acceptable to professionals and public, and of interest even to cautious asylum doctors. Shifting from simple therapeutic bathing, more risky methods evolved, such as combining bathing plus electricity in an "electric bath".[91] This was believed to stimulate stuporose patients and to help excretion of toxins in schizophrenia. Using baths specially constructed from earthenware or wood, with a large flat copper electrode covered with towelling at each end connected to a battery, the procedure was considered safe. Twenty-two-year-old Annie H reportedly benefitted from electric baths, then died suddenly after a treatment. According to the Board, procedures had been followed correctly, staff supervised the bathing and applied the correct current. At post-mortem Annie was found to have "status lymphaticus", characterised by large thymus, thyroid and lymph glands, and bone marrow hyperplasia. The coroner concluded that her death was due to sudden paralysis of the heart due to status lymphaticus, unrelated to the bath.[92]

But what was status lymphaticus? Detected at post-mortem, usually after a sudden death when under medical care, its incidence increased in parallel with the use of anaesthetics. It was a convenient post-mortem diagnosis. For bereaved relatives, scientific explanations were more acceptable than "a visitation of God" in an increasingly secular society. It also provided a way for coroners to justify a verdict of death from natural causes, much to the relief of the medical profession. The existence of status lymphaticus was debated during the first half of the twentieth century, then disappeared from the medical corpus.[93] In reality, it never existed. It deflected blame for medical failure onto the patient. It was a diagnostic label created to fulfil professional and social needs. In this instance, it primarily protected the medical profession. Post-mortem findings were probably extremes of normal, modified by age, and mis-interpreted as abnormal, but with credibility compounded by the ferocious search for physical aetiologies.[94]

NATURE AND NURTURE: BIOLOGICAL, SOCIAL AND PSYCHOLOGICAL

In their style of pragmatic and cautious consideration, psychiatrists in England tried to fathom out which vulnerabilities predisposed to mental breakdown, and why people responded differently to similar hazards, such as infective organisms, social circumstances, alcohol, or war stresses. In their clinical practice, according to Loughran, they took a "magpie approach", choosing apparently useful aspects of particular theories without any one predominating.[95] Meyer's work also advocated a combined biological, psychological and social ("bio-psycho-social") approach to mental disorders, and looked beyond single issues and promoted an eclectic approach to treatment.[96] There was little consensus on the relative contributions of heredity, brain disease, infection, psycho-social, spiritual and other medical and non-medical factors to causing mental disorders. Debates on causes of mental disorder in civilian patients dovetailed with those concerning aetiology of shell shock—commotion, emotion or both—which continued throughout the war.[97] Baffled by the lack of clarity on causation of mental disorders, the Ministry of Pensions asked the Board for a simple rule to help clerical staff determine pension eligibility for mentally disturbed soldiers: the Board declined to provide one.[98]

Prominent biological theories of heredity included "degeneration", a downwards movement of health and wellbeing of individuals, families and society. Degeneration theories had punctuated Western philosophy, politics and religion for centuries,[99] and according to George Rosen, ideas included that once degeneracy set in, "the various generations of a family went inexorably to their doom."[100] Bénédict Morel introduced his *Dégénérescence* hypothesis in the 1850s, using it to explain mental and social disturbances.[101] The theory gained ground, among public, politicians, physicians and scientists including the influential psychiatrist Henry Maudsley who regarded degeneration as a threat to the prevailing culture of the British Empire and to European "civilisation".[102] As well as being founded on dubious scientific evidence, degeneration had racist and eugenic interpretations.

Benjamin Seebohm Rowntree proposed an alternative causal explanation for the numerous problems experienced by working class people: poverty.[103] Since poverty tended to affect whole families, it complicated differentiating between nature and nurture, intrinsic and extrinsic causes. In contrast to poverty being a primary cause, degeneration provided excuses, convenient for the elite, for failures of society. Blaming the constitution of the individual rather than intervening to alleviate poverty assuaged the consciences of the ruling classes. Degeneration theory, by its message of inevitable decline, could also discourage public interest in people in asylums whose problems were attributed to it. It added to stigma and gave a sense of hopelessness, a lost cause.

Degeneration had other effects on attitudes and practices in asylums. It was a reassuring and comforting "scientific" explanation for psychiatrists who failed to cure their patients. Nevertheless, many psychiatrists were also aware that theories of degeneration or heredity did not always hold: children of insane parents did not necessarily become insane or show other predicted decline or deficits.[104] Ideas of degeneration or heredity, or as Bill Bynum characterised it, a "concept of progressive hereditary degeneration",[105] did not deter psychiatrists from treating their patients labelled in this way, nor did it preclude rehabilitation, discharge or normal life events, as in the case of Dorothea S, a 33-year-old a single woman from Islington who assisted her mother Adelaide to run a boarding house before her admission to Colney Hatch.[106] Discharged after 18-months, labelled as suffering from "Mental Stress. Insane Heredity", three months later she married George M, a clerical worker, one of the residents of the boarding house.[107]

Although degeneracy and hereditary labels were ignored in terms of prognosis and treatment for individuals, according to Richard Walter, in his essay "What became of the degenerate?", eugenicists "adopted many of the claims of the devotees of degeneration."[108] Eugenics encouraged the reproduction of people with "desirable" traits, and discouraged reproduction of those with "undesirable". Eugenic proposals included sterilising the "unfit", such as insane people.[109] The war added other dimensions to the degeneration debate: if British soldiers were not degenerate, why did so many succumb to shell shock? Conversely, if they were degenerate, how did they win the war? Edward Shorter argued that degeneration theories were being discredited within psychiatry before the war,[110] although in England psychiatrists had never unanimously accepted them. Daniel Pick argued that the war "put paid to the dominance of *dégénérescence* within psychiatry and shifted the language of debate."[111] Nevertheless, the Board received the following statement before it was put to a meeting of the Board of Guardians at Sevenoaks in Kent in 1918:

> The War has taken an appalling toll on the lives of the noblest and best of our manhood, yet, today, too little or nothing is being done to safeguard the Race from the menace of the weak and dependent who constitute an ever growing financial burden on the Ratepayers, who, in themselves, are becoming yearly less able to bear the strain.[112]

The Board of Control stood its ground against eugenic proposals, including from psychiatrists, to sterilise insane patients, and against public opinion which surfaced advocating for it.[113] The war may have undermined degeneration theories, but related ideas around eugenics continued.

Biological and degeneration theories had the potential to profoundly affect the wellbeing of patients, but over-enthusiasm in that direction was tempered by the conservative culture of the medical profession and ideas on causes and treatment of mental disturbance arising from new mind-focussed disciplines. Concepts of psychology, psychoanalysis, and suggestive therapies were expounded by new professional groupings.[114] Some psychiatrists, such as Bernard Hart, medical superintendent of a private asylum and lecturer at University College Hospital, London, advocated for their methods as integral to the practice of psychiatry.[115] Lomax also recommended a psychological approach, such as placating and reasoning with patients to modify their behaviours.[116] At a basic level of psycho-social treatment, asylum staff were meant to demonstrate exemplary conduct to help correct patients' behavioural disturbances. While some staff used psychological skills acquired from experience, such as to diffuse a difficult ward situation, more widespread use of psychological methods would require more, and better trained, staff.[117]

Psychoanalysis gave new perspectives on causes and treatment of mental distress. It became better known in England concurrent with the war. Sigmund Freud's theories were translated into English by Ernest Jones, his disciple in England.[118] Carl Jung's British followers began promoting his views, arguing that his more optimistic and less sexually oriented conception of the unconscious was preferable to Freud's. However, mid-war, the *JMS* gave an airing to French zoologist Yves Delage who likened Freud's theories to an army or infectious disorder:

This new affection, which threatens to invade France, had its birth in Austria, at Vienna, some twenty years ago. Its progress, at first very slow, soon became rapid, and the spread of the evil generally now knows no pause....it would be imprudent to allow ourselves to be lulled to sleep under a delusive sense of security.[119]

Mercier also ridiculed Freud's theories of sexual excess, repressed complexes and infantile sexual longings, and asserted: "I do not hold that there is only one cause of mental disease. If I did so hold, I should be little better than a psycho-analyst."[120] Some doctors found psychoanalytic theories meaningful in their private work and when working with shell-shocked patients, such as WHR Rivers whose broadly psychological approach included catharsis, re-education, faith and suggestion.[121] However, as with much of psychiatric practice, clinicians used different methods. Lewis Yealland, for example, in contrast to Rivers, advocated a "disciplinary" and physical approach to shell shock and administered electric shocks.[122] More widely, psychoanalytic concepts and methods gained popularity mainly among the educated lay public.[123] Psychological and psychotherapeutic processes were far-removed from asylum practices even though they fitted with ideals of practice recommended by psychiatrists, that treatment for insanity must be humane and "individual".[124]

TREATMENTS: MORAL AND MEDICAL, RESTRAINT AND SECLUSION

Within the asylums, despite psychiatric recommendations for treatment to be individual and commenced as early as possible, just as for physical illnesses,[125] achieving this was beyond imagination. With the country's military needs taking precedence asylums were short staffed, losing the precious commodity of staff time to build therapeutic relationships and use their existing psychological skills to manage the most difficult, and potentially dangerous, patients. Lomax wrote: "To crowd lunatics into asylums is worse than useless unless we have some recognized principles of treating them when once we have got them there".[126] At the Cobb Inquiry, one former patient said: "If a man gets better it is in spite of the treatment, not because of it".[127] Another declared that in the asylum where he was admitted "There was no mental treatment at all".[128]

"Moral" treatment, which emphasised achieving mental and physical well-being, emerged as an ideal way of treating psychiatric disturbance, but it was never adopted widely. It was particularly hard to implement in larger, impersonal, overcrowded and inadequately staffed asylums. The method was attributed to William Tuke, the non-medical founder of the York Retreat. Despite support from psychiatrists, Bynum argued that "Professional, social, and economic considerations coloured their own judgments and tempered the enthusiasm they showed towards moral therapy". They were prepared to adopt features of it into their own therapeutic programmes, but not to jettison their medical models.[129] Alongside medical models and some practices inspired by moral treatment, asylums used many other approaches including careful attention and watchfulness, dealing with "dirty habits" (incontinence), and preventing physical injury or suicide, or death due to "maniacal exhaustion, an ending which is looked upon in asylums as being something of an opprobrium to those who have had charge of the case".[130]

Curative medications were generally unavailable for psychiatric and physical disorders. The psycho-pharmacopoeia was limited. Iron, quinine, arsenic, and strychnine were used as tonics.[131] A range of sedatives were available, with lack of consensus on whether to use them, which ones, and at what dosage.[132] Suggested drug treatments were often accompanied by warnings of their limited usefulness and toxicity.[133] Relying on imported medication, which was sometimes delayed at the docks during the war,[134] could have benefits and drawbacks for patients.

Laxatives were an ancient remedy for mental disturbance still within the psycho-pharmacopoeia. John Haslam, an eighteenth-century physician, referred to laxatives as "cathartics", the cleansing process of catharsis referring to purging bowels or mind.[135] They were also used to sedate, in the sense that profuse diarrhoea would temporarily weaken a patient, rendering him less liable to aggressive outbursts. Some doctors prescribed tiny doses of the laxative croton oil, up to 1 minim, the volume of a single drop of water, for constipation in patients who would not, or could not, cooperate with taking medication.[136] However, the tiny volume also made croton oil liable to misuse, easy for staff to dispense on a whim or conceal in food or drink. Weatherly and Lomax alleged that potent laxatives, particularly croton oil, were given punitively without the dose being documented.[137] The Cobb Inquiry investigated this allegation. It obtained records of purchases of croton oil at several asylums during

1919. Prestwich, where Lomas had worked, purchased around 6500 minims, compared to 480 minims at Colney Hatch and none at other asylums.[138] Although drug purchases depended upon how much the asylum had in stock, this was unlikely to account for the enormous differences. Neither could asylum size nor different types of illness or symptoms account for it, adding weight to the suspicion that some asylums used croton oil to punish, exhaust and sedate. Punitive practices may have been deliberately malicious, but could also have reflected lack of training and a despairing staff body who could not cope with the demands placed upon them (see Chapter 4).

Lomax agreed with psychiatrist William Stoddart that hefty sedation was "a refined substitute for hitting [the patient] on the head with a club."[139] Another term for using medication to calm disturbed behaviour was "chemical restraint", with controlling effects comparable to "manual restraint" which required person to person contact or "mechanical restraint" which required equipment. Manual and chemical methods were usually initiated by ward staff in response to a crisis. These methods were not formally monitored but there were guidelines to ensure safety of both parties: "A violent patient must be overcome by weight of numbers and never by blows or any such form of retaliation" wrote Stoddart.[140] However, unregulated and transitory, chemical and manual restraint could be secretive, abusive and punitive, and manual restraint could cause severe injuries (see Chapter 8).

By the war, early forms of mechanical restraint such as chains and shackles had been replaced by devices usually of cloth or leather, such as straitjackets and strong dresses made of very thick material and fastened at the back with sleeves which could be tied to the patient's torso. Jane Hamlett and Lesley Hoskins, in their study of asylum clothing, explained that restraint in a strong dress was "theoretically, a means of management and a treatment rather than a punishment but it did mark out 'difficult' patients and was certainly open to overuse or abuse by ward staff."[141] Mechanical restraint could be applied for prolonged periods and was known to be used punitively, hence it was monitored by the Board under the Lunacy Act.[142] A senior staff member needed to authorise the procedure, to document the reasons for using it and the duration of use.[143] Another method of control was seclusion, with reasons for monitoring similar to those for mechanical restraint. Lomax and Stoddart disapproved of restraint and seclusion generally, and instead advocated taking a disturbed patient out of doors to calm down, giving him a foot-ball,[144] or "turning him into the garden by himself and keeping him there till his aggressiveness has blown over".[145] Restraint and seclusion methods were commonplace during the war, as they were less labour intensive for staff than finding out the cause of a patient's restlessness, or providing social or psychological calming alternatives.[146]

Some asylums used either mechanical restraint or seclusion, some both, others neither.[147] Some differences in recorded usage may be accounted for by furtive completion of records.[148] At Claybury, for example, medical superintendent Robert Armstrong-Jones reported to his committee that when patient Harriet R was wrapped in a wet blanket, a recognised means of mechanical restraint, "her limbs had been quite free to move, and therefore the case had not been entered in the register",[149] despite rules that the reasons for using it had to be documented rather than the outcome of doing so. Soon after this, the Board inspected Claybury and commended it for not using mechanical restraint.[150] This sequence of events suggests that using methods of which the Board disapproved, encouraged deception, left the Board unaware of the extent of their use, and maintained appearances of good practice. Weatherly reflected on restraint procedures: "Whenever I see in the reports of the Commissioners the statement, "We are glad to see that there is no record of mechanical restraint," I often wonder what substitute has been used".[151] He also wrote:

> Nothing, to my mind, is worse than to see a suicidal patient struggling with two or three nurses or attendants, and I have often been told by such patients how much they appreciated the kindly supervised mechanical restraint that I had ordered.[152]

Perhaps self-congratulatory, and although his opinion was contrary to the Lunacy Act and the official standpoint of the Board, others agreed with him that the type of restraint was not as important as using it humanely.[153] Another method of mechanical restraint which by-passed official gaze was to sit particularly difficult patients against a wall with a heavy table pushed close in front of them, without amusement or employment, only allowing them out to use the lavatory. In this way, one attendant could observe several difficult patients. Lomax described this as a "brutalizing form of restraint", "an inhuman device to save attendants trouble".[154] Established practices which made life easier for the staff persisted even when condemned as cruel: placing patients "behind the table" continued at Prestwich into the 1950s, according to a staff member witness speaking in an oral history interview.[155]

Seclusion was meant to provide "time-out", a cooling-off period for extremely disturbed people, but it could also be used punitively, resembling solitary confinement in prisons. Some seclusion rooms were padded, and many were unheated and lacked light and ventilation. Furniture was attached to the floor to prevent it being used to harm self or others. Each room generally had an observation window or peep hole in the door which was openable only from the outside.[156] Lomax advocated having an attendant always outside the door to avoid the patients' "horror of loneliness and darkness which make them worse."[157] In an autobiographical account of his experience in an Australian asylum, Mr. D Davidson described his isolation in a "cell" with an "eye-hole" through which a tall man occasionally squinted at him. Davidson linked his isolation and observation to the worsening of his terrifying beliefs that he would be tortured and killed.[158] Another patient, James Scott, wrote about "padded cells", and drew one with a patient naked inside (Fig. 3.5). It is unclear whether the "hideous" sounds he referred to were the reason for, or outcome of, the seclusion:

> The padded cells in an asylum are the most dreadful places imaginable; and the sounds which emanate from them, customarily, are hideous. I fervently ask the Almighty to spare me from ever again hearing such soul haunting noises, blasphemies, obscenities, cries and moans, as those which I so often heard during my four years imprisonment in the awful institution of which I am now disclosing the secrets.[159]

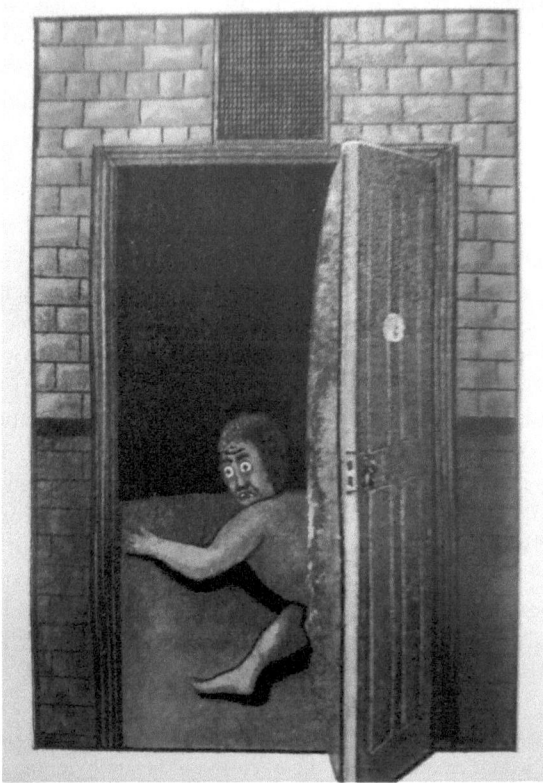

Fig. 3.5 James Scott's drawing of a seclusion room (James Scott, *Sane in Asylum Walls* [London: Fowler Wright, 1931], facing p. 102) (Copyright: owner sought but not found)

RECOVERY, CONVALESCENCE AND DISCHARGE

Despite inadequate and harsh treatment in asylums, a proportion of patients recovered sufficiently to be discharged. However, in 1916, Weatherly reminded his readers that "the recovery-rate of mental diseases is…no higher than it was in the 'seventies' of the last century."[160] The annual recovery and discharge rate from lunacy institutions declined, from around 40 per cent of admissions between 1889 and 1905, to 32 per cent by 1914, and 27 per cent in 1918 (Table 3.2). In 1913,

Table 3.2 Rates of recovery, 1878–1919, across all lunacy institutions in England and Wales

Years	Men: % of annual admissions	Men: % of total resident	Women: % of annual admissions	Women: % of total resident
1878–1882	36.1	10.6	43.7	11.4
1883–1887	35.6	9.7	44.5	10.6
1888–1897	35.3	9.8	42.5	10.4
1898–1902	34.7	9.2	40.4	9.3
1903–1907	33.6	8.2	40.6	8.9
1908–1912	30.8	6.6	37.7	7.6
1913–1917	29.1	5.7	35.9	6.7
1918	22.8	5.2	30.9	6.5
1919	25.0	6.5	38.0	8.4

Source Sixth Annual Report of the Board of Control, for the Year 1919 (London: HMSO, 1920) Appendix A, 22–23.

about 10,000 people were discharged, but some of them were classed as "relieved" (somewhat better) or "not improved", rather than "recovered". Recovery data are not straightforward, partly because the Board sometimes used the term synonymously with discharge. Data on recovery rates were also presented in two ways: as a proportion of the number of admissions in any one year and compared to the total asylum population (Table 3.2).[161] The first gave a far more optimistic view than the second. These data are also difficult to interpret because numerous factors contributed to the changing discharge rates, such as admissions of more patients like Lily, with disturbed behaviour due to underlying physical illness, and bed shortages so that only the most unwell were admitted. Overcrowding and understaffing hindered staff-patient therapeutic relationships, reinforced custodial practices and minimised occupational and social treatments, all of which had the potential to affect recovery. Other less well-founded explanations for reduced recovery included that mental disorders were becoming more incurable and that clinicians were getting better at detecting insanity making them reluctant to discharge patients until all their symptoms had resolved.[162] These explanations, convenient and credible to the leadership, exonerated the medical officers from failing to cure their patients while praising their expertise.

Although discharge became increasingly unlikely with longer duration of admission,[163] some discharges occurred after many years, such as for Ida D (Fig. 3.6[164]). Ida was a single 38-year-old cork cutter who lived with her widowed mother in Whitechapel.[165] She was admitted to Colney Hatch in 1914 with a one-month history of mental disturbance. She was discharged "not improved" in 1951, 37 years later.[166] This preceded Ministry of Health policies on closing institutions and developing community care, suggesting that the discharge initiative came from the asylum itself or from friends or a charity outside the institution. Contrary to stereotypical assumptions, age was no bar to discharge, either for Ida after her long admission or for Albert A in 1914 (Fig. 3.6[167]). Albert was a 73-year-old widowed, former horse cab driver from Stoke Newington then working as a messenger.[168] He was admitted to Colney Hatch with his "first attack" of insanity attributed to alcohol and arteriosclerosis. Four months later, shortly before war broke out, he was discharged to the care of his son.[169] Despite overall poor discharge rates,

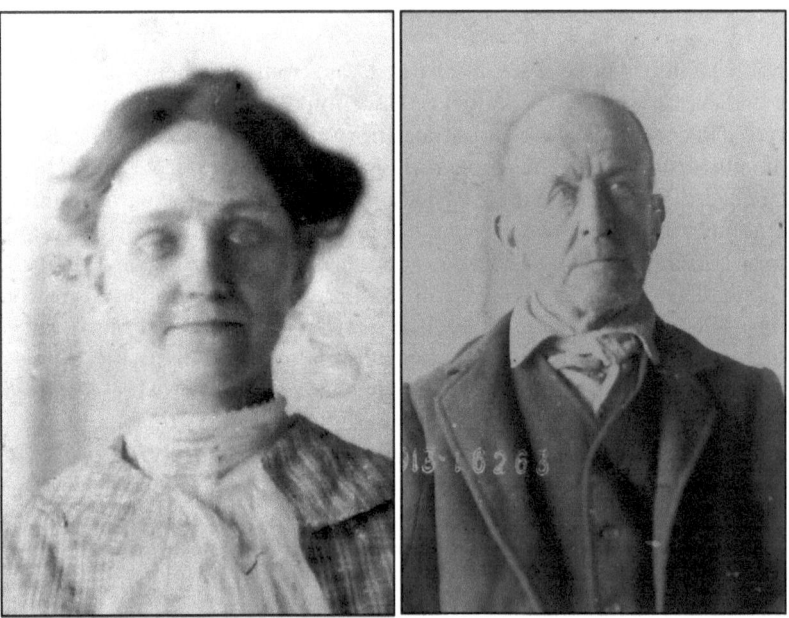

Fig. 3.6   Discharged contrary to expectations: Ida D and Albert A (Photographs of female patients 1908–1918 H12/CH/B/18/003 and male patients 1908–1920 H12/CH/B/19/003 at Colney Hatch, LMA)

the stories of Ida and Albert go some way to counteracting the impression of inevitable and permanent long-term confinement, even for patients considered to have an unfavourable outlook.[170]

As with other aspects of psychiatric care, asylum doctors aspired to the clinical methods of their colleagues who treated patients with physical illness or injury. In this case, a period of convalescence (from Latin, *con valescere*, to grow strong or well) was a frequent part of medical and surgical practice to enhance recovery. The concept of convalescence was widely understood including outside medicine, such as for national and economic health; Winston Churchill used it to describe the country's post-war recovery.[171] Some asylums had convalescent wards in the main hospital, others had villas set aside in the grounds for that purpose. Unfortunately, detached villas were particularly vulnerable to being taken over for other purposes during the war, compounding the staffing and over-crowding challenges which impinged on therapeutic social interactions integral to the process of rehabilitation.

Convalescence, as many other aspects of asylum life, has been criticised by social scientists and historians. Stephen Soanes summarised views of Erving Goffman, Andrew Scull and others, that convalescence was part of a system of control, an extension of the ward system, a disciplinary mechanism, and that it "had a subordinate and perhaps deceptive place in the asylum, as classification that pointed to imminent release, but actually formed part of a primarily carceral institution."[172] This criticism ignored the imperative to discharge as many patients as possible in order to vacate beds to allow new admissions. It also failed to take into account the extraordinarily slow pace of recovery from mental breakdown, to rebuild self-confidence and self-esteem, deal with fear of relapse, and rebuild fractured social and employment relationships, hurdles recognised by some asylums which did provide convalescence.[173]

Alongside convalescence, the asylums had the option of granting a patient up to four weeks trial leave to help identify their needs prior to full discharge, aiming to prevent "early relapses—so vexatious and dispiriting to the authority concerned".[174] Patients were described as being "on trial", a term with ambiguous judicial connotations. Hubert Bond, a senior member of the Board, advocated that asylums should follow the Lunacy Act, which permitted them to provide a monetary allowance for each patient during leave.[175] This could relieve financial stress and might help create a successful outcome. Despite these ideals, asylums varied in their approach to trial leave, from none,[176] to leave plus allowance.[177]

Some asylums would not provide the allowance, viewing it as unnecessary, or extravagant, even though many patients had no other financial support at that time.[178] During the war, austerity meant that the London County Council did not enforce the recommendation,[179] despite the risk of that impeding outcome.

To promote successful discharge, Bond also encouraged "after-care". The Mental After Care Association (MACA), was founded in 1879 by Henry Hawkins, chaplain at Colney Hatch. MACA mainly provided clothing, tools to help patients restart their trade, a place in a cottage home for convalescence, and assistance finding employment,[180] tailoring its support to individual needs.[181] It worked closely with local Guardians, who often had long-term knowledge about a family.[182] MACA described itself as a "unique charity...doing work untouched by any other Association",[183] but it was relatively small, its resources only stretching to about 600 discharges each year, mainly in the London area.[184] Bond encouraged medical superintendents to inform MACA of impending discharges, with the patients' agreement, and MACA liaised constructively with medical superintendents, even after discharge.[185]

Bond wanted MACA to serve all patients who were likely to benefit from its support in the course of their discharge from a public asylum.[186] However, there was diversity of opinion. Not all asylum committees agreed with Bond. One in Berkshire considered it inadvisable to have a dedicated "after-care committee" because

> when patients are discharged...they do not in any way wish to be considered as in need of after-care or different from their fellows....in many cases it is obviously to their advantage, that their residence in a Mental Hospital should be forgotten.[187]

This opinion contradicted MACA's experience. For example, in the employment-seeking advertisements which it placed in newspapers on the patients' behalf, it often stated: "Has been mentally ill, now perfectly well and strong".[188] This honesty did not preclude former patients from obtaining work, although not all placements lasted, due to employer, employee, or wider social factors.[189] Philanthropic donations also indicated public sympathy, rather than ostracism, towards people recovering from mental disorder, however, MACA's focus on London does not allow judgement about generosity or attitudes elsewhere. Despite donations, without statutory support, MACA lacked the means to satisfy demand for its services. In Bond's understanding, after-care helped prevent relapses, so was "economically worthy of generous support"[190] and the Board requested funding for it in its proposals to the Reconstruction Committee in 1917.[191] The evidence that after-care could benefit patients and that MACA received public support for its work, raises questions about the attitudes and understanding of those people running the asylums who opposed it.

MACA was necessarily selective about whom it supported, but many of those it helped remained well.[192] Recipients were generally grateful, and some reimbursed the charity all that it had spent on them.[193] Some case studies are preserved in the MACA archive, but it is unclear if they form a representative sample or a successful-outcome sample. Nevertheless, they provide insights into the diverse and personal support given, and a few are therefore worthy of mention here. One, Norman B, a 36-year-old electrical engineer who worked well in the asylum engineer's workshop during his admission, wanted to be a ship's engineer. With some financial support from MACA, and their letters to potential employers, he got work on board a ship, and went to Ceylon (Sri Lanka).[194] Another, Annie Sh, was also helped by MACA. Her asylum admission was precipitated by her husband's marital infidelity. With MACA's help, Annie obtained a legal separation from him, custody of their three children and 15 shillings a week to support them.[195]

MACA also accepted a referral for George C who needed new clothes and sought work as a baker. It provided some clothing from its own store with the rest made-to-measure. It placed an advert in the *Daily Chronicle*: "Bakers.- Respectable young man, 20, seeks situation as assistant; experienced; good references."[196] George found a job quickly, but found the work too onerous, so left and enlisted with an infantry battalion in August 1914. Perhaps unsurprisingly, five months later he absconded, before embarking for France.[197] George's account is a reminder of the situation of many men who enlisted shortly after discharged from asylums. Later in the war, some recruiting offices requested the names of recovering patients and expected them to register for military service before leaving the institution.[198] Likewise, and contrary to Board recommendations, there was a drive to recruit young men registered as mental defectives.[199] Recruitment officials ignored advice from the men's own doctors that they were unsuitable to serve,[200] and a leader in the *Times* commented that physically fit men "were passed for service in the Army, when they were more fitted to be certified for asylums."[201] These criticisms point to

Army recruitment officers paying little attention to existing understanding of mental disorders and the psychological resilience servicemen required. Such recruitment practices arguably contributed to the catastrophe of shell shock.

But, returning to George C, his story has a happy ending. He survived the war and appears to have had a satisfactory life thereafter. In 1936, 22 years after his discharge from the asylum, he sent Christmas greetings to his former MACA worker, Miss Vickers, indicating his gratitude to her.[202]

CONCLUSIONS

Treating patients with mental disorder, the *raison d'être* of the asylum, was fraught with tensions. Understanding about mental disorders—their causes, classification, course and treatment—was subject to a mismatch between scientific evidence, opinions and practices. Psychiatrists were presented with contradictory hypotheses and information, with the significance of each difficult to evaluate. Psychiatrists in England, as a group, were at odds as to what to believe. Although they did little research, they questioned what was presented to them, from the UK and abroad. Much discussion appeared in the *JMS*, which was published regularly through the war. Caution and healthy scepticism and acknowledgement of the risk of harm from adopting new practices too readily, created a safety mechanism when faced with radical options. However, these collective traits were also associated with inertia, and lack of innovation when the opportunities arose for making other, constructive changes.

Psychiatrists were trained, as were their medical contemporaries, to improve the lives of their patients, preferably to cure them. There was a sense of frustration that scientific advances in other medical disciplines surpassed those in their own. The overlap in symptoms between physical and mental disorders and the discovery of invisible causes of physical illnesses reinforced beliefs that mental and physical disorders had similar causes. This gave asylum doctors hope of scientific breakthroughs for the most severe forms of insanity. Lack of clinically useful discoveries, demoralising on the one hand, spurred some doctors on to persist with research, determined to achieve better for their patients. Various aspects of the lunacy system militated against this, such as geographical and intellectual isolation of asylums from teaching hospitals and universities, a lack of scientific expertise and heavy clinical responsibilities which gave no time for research. The paltry sum of money allocated for psychiatric research compared to that for physical illnesses was disproportionate to the challenge. It is arguable that heredity and degeneration hypotheses associated with negativity and inevitability about mental disorders may have deterred potential funders from sponsoring research. To achieve research-based improvements in clinical practice also required collaboration across professions and organisations—legal, medical, academic, asylum and governmental. That collaboration was absent before, during and after the war.

The Lunacy Act contributed to hindering asylum doctors from adopting patient-centred good medical practices expected of their counterparts in general hospitals. They were not allowed to offer out-patient treatment, to admit voluntary patients, or to decide who should be admitted to their beds, or at what stage of their illness. The Act did not serve the needs of many mentally unwell people. Convalescence, integral to treatment of physical illness and injury, was incorporated into some asylum regimes, but outside the asylum walls support was limited, mainly to that provided by MACA in the London area. MACA's work supported the notion of some public sympathy towards people seeking to resume their normal lives following an asylum admission.

Falling discharge rates (and high death rates; see Chapter 7) indicate declining standards in the asylums before the war. Pressures on the asylums during the war, particularly of overcrowding with a depleted staff, added to untherapeutic environments associated with more custodial care, some punitive practices, and a fall in therapeutic interventions. Overall, the impression given is of asylum practices pulled in all directions by scientific, legal, social, economic, military and other factors, sometimes floundering in uncertainty and at other times knowing what should be done but hampered by internal and external constraints. The voice of the patient and his family was missing. There is evidence that clinical practice was associated with a degree of self-justification by the medical and lay leadership, and that deception may have hidden harsh practices and affected statistics, possibly contributing to a more positive image of the asylums than they deserved.

NOTES

1. Colney Hatch H12/CH/B/16/003 Case notes of female patients who died 1918–1919 LMA.
2. Anon. *The LCC Hospitals: A Retrospect* (London: LCC, 1949), 46.
3. Committee on the Administration of Public Mental Hospitals (Chairman: Sir Cyril Cobb) (Cobb Inquiry), 16 March 1922 Charles McCarthy Q:811, MH 58/219 TNA.
4. John Keay, "Presidential Address on the War and the Burden of Insanity," *Journal of Mental Science (JMS)* 64 (1918): 325–44, 341.
5. Tom Williams, "The Management of Confusional States with Special Reference to Pathogenesis," *JMS* 63 (1917): 389–400.
6. WA Cramond, "Psychiatry and Old Age: The Psychiatric Hospital and the Aged Patient," *Nursing Mirror*, 17 March 1961, xi–xii.
7. Colney Hatch H12/CH/B/18/004 Photographs of female patients admitted and discharged 1918–1920 LMA; Annual Report: Barony Parochial Asylum at Woodilee, Dunbartonshire, 1901–1902, HB30/2/12A19 NHS Greater Glasgow Archives.
8. Claybury LCC/MIN/00948 Meeting, 3 January 1918, 286 LMA.
9. Colney Hatch H12/CH/B/16/003 Case notes of female patients who died 1918–1919 LMA.
10. German Berrios, "British Psychopathology Since the Early 20th Century," 232–44, in *150 Years of British Psychiatry 1841–1991*, ed. German Berrios and Hugh Freeman (London: Gaskell, 1991), 232–33.
11. German Berrios, "Delirium and Confusion in the 19th Century: A Conceptual History," *British Journal of Psychiatry* 139 (1981): 439–49, 446; Edward Younger, *Insanity in Everyday Practice* (London: Baillière, Tindall and Cox, 1914), 36.
12. Berrios, "Delirium": 439.
13. Colney Hatch H12/CH/B/22/015 Autopsy book for female patients 1918–1919 LMA.
14. R Percy Smith, "Mental Disorders in Civilians Arising in Connexion with the War," *Proceedings of the Royal Society of Medicine (Proc RSM)* 10 (1917): Section of Psychiatry, 1–20, 11–12, 20.
15. JM Winter, "The Impact of the First World War on Civilian Health in Britain," *Economic History Review* 30 (1977): 487–507, 503; Reconstruction Committee, letters to BoC, 14 August 1916 and 2 January 1917 MH 51/687 TNA; Pat Thane, *Divided Kingdom: A History of Britain, 1900 to the Present* (Cambridge: Cambridge University Press, 2018), 56–57.
16. Edgar Jones, Robin Woolven, Bill Durodié, and Simon Wessely, "Civilian Morale During the Second World War: Responses to Air Raids Re-Examined," *Social History of Medicine* 17 (2004): 463–79.

17. Hazel Croft, "Rethinking Civilian Neuroses in the Second World War," 95–116, in *Traumatic Memories of the Second World War and After*, ed. Peter Leese and Jason Crouthamel (London: Palgrave Macmillan, 2016).
18. BoC, Patients Admission Registers: Rate aided admissions, 1914–1918. Forty-nine names collected at random from admission registers. MH 94/48–53 TNA.
19. Colney Hatch H12/CH/B/16/002 Case notes of female patients who died 1916–1917 LMA; Rate-aided admissions, to asylums, hospitals, licenced houses (excluding idiot institutions) 1915 MH 94/50 TNA; Colney Hatch H12/CH/B/18/003 Photographs of female patients admitted and discharged 1908–1918 LMA.
20. Pamela Michael, *Care and Treatment of the Mentally Ill in North Wales 1800–2000* (Cardiff: University of Wales Press, 2003), 119.
21. Harry Bernstein, *The Invisible Wall* (London: Hutchinson, 2007), 168.
22. Vera Brittain, *Testament of Youth* (1933; London: Virago Press, 1982).
23. Claybury, Female patient case notes 1917, Redbridge Heritage Centre.
24. England and Wales Register 1939, https://www.ancestry.co.uk/search/collections/1939ukregister/.
25. Eunice Winters (ed.), *The Collected Papers of Adolf Meyer*, vol. 2. (Baltimore: John Hopkins, 1951), 250, quoted in Edward Shorter, *A History of Psychiatry* (New York: Wiley, 1997), 90.
26. Colney Hatch H12/CH/B/18/004 Photographs of female patients admitted and discharged 1918–1920 LMA.
27. Tracy Loughran, *Shell-Shock and Medical Culture in First World War Britain* (Cambridge: Cambridge University Press, 2017), 60.
28. Ernest Jones, in discussion on: Charles Mercier, "The Concept of Insanity," *Proc RSM* 7 (1914): Section of Psychiatry, 3–14, 13; Younger, *Insanity*, 4.
29. Lunacy Act 1890 section 341.
30. Mercier, "Concept of Insanity": 3–4.
31. John Turner, "The Classification of Insanity," *JMS* 58 (1912): 9–25, 10.
32. Younger, *Insanity*, 5.
33. Peter Bartrip, "A Talent to Alienate: The 2nd Earl (Frank) Russell (1865–1931)," *Russell: Journal of Bertrand Russell Studies* 32 (2012): 101–26; Voluntary Mental Treatment Bill. *Hansard* HL Deb, 22 July 1914, vol. 17, cc.89–92.
34. For example, the form of a delusion, as a fixed, false belief, can point to specific types of disorder. Delusions can be experienced with variable content. One patient experienced delusions during the war about "abusive Marconigrams", being a spy and his thoughts being discovered by X-rays; Younger, *Insanity*, 48; Smith, "Mental Disorders in Civilians".
35. Jack Drescher, Carol North, and Alina Suris, "Out of DSM: Depathologizing Homosexuality," *Behavioral Sciences* (Basel) 5 (2015): 565–75.

36. Lunacy Law (Committal of Sane Persons). *Hansard* HC Deb, 28 February 1910, vol. 14, c.562.

37. Richard Rows, "Clinics and Centres for Teaching," *JMS* 60 (1914): 674–81.

38. David Healy, Margaret Harris, Fiona Farquhar, Stefanie Tschinkel, and Joanna Le Noury, "Historical Overview: Kraepelin's Impact on Psychiatry," *European Archives of Psychiatry and Clinical Neuroscience* 258 (Suppl. 2) (2008): 18–24.

39. Mercier, "Concept of Insanity": 14.

40. Havelock Ellis, "A Criticism of Kraepelin," *JMS* 60 (1914): 523–26.

41. James Anglin, "Presidential Address, Delivered at the Seventy-Fourth Annual Meeting of the American Medico-Psychological Association, Chicago, Ill., June 4th–7th, 1918," *JMS* 65 (1919): 1–16, 1.

42. William Ford Robertson, "Vaccine Treatment in Asylums," *JMS* 60 (1914): 17–30.

43. Bernard Hollander, *The First Signs of Insanity: Their Prevention and Treatment* (London: Stanley Paul and Co, 1912), 143; Charles Mercier, *A Textbook of Insanity* (London: George Allen and Unwin, 1914), 14.

44. Jennifer Wallis, *Investigating the Body in the Victorian Asylum: Doctors, Patients, and Practices* (London: Palgrave Macmillan, 2017), 1–6.

45. Robert Mccarrison, "The Ductless Glands," *Lancet* 28 March 1914, 931; Rupert Farrant, "The Causation and Cure of Certain Lunacies," *Lancet* 24 June 1916, 1260–61.

46. Ngram viewer, "Pull Yourself Together," https://books.google.com/ngrams.

47. Montagu Lomax, *The Experiences of an Asylum Doctor* (London: Allen and Unwin, 1921), 88.

48. Commissioners in Lunacy, Tables xvii (male), xviii (female): causes of first admissions, excluding to idiot establishments, 1907–1911 MH 51/687 TNA.

49. E.g. Sebastian Barry, *The Secret Scripture* (London: Faber and Faber, 2008); Maggie O'Farrell, *The Vanishing Act of Esme Lennox* (London: Headline Review, 2006); Younger, *Insanity,* 105–8; David Jones, "Moral Insanity and Psychological Disorder: The Hybrid Roots of Psychiatry," *History of Psychiatry* 28 (2017): 263–79.

50. Mental Deficiency Act, 1913 section 2.

51. Lomax, *Experiences*, 55; Cobb Inquiry, 16 February 1922 Dr. Bond Q:99–102, MH 58/219 TNA.

52. Cobb Inquiry, 24 February 1922 Dr. Perceval Q:362; 16 February 1922 Dr. Bond Q:99–100, 109; MH 58/219 TNA.

53. Cobb Inquiry, 24 March 1922 Lionel Weatherly Q:1581, MH 58/219 TNA.

54. Cobb Inquiry, 16 March 1922 Nurse Jane Dagg Q:952, 957, MH 58/219 TNA.
55. Cobb Inquiry, 24 March 1922 Lionel Weatherly Q:1597; 16 March 1922 Herbert Ellis JP Q:902, MH 58/219 TNA.
56. Hugh Freeman, "Psychiatry in Britain c.1900," *History of Psychiatry* 21 (2010): 312–24, 316–17.
57. Since 1963, *British Journal of Psychiatry*.
58. Robertson, "Vaccine Treatment"; Harold Gettings, "Dysentery Past and Present," *JMS* 60 (1914): 39–56; DJ Jackson, "The Clinical Value and Significance of Leucocytosis in Mental Disease," *JMS* 60 (1914): 56–72; Patrick O'Doherty, "Some Features of the Recent Outbreak of Enteric Fever at Omagh District Asylum," *JMS* 60 (1914): 76–81.
59. H Wolseley-Lewis and RH Cole, "The Amendment of Lunacy Legislation," *Lancet* 26 January 1918, 163.
60. James Whitwell, "The Administration of Bromide," *Lancet* 5 January 1918, 35; EW Adams, "The Administration of Bromide," *Lancet*, 12 January 1918, 8; Maurice Craig, "The Administration of Bromide," *Lancet* 19 January 1918, 119.
61. Lionel Weatherly, "Sexual Perversion," *Lancet* 22 June 1918, 884–85; Brian Donkin, "Sexual Perversion," *Lancet* 13 July 1918, 56.
62. George Savage, "The Presidential Address, Delivered at the Opening Meeting of the Section of Psychiatry of the Royal Society of Medicine, on October 22nd, 1912," *JMS* 59 (1913): 14–27, 27.
63. Freeman, "Psychiatry in Britain": 321.
64. JL Wheatley, Town Clerk, Cardiff, letter to Commissioners in Lunacy: State aid for research into mental diseases and mental defect, 13 December 1912 MH 51/78 TNA.
65. BoC, Research Committee, minutes, 30 July 1914, 13 MH 51/82 TNA.
66. BoC W/FM, 2 December 1914, 268 MH 50/43 TNA; BoC correspondence with Dr. J Shaw Bolton, MS, Wakefield Asylum, 25 March, 27 March, 4 December 1914, MH 51/79 TNA.
67. Henry Harris, *National Health Insurance in Great Britain, 1911 to 1921* (Washington, DC: Government Printing Office, 1923), 10; BoC, Research Committee, minutes, 30 July 1914, 5 MH 51/82 TNA.
68. Dean of Faculty of Medicine, University of Manchester, letter to BoC 4 April 1914 MH 51/80 TNA; Sidney Coupland, BoC, "Report on Replies to Circular Letter re: Scientific Research," 1914 MH 51/81 TNA.
69. *First Annual Report of the Board of Control, for the Year 1914* (London: HMSO, 1916) (*BoC AR 1914*), Part 1, 61–62; Lewis Bruce, "The Complement-Deviation in Cases of Manic-Depressive Insanity," *JMS* 60 (1914): 177–84.

70. Keay, "War and the Burden of Insanity": 341.
71. Oliver Sacks, *Awakenings* (New York: Summit Books, 1973).
72. Harold Pinter, *A Kind of Alaska: A Play*, in *Other Places* (London: Methuen, 1982).
73. NPAS Johnson, "The Overshadowed Killer: Influenza in Britain in 1918–19," 132–155, in *The Spanish Influenza Epidemic of 1918–19*, ed. Howard Phillips and David Killingray (London: Routledge, 2003), 139; The relationship was clarified in 1982: RT Ravenholt and William Foege, "1918 Influenza, Encephalitis Lethargica and Parkinsonism," *Lancet* 16 October 1982, 860–64.
74. BoC circular, Evidence of Syphilis. Replies from County and Borough Mental Hospitals, 2 August 1928 MH 51/539 TNA.
75. Keay, "War and the Burden of Insanity": 337.
76. Younger, *Insanity*, 56.
77. Younger, *Insanity*, 15.
78. M Fitzmaurice-Kelly, "Salvarsan in General Paralysis of the Insane and Tabes," *JMS* 59 (1913): 498–502.
79. George Schrøder and Hj. Helweg, "Some Experiments on Treatment of Dementia Paralytica with Subdural Injections of Neosalvarsan," *JMS* 65 (1919): 24–36.
80. Younger, *Insanity*, 88–89.
81. Claybury LCC/MIN/00945 Meeting, 12 November 1914, 231; LCC LCC/MIN/00581 Meeting, 26 October 1915, 56 LMA.
82. Colney Hatch LCC/PH/MENT/04/016 Lists of patients admitted, died and recommended for discharge 1911–1917 LMA.
83. Colney Hatch: H12/CH/B/17/002 Case notes of male patients who died in 1917; H12/CH/B/23/013 Autopsy book for male patients 1916–1918 LMA.
84. Shorter, *History of Psychiatry*, 379fn9, citing *Psychiatrisch-Neurologische Wochenschrift*, 4 January 1919.
85. William Halsted, "The Results of Operations for the Cure of Cancer of the Breast Performed at the Johns Hopkins Hospital from June, 1889, to January, 1894," *Annals of Surgery* 20 (1894): 497–555; Stefano Zurrida, Fabio Bassi, Paolo Arnone, Stefano Martella, Andres Del Castillo, Rafael Ribeiro Martini, M. Eugenia Semenkiw, and Pietro Caldarella, "The Changing Face of Mastectomy (from Mutilation to Aid to Breast Reconstruction)," *International Journal of Surgical Oncology* (2011): 1–7, 2. Article ID: 980158, https://dx.doi.org/10.1155/2011/980158.
86. Shorter, *History of Psychiatry*, 111–12.
87. Gerald Grob, "The Rise and Decline of Tonsillectomy in Twentieth-Century America," *Journal of the History of Medicine and Allied Sciences* 62 (2007): 383–421, 387.

88. Thomas Bewley, *Madness to Mental Illness: A History of the Royal College of Psychiatrists* (London: RCPsych Publications, 2008), 47; Andrew Scull, "Focal Infection," 79–81, in *A Century of Psychiatry*, ed. Hugh Freeman (London: Mosby, 1999).
89. BoC W/FM, 16 September 1914 MH 50/43; 31 March 1915, 383 MH 50/44 TNA.
90. Younger, *Insanity*, 46; William Stoddart, *Mental Nursing* (London: Scientific Press, 1916), 79.
91. Stoddart, *Mental Nursing*, 78–79.
92. BoC W/FM, 17 June 1914, 97 MH 50/43 TNA; *BoC AR 1914*, Part 1, 30.
93. H Dodwell, "'Status Lymphaticus,' the Growth of a Myth," *BMJ* 16 January 1954, 149–51.
94. Ann Dally, "Status Lymphaticus: Sudden Death in Children from 'Visitation of God' to Cot Death," *Medical History* 42 (1997): 70–85.
95. Loughran, *Shell-Shock*, 54.
96. Jack Pressman, *Last Resort: Psychosurgery and the Limits of Medicine* (Cambridge: Cambridge University Press, 1998), 19, 84.
97. Frederick Mott, "War Psycho-Neurosis," *Lancet* 2 February 1918, 169–72; Hudson Bury, "Remarks on the Pathology of War Neuroses," *Lancet* 2 July 1918, 97–99.
98. Ministry of Pensions, letter to BoC, 25 July 1917 MH 51/694 TNA.
99. Daniel Pick, *Faces of Degeneration: A European Disorder, c.1848–c.1918* (Cambridge: Cambridge University Press, 1989), 18–19.
100. George Rosen, *Madness in Society: Chapters in the Historical Sociology of Mental Illness* (Chicago: University of Chicago Press, 1980), 255.
101. Bénédict Morel, *Traité des Dégénérescences Physiques, Intellectuelles et Morales de L'espèce Humaine et des Causes qui Produisent ces Variétés Maladives* (London: H. Baillière, 1857).
102. Henry Maudsley, "Considerations with Regard to Hereditary Influence," *JMS* 8 (1863): 482–512 and 9 (1864): 506–30; Younger, *Insanity*, 53; Pick, *Faces of Degeneration*, 9, 13.
103. Benjamin Seebohm Rowntree, *Poverty: A Study of Town Life* (London: Macmillan, 1902), 304–5.
104. Mercier, *Textbook of Insanity*, 44.
105. William Bynum, "Alcoholism and Degeneration in 19th Century European Medicine and Psychiatry," *British Journal of Addiction* 79 (1984): 59–70, 59.
106. Census 1911, https://www.ancestry.co.uk/cs/uk1911census.
107. Colney Hatch LCC/PH/MENT/04/016 Lists of patients admitted, died and recommended for discharge 1911–1917 LMA; Census 1911, https://www.ancestry.co.uk/cs/uk1911census; London Church of England marriage banns, 1754–1932, https://www.ancestry.co.uk/search/collections/lmamarriages/, 28 June 1914.

108. Richard Walter, "What Became of the Degenerate? A Brief History of a Concept," *Journal of the History of Medicine and Allied Sciences* 11 (1956): 422–29, 427.

109. Robert Armstrong-Jones, "The Eighth Annual Report of the Board of Control for the Year 1921," *Eugenics Review* 15 (1923): 426–32.

110. Shorter, *History of Psychiatry*, 98.

111. Pick, *Faces of Degeneration*, 17.

112. BoC, Resolution from the Sevenoaks Board of Guardians: "Motion to be Proposed by Mrs Pearce-Clark" April 1918 MH 51/667 TNA.

113. BoC, W/FM, 31 January 1917, 39, discussion about letter from Sir George Savage, MH 50/45; BoC response to Resolution from the Sevenoaks Board of Guardians: "Motion to be Proposed by Mrs Pearce-Clark" April 1918 MH 51/667 TNA.

114. British Psychological Society, timeline 1901–2009, https://www.bps.org.uk/sites/bps.org.uk/files/History%20of%20Psychology/Timeline%20of%20the%20BPS%201901%20to%202009.pdf; London Psychoanalytical Society, founded by Ernest Jones, 1913; RD Hinshelwood, "Psychodynamic Psychiatry Before World War 1," 197–205, in *150 Years of British Psychiatry*, ed. Berrios and Freeman, 202.

115. Bernard Hart, *The Psychology of Insanity* (Cambridge: University Press, 1912).

116. Lomax, *Experiences*, 83.

117. Hanwell H11/HLL/C/06/006 Male attendants' fine book 1914–1935 LMA; Lomax, *Experiences*, 83.

118. Ernest Jones, *Papers on Psycho-Analysis* (London: Bailliére, Tindall and Cox, 1913).

119. Yves Delage, "*Psychoanalysis, a New Psychosis. Une Psychose Nouvelle: La Psychoanalyse. Mercure de France*, September 1st, 1916," *JMS* 63 (1917): 61–76.

120. Charles Mercier, "Diet as a Factor in the Causation of Mental Disease," *JMS* 62 (1916): 505–29, 529.

121. William HR Rivers, "The Repression of War Experience," *Lancet* 2 February 1918, 173–77, 174–76.

122. Loughran, *Shell-Shock*, 158.

123. Dean Rapp, "The Early Discovery of Freud by the British General Educated Public, 1912–1919," *Social History of Medicine* 3 (1990): 217–43.

124. Hollander, *First Signs*, 5.

125. Hollander, *First Signs*, 5; Grafton Elliott Smith and Tom Pear, *Shell Shock and Its Lessons* (Manchester: University Press, 1917), 109.

126. Lomax, *Experiences*, 39.

127. Cobb Inquiry, 30 March 1922 Edward Mason Q:2056, MH 52/220 TNA.

128. Cobb Inquiry, 16 March 1922 Charles McCarthy Q:836, MH 52/219 TNA.

129. William Bynum, "Rationales for Therapy in British Psychiatry: 1780–1835," *Medical History* 18 (1974): 317–34, 331–32.

130. Younger, *Insanity*, 37–39.

131. Younger, *Insanity*, 71.

132. Younger, *Insanity*, 40.

133. Maurice Craig and ED Macnamara, "Treatments of Mental Disorders," 484–97, in *The Practitioner's Encyclopaedia of Medical Treatment*, ed. W Langdon Brown and J Keogh Murphy (London: Oxford University Press, 1915), 489.

134. Claybury LCC/MIN/00946 Meeting, 8 July 1915, 168 LMA.

135. Shorter, *History of Psychiatry*, 196 and 379fn18 citing John Haslam, *Observations on Madness and Melancholy* (London: Callow, 1809).

136. 1 minim = 1/480 fluid ounce = 60 mm³ = one drop of water; PP Laidlaw, "Purgatives and Cholagogues," 722–30, in *Practitioner's Encyclopaedia of Medical Treatment*, ed. Langdon Brown and Keogh Murphy, 726.

137. Lomax, *Experiences*, 100; Cobb Inquiry, 24 March 1922 Lionel Weatherly Q:1677–79, MH 52/219 TNA.

138. Ministry of Health, *Report of the Committee on Administration of Public Mental Hospitals* Cmd. 1730 (London: HMSO, 1922) Annotated draft 112, 114–17 MH 52/222 TNA.

139. Lomax, *Experiences*, 96.

140. Stoddart, *Mental Nursing*, 38–39.

141. Jane Hamlett and Lesley Hoskins, "Comfort in Small Things? Clothing, Control and Agency in County Lunatic Asylums in Nineteenth- and Early Twentieth-Century England," *Journal of Victorian Culture* 18 (2013): 93–114, 98.

142. Lunacy Act 1890 section 40.

143. BoC circular concerning record keeping: Form 9: seclusion and mechanical restraint. 6 May 1922, 607C MH 51/240 TNA.

144. Lomax, *Experiences*, 84.

145. Stoddart, *Mental Nursing*, 38–39.

146. Lomax, *Experiences*, 96–97.

147. *BoC AR 1914*, Part 2, Three Counties Asylum 16 June 1914, 196; Long Grove Asylum 11 December 1914, 278.

148. Cobb Inquiry, 24 March 1922 Lionel Weatherly Q:1684 MH 52/219 TNA.

149. Claybury LCC/MIN/00947 Meeting, 22 June 1916, 146–47 LMA.

150. Claybury LCC/MIN/00947 Meeting, 23 November 1916. Between pp. 273–74 LMA.

151. Lionel Weatherly, *A Plea for the Insane: The Case for Reform in the Care and Treatment of Mental Diseases* (London: Grant Richards Ltd, 1918), 33.
152. Lionel Weatherly, "The Management of Lunacy Patients," *Lancet* 21 September 1918, 405–6.
153. Weatherly, *Plea for the Insane*, 33.
154. Lomax, *Experiences*, 47–48.
155. John Hopton, "Prestwich Hospital in the Twentieth Century: A Case Study of Slow and Uneven Progress in the Development of Psychiatric Care," *History of Psychiatry* 10 (1999): 349–69, 362.
156. Lomax, *Experiences*, 46.
157. Lomax, *Experiences*, 83.
158. D Davidson, *Remembrances of a Religio-Maniac* (Stratford-on-Avon, UK: Shakespeare Press, 1912), 50–51.
159. James Scott, *Sane in Asylum Walls* (London: Fowler Wright, 1931), 98, and picture facing p. 102.
160. Lionel Weatherly, "The Work of the Registered Hospitals for the Insane," *Lancet* 5 August 1916, 248.
161. *Sixth Annual Report of the Board of Control, for the Year 1919* (London: HMSO, 1920) Appendix A, 22–23.
162. Anon. "Asylum Reports: *London County Council, 1914*," *JMS* 62 (1916): 627–34, 632.
163. BoC, Patients admission registers: Rate aided admissions, 1913–1918 MH 94/48–53 TNA.
164. Colney Hatch H12/CH/B/18/003 Photographs of female patients admitted and discharged 1908–1918 LMA.
165. Census 1911, https://www.ancestry.co.uk/cs/uk1911census.
166. BoC, Patients admission registers: Rate aided admissions, 1914 MH 94/49 TNA.
167. Colney Hatch H12/CH/B/19/003 Photographs of male patients admitted and discharged 1908–1920 LMA.
168. Census 1911, https://www.ancestry.co.uk/cs/uk1911census.
169. Colney Hatch: H12/CH/B/13/066 Case book for male patients admitted 1912–1914; LCC/PH/MENT/04/016 Lists of patients admitted, died and recommended for discharge 1911–1917 LMA.
170. Peter Barham, *Forgotten Lunatics of the Great War* (New Haven and London: Yale University Press, 2004), 3.
171. Stephen Soanes, "Rest and Restitution: Convalescence and the Public Mental Hospital in England, 1919–39" (PhD thesis, University of Warwick, 2011), http://wrap.warwick.ac.uk/54604/1/WRAP_THESIS_Soanes_2011.pdf, 6.
172. Soanes, "Rest and Restitution": 21.

173. Claybury: Female Patient Case Notes 1917, Louise F. Redbridge Heritage Centre.
174. C Hubert Bond, "After-Care in Cases of Mental Disorder, and the Desirability of Its More Extended Scope," *JMS* 59 (1913): 274–86.
175. Lunacy Act 1890 section 55 (1) (2).
176. *BoC AR 1914*, Part 2, Whittingham Asylum 28 February 1914, 252.
177. *BoC AR 1914*, Part 2, Claybury Asylum 27 June 1914, 269.
178. LCC LCC/MIN/00580, Meeting, 27 July 1915, 698 LMA; *BoC AR 1914*, Part 2, Derbyshire Asylum 8 July 1914, 216; Severalls Asylum 27 October 1914, 227.
179. LCC LCC/MIN/00580, Meeting, 27 July 1915, 698 LMA.
180. Anon. "The After-Care Association," *JMS* 60 (1914): 343–45.
181. *Report of the Council, After Care Association* (1914): 5, SA/MAC/B.1/27 WL.
182. MACA, Annie S, SA/MAC/G.3/14 WL.
183. *Report of the Council, The Mental After Care Association for Poor Persons Convalescent or Recovered from Institutions for the Insane* (1915): 3, SA/MAC/B.1/28 WL.
184. *Report of the Council, The After Care Association for Poor Persons Discharged Recovered from Asylums for the Insane* (1914): 4, SA/MAC/B.1/27 WL.
185. MACA, Ernest C, SA/MAC/G.3/17 WL.
186. *BoC AR 1914*, Part 1, 10: Discharged recovered: 7487; Discharged not recovered: 2605.
187. Berkshire Mental Hospital, "Interim Report of the House Sub-committee on the Report of the Departmental Committee of Inquiry Dated 1922 and the Recommendations of the Board of Control Resulting from the Inquiry," 25 May 1923 MH 51/686 TNA.
188. *Daily Telegraph*, 24 August 1916, SA/MAC/G.3/5 WL; *Nursing Mirror*, 26 November 1921, SA/MAC/G.3/8 WL.
189. MACA, Florence H, SA/MAC/G.3/5 WL.
190. Bond, "After-Care": 282–83.
191. BoC, letter to Reconstruction Committee, 9 February 1917 MH 51/687 TNA.
192. *Report of the Council, After Care Association* (1914): 6, SA/MAC/B.1/27 WL.
193. *Report of the Council, Mental After Care Association* (1915): 5, SA/MAC/B.1/28 WL.
194. MACA, Norman B, SA/MAC/G.3/3 WL.
195. MACA, Annie Sh, SA/MAC/G.3/14 WL.
196. MACA, George C: *Daily Chronicle*, 16 June 1914, SA/MAC/G.3/4 WL.

197. *Police Gazette*, 19 January 1915, https://www.ancestry.co.uk/search/collections/ukpolicegazettes/.
198. Claybury LCC/MIN/00947 Meeting, 30 March 1916, 70, Ilford Tribunal letter to VC, 28 March 1916 LMA.
199. BoC W/FM request from Clerk of Smethwick Council, 11 October 1916, 289; 22 November 1916, 338 MH 50/44 TNA.
200. BoC, "Notes of Some Typical Mental Cases for Special Consideration," July 1917 MH 51/694 TNA.
201. Anon. "Lunacy During the War," *Times*, 6 September 1919.
202. MACA, George C, SA/MAC/G.3/4 WL.

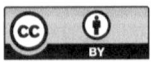

CHAPTER 4

Personnel: Staffing the Asylums and Serving the Colours

INTRODUCTION

A parliamentary select committee in 1911 discussed a London County Council (LCC) survey of its asylum staff. It showed that they did not become insane any more than members of the general public despite their proximity to insane people day after day. This finding surprised the committee. It challenged their assumptions about the transmissibility of insanity. The LCC explained that their staff were "specially selected for their mental and physical fitness",[1] and were therefore resilient, but the Medico-Psychological Association (MPA) challenged the ease of appointing suitable staff: asylums needed more staff who were "in sympathy with the insane" and who did not behave like "warder to convict".[2]

In 1914, the LCC employed 3500 staff across its ten asylums.[3] They were appointed with the aim of supporting patients who required medical, psychological and social forms of treatment to allow them to have the best possible quality of life, either long-term in the asylums, or by recovering and returning to the community. In addition to doctors and male ward attendants on the men's wards and female nurses mainly on the women's wards, there were shoemakers, tinsmiths, tailors, upholsterers and other artisans who worked alongside clergy, kitchen and laundry workers, and other who maintained buildings, farm, gardens and cemetery.[4] Sometimes whole families worked at an asylum, such as the Mingays

© The Author(s) 2021   117
C. Hilton, *Civilian Lunatic Asylums During the First World War*,
Mental Health in Historical Perspective,
https://doi.org/10.1007/978-3-030-54871-1_4

at Colney Hatch, who fulfilled roles of porter, organist, ward attendant and work-mistress responsible for finding and supervising daily activities for women patients.[5] This chapter seeks to explore the experiences of the staff, the challenges facing them, and how they coped. Many staff lived on the asylum estate. Some had their rooms adjacent to wards, others lived in nurses' homes, and others in staff cottages with their families. All were subject to strict disciplinary rules, in a similar way to their patients. Some had formal professional qualifications, others did not. The majority were low in the ranks of the hierarchical system of asylum management which threaded through from government, via the Board of Control ("the Board") and into the asylums. Staff life changed during the war, associated with many male staff serving the Colours, new gender roles, and the hardships of civilian life which were particularly intense in the asylums.

THE STAFF ON THE ASYLUM FRONT LINE

In 1914, Viscount Wolmer MP asked Prime Minister Herbert Asquith whether he was aware of unrest among asylum staff in various parts of the country. Asquith informed the House of Commons that "there is no widespread unrest, though some dissatisfaction does undoubtedly exist."[6] This did not bode well for future stressful circumstances. The Board realised that wartime changes would cause staff anxiety and inconvenience, but they were sure that these "would be cheerfully borne" and not detrimental to patients.[7] In 1915, psychiatrist Sir James Crichton Brown said about wartime asylum staff:

> They have been left short-handed, they have had double duty thrown upon them, they have had to work overtime, they have had a most anxious and wearing experience,...their wages have been practically reduced, for the purchasing power of a sovereign is not now what it was twelve months ago.[8]

Some staff responded to the pressures of work and deprivation in unprofessional ways. The minutes of Colney Hatch asylum's lay management, or "visiting", committee (VC) recount how Nurse Hammond found Nurse Laycock in a ward storeroom drinking the patients' milk and Nurse Davies holding a cup of milk under her apron. Nurse Hammond reported her colleagues to a more senior nurse. Later that day, someone ransacked

Nurse Hammond's bedroom, and she was assaulted on a dark corridor, covered with a wet sheet then ducked in a bath of cold water. The alleged milk-thieves were summoned to the medical superintendent who was put in the invidious position of having to get to the root of the dispute. Numerous other allegations emerged including food being misappropriated and patients being dragged by the hair and hit by senior staff. Many of the backlog of accounts were inconsistent or contradictory, suggesting staff covering up or blaming each other in the context of a malfunctioning ward team. All three nurses resigned.[9]

Staff were expected to conform to strict regimes of discipline and control, imposed on them in both employment and personal spheres, a pattern common in "total institutions".[10] There were many ways in which VCs could detect infringements of rules, some simpler ones being to install "time clocks" which required staff to "peg in" their key to monitor punctuality, or using electric "tell-tale clocks" to make sure they did not fall asleep on night duty.[11] At a minimum, disobedience or a lapse of behaviour meant that the accused appeared before the VC or medical superintendent to account for their deeds. Internal inquiries gave staff no right of representation or appeal or other safeguards, risking unjust penalties. Being admonished by the medical superintendent or the VC chairman, and having their misdemeanour entered into a register of staff offences was humiliating,[12] but some misdemeanours were associated with severe penalties, such as being demoted, instantly dismissed, or prosecuted.[13] In 1916, Hanwell VC dismissed an attendant of long-standing "For ~~taking patients meat~~ neglecting to give to the Patients part of the meat issued".[14] The hand-written, altered entry in the harshly named "fine book", was compatible with reducing the allegation from criminal, which required a police investigation, to a misdemeanour which allowed dismissal. The latter was more convenient for the VC, and it was kinder to staff who, although losing their job and forfeiting their superannuation contributions, did not acquire a criminal record.[15] Dismissal removed the offender, and their threat to the asylum's reputation, but provided little stimulus for the leadership to learn from events, or consider systemic problems within their asylum, to prevent further transgressions. Dedicated staff were sometimes dismissed for a genuine error of judgement, although occasionally wartime constraints militated in their favour, such as for an attendant at Claybury of 14 years standing with a previous good work record, under whose watch a patient committed suicide: he remained in post because the medical superintendent had "no better man to replace him with."[16]

Entries in Hanwell's fine book were few and far between compared to the number of staff employed, suggesting that most staff behaved according to expectations of the leadership. However, the data need to be interpreted cautiously as the entries indicate the staff caught and their misdemeanours judged appropriate for recording in the book, rather than the total number of subversive or aberrant staff whose behaviours passed unnoticed. Occasionally, alongside many reprimands for breaking rules, such as giving ward keys to a patient, or playing draughts or ball games with other staff while on duty, praise was put on permanent record: Joseph Taylor was "Commended for action taken whereby a patient's life was saved".[17] This type of entry was unusual, as staff were assumed to be dedicated and kind, and they received little, if any, praise. Bedford Pierce, medical superintendent at the York Retreat, criticised his colleagues who did not encourage their VCs to show appreciation to their staff whose work was arduous and pay "miserably poor".[18]

Regarding staff personal lives, the VC kept a close eye on comings and goings and regulated their staff in many ways: even matron had to seek permission to have a guest staying in her quarters.[19] Some asylums stipulated times for staff to go to bed and to get up.[20] Resident day staff were generally allowed out of the asylum between 8 and 10 p.m.,[21] after the night staff came on duty, although that freedom was regulated almost as stringently as parole for patients. Similar to patients, leave could be given as a reward, or withdrawn as punishment, such as happened to two nurses caught stealing fruit at Napsbury.[22] Staff were also disciplined if they mis-used their freedom, such as returning later than their night-pass permitted.[23] Eliza Maidman, a laundry-maid at Colney Hatch for over 25 years who lived-in,[24] had a pass to leave the asylum for an evening. It expired at 10 p.m., but she arrived back at 5.35 a.m. the following morning. Summoned to the VC to account for her behaviour, she stated that she was delayed by a Zeppelin raid. With heavy raids just north of London, the VC did not question her further.[25] Her determination to return in time to start work the following morning was admirable. She was loyal to her asylum—her home, workplace and community— and appeared accepting of its rules. It is disconcerting that, just as praise for Joseph Taylor was found in the fine book, an investigation into suspected misdemeanours was the route into discovering a staff member's commitment.

Sometimes VCs showed compassion to staff in difficulty, such as giving paid leave to a member of staff to care for her sick husband who was also an employee of the asylum.[26] At other times, compassion was wanting. When Nurse Gertrude Stephens, a single woman, was pregnant, the rules gave her no choice but to resign from her job. Her child was stillborn. Since she was no longer employed by the asylum, she asked, as she was entitled to do, for her superannuation payments to be returned to her.[27] The VC refused, on the grounds that her services were terminated "by reason of her own misconduct." She had no job, no child and no money to tide her over.[28] A comparable sort of callousness was shown towards a 19-year-old woman who had received an offer of work at Colney Hatch. Mid-war, she travelled from Ireland to take up her post, but probably due to head lice, she was rejected, and sent away penniless. She sought shelter in a convent. Since she was not the first to reach the nuns in similar circumstances, they relayed her story to a magistrate. He wrote to the medical superintendent saying that she had been "thrown to the wolves by one of [her] own sex".[29]

Other asylum rules concerned staff who wanted to marry. Female staff were expected to leave their job on marriage. However, with difficulty recruiting staff and soaring hasty marriage rates, particularly of soldiers tying the knot with their sweethearts before departing to the war front or while on leave,[30] compromises were needed. In this case, married nurses could return to asylum work, but only to temporary positions,[31] giving them little job security.[32] Male staff who wanted to marry also faced challenges, associated with limited married accommodation in the asylum grounds.[33] They too had to seek consent from the asylum leadership, with permission usually only being granted to those who had given 5 years' service, seniority giving priority for coveted accommodation. Similar marriage rules applied to doctors: without permission from the medical superintendent, doctors who married could be dismissed and forfeit their superannuation payments, even if the marriage took place while they were on military service.[34] Strict rules, about where staff lived, on- or off-site, began to change, in some places, before the war.[35] This was partly due to insufficient and unsuitable nurses' homes, such as one with only 2 baths for 79 nurses which gave nurses no option but to bathe on the wards.[36] More asylums permitted living-out during the war, influenced by the demands of temporary attendants who were concerned about the well-being of their own families in the event of an air raid.[37]

Regarding the work undertaken on the wards, the select committee in 1911 described it as "irksome", and Neil Brimblecombe, in his study of asylum nursing until 1910, described it as hard and often unpleasant.[38] The type of work, often with an 80-hour working week on a two-shift per day rota, combined with a punitive style of asylum leadership and strict discipline, probably contributed to the high turnover of asylum staff, in some places over 75 per cent annually. This resulted in an inexperienced workforce, potentially detrimental to patients, and with further recruitment being time consuming for the leadership.[39] The select committee recommended reducing the hours of work,[40] but the Board disagreed, arguing that more changes in staff through the day would be disruptive to patients.[41] The Board's stance altered, however, and by 1914 it considered an 80-hour week too onerous.[42] Around the same time, the LCC tried to implement a 66-hour week for ward staff. This was close to the 60-hour week worked by asylum staff in jobs off the wards, but still more than the typical working week of 50 hours in most industrial and agricultural labour sectors.[43] The LCC began to envisage benefits accruing from fewer hours, such as staff being less exhausted and therefore able to work more therapeutically with the patients, a change which might also encourage staff retention and recruitment. More staff, however, would be expensive.

Alongside challenges from the type and hours of ward work and asylum culture and accommodation, terms of employment were problematic and required improvement to secure the best possible staff.[44] The staffing situation was similarly "critical" in Scottish asylums. There, recommendations were made to relax over-rigid discipline and "systematic petty tyranny", and to improve accommodation, conditions of service, pay, and pension rights to match the higher standards achieved by other public bodies, notably the Prison Service.[45] However, the LCC was complacent when it came to improving these employment conditions, as were some VCs who appeared out of touch with their staff.[46] Harsh discipline and hierarchical management were unlikely to foster a trusting relationship between seniors and juniors[47] and the punitive culture aroused apprehension and "a general feeling of insecurity" among staff.[48] These factors probably also encouraged dishonesty and concealment, with inconsistent and contradictory reporting of incidents, such as the events around the milk-thieves. As the war edged on, little was done to remedy staff working conditions. Staff suffered high rates of sickness and absence, and many resigned.[49] They did not become insane, but constituted a fragile body of workers. One temporary wartime attendant summarised his experience: "I was only there for a month – I could not stand it any longer."[50]

HIERARCHIES

Most staff were low in the ranks of the pervasive, almost feudal asylum hierarchy. The pecking order placed the medical superintendent at the top. He (there were no women in this role in the public asylums) had often climbed the medical career ladder in the same institution. Under him came the asylum "officers" including other doctors (hence known as "medical officers"), and senior staff in all disciplines, including matron, chaplain, steward (responsible for managing supplies, stores, staffing and day-to-day operation of the asylum) and farm bailiff. Below them came the main body of staff, then the probationers and finally the patients. Salaries and size of accommodation reflected the hierarchy. The medical superintendent at Colney Hatch received an annual salary of over £1000.[51] Required to live on site by the Lunacy Act,[52] he usually had a substantial house demonstrating his status within the asylum (Fig. 4.1). Its grandeur partly compensated for the freedom given to his medical and surgical colleagues of similar seniority who could choose their homes in more fashionable locations.

Junior doctors fared better than senior nurses, indicative of the overall medical hierarchy. A temporary assistant medical officer earnt about £300 a year, while matron's starting salary was around £100 plus emoluments.[53] The head attendant, who might have a cottage in the grounds if married, received about £80 plus £50 emoluments plus overtime. He might also be eligible for bonuses, such as the "war bonus" to help cover steep price rises.[54] The pay-roll at Colney Hatch showed that Miss Mingay, the work-mistress, received £46 plus £47 emoluments, and female probationer nurses earnt £20 plus board, lodging, laundry and uniform.[55] Although difficult to compare directly, for most staff, pay combined with emoluments was roughly equivalent to salaries of agricultural or factory labourers or domestic servants,[56] ranking their "worth" as employees among the lower tiers of the working class.

During the war, the VCs accorded the most junior ward staff, alongside temporary staff of almost all disciplines, a status only minimally higher than that of patients.[57] Also like the patients, junior and temporary staff were expected to be uncritical of asylum practices, or "to obey the 'God

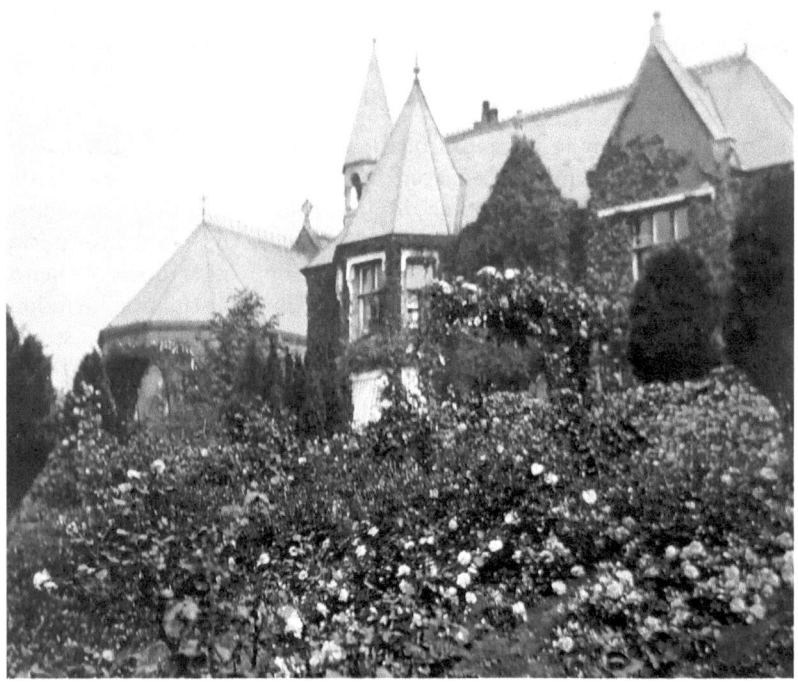

Fig. 4.1 The medical superintendent's house at Claybury, photographed from the rose garden, before 1917. The chapel is behind the house, to the left (Armstrong-Jones collection, Royal College of Psychiatrists' Archives)

of things as they are,' not of 'things as they should be'", in the words of Montagu Lomax, whose book about his wartime asylum work subsequently triggered the Cobb Inquiry into asylum practices.[58] With the risk of being dismissed for criticising the authorities, Lomax was aware that he had to take a difficult ethical decision: either to complain and risk being dismissed, or to continue to observe while part of the asylum system for long enough to write about his experiences at a later date.[59]

For ward staff, a practical demonstration of their place in the hierarchy was provided by the quality of their uniforms which could be little better than the clothing supplied to patients: when one attendant left Colney Hatch wearing his second-hand uniform, the VC was not concerned as it "would only have been fit to put in the rag bag".[60] Ward staff, however, regarding themselves as higher in the hierarchy than the patients, took it upon themselves to demonstrate their superiority and power over those in their charge. One way to do this was for ward staff to carry huge bunches of keys, sometimes 30 or more; the Board doubted that so many different locks were "really necessary" for security.[61] Monitoring ward staff, such as by them pegging in or recording their activities in registers, did not give oversight of the quality of their practice: behind locked doors on wards, staff were often unsupervised with their patients. One former patient observed that attendants had "almost unlimited power in dealing with patients unbeknown to the doctor"[62] and another commented: "The Visiting Committee are only a bit of eyewash; the attendants govern the asylum".[63] It is conceivable that ward staff, treated with little respect by their seniors in an authoritarian culture which did little to encourage kindness, would model their behaviours towards patients on the harsh and punitive ways in which they were treated.[64] The behaviour of seniors as models was particularly important for staff who had little formal training for the roles and responsibilities which they were expected to undertake. This would not foster practices which matched ideals of humane and attentive asylum care as promoted by forward-thinking psychiatrists and a wishful-thinking Board.[65]

GENDER, STATUS AND STAFF EDUCATION

The Lunacy Act ruled on gender segregation in asylums. It forbade any "male person" from having "personal custody" of any female patient,[66] so attendants provided day-to-day care for male patients, and nurses for female patients. Of necessity, since most doctors were male, they were permitted to work with male and female patients, chaperoned on their rounds where appropriate.[67] Culture also influenced practices and debates on gender and ward staffing. In Scotland, but not in England or Wales, asylums encouraged female nurses to care for male psychiatric patients. One Scottish medical superintendent, George Robertson, later professor of psychiatry in Edinburgh, spoke about women's "mothering instincts, and natural gifts for the nursing and care of male patients", as in general hospitals. Women, he said, could manage disturbed men, because they used persuasion rather than a "show of force":

> Excited patients who are ready to fight any man who comes near them will
> often do anything they are told by a nurse, and they will become calm if
> they receive a word of sympathy from her....it is absurd to assume that all
> feelings of chivalry and honour die in a man because he suffers from some
> derangement of the mind.[68]

Relatives also liked women nursing their menfolk as they feared less
violence from them.[69] South of the border, many VCs considered it
improper for women to nurse men and preferred male staff who could use
their physical prowess to control patients if necessary. This contributed
to propagating unwholesome images of asylums and mental disorders as
synonymous with violence.

Asylum nursing in England not only differed from that in Scotland
but it also contrasted with the model of "general" nursing for physical disorders and injury. General nursing was a respectable vocation for
middle class women, developed by Florence Nightingale, the pioneering
leader of modern nursing, and professionalized through education and
organisation. Practices of asylum nurses had some commonalities with the
Nightingale tradition, whereas attendants tended to adopt their model
of care from military orderlies. Nevertheless, the low status of asylum
ward staff made them uneasy that their better trained and middle class
general nursing colleagues might take over some of their roles and
responsibilities.[70]

Military demands dramatically reduced the availability of attendants,[71]
necessitating further consideration of nurses filling their posts.[72] There
were practical and moral considerations. In many asylums there were
barely sufficient nurses to staff the female wards, let alone the rest of
the asylum. Much discussion focussed on whether nurses should bathe
insane men or if work with disturbed men was suitable for younger
nurses, and what might be done in asylums where ward staff had their
bedrooms on or adjoining the wards, an arrangement which aimed to
facilitate them responding to an emergency at night.[73] Taking a lead from
general nursing where women nursed physically incapacitated men, some
VCs introduced nurses onto their male infirmary wards where the patients
were also physically unwell, and onto wards "occupied mainly by senile
cases".[74] Some asylums encouraged nurses to volunteer to work on the
male wards, elsewhere they were dismissed if they refused orders do so.[75]

Until the war, domestic service was the likely previous employment
experience of women taking up posts in asylums.[76] During the war,

with the wide range of employment opportunities available to women, some entered the asylum service having worked in day nurseries, hospitals, shops, munitions and other industries.[77] This gave them more skills and experiences of industrial-scale organisations and employment rights, which they used to further their own careers. When, for example, VCs told nurses that they could not be spared to undertake nursing of soldiers because of asylum staffing needs, they left anyway.[78] In the LCC's opinion "something should be done speedily" to make it worthwhile for women to remain on the asylum staff, rather than to move into jobs regarded as more glamorous or lucrative.[79] Gender had other implications for the asylums during the war years, as although more women than men were employed in lower ranks of asylum work, they were few and far between in the higher tiers. A few were appointed to roles which required specific training or expertise, such as doctors or pharmacists,[80] but more affluent women, who traditionally took on voluntary roles, remained under-represented: only six of 25 members of the LCC asylum committee were female.[81]

Other forces which shaped asylum practices included the trade unions. They favoured gender segregation in asylums as they feared that employing women in male roles might jeopardise jobs for men, and that since women received lower pay, VCs might maintain their wartime female workforce indefinitely as a cheaper option.[82] Women usually earnt about 20 per cent less than men for the same job, and only men were entitled to long-term service bonuses after five and ten years. The salary difference created unrest among women staff. Rarely, as in the case of experienced female agricultural workers on the asylum farms, they received the same wages as men, but capped so as not to exceed them.[83] The LCC ignored trade unions' war time requests about equal pay and stalled negotiations until after the war, on the grounds that such decisions warranted a government committee to consider the principles underlying it.[84] The LCC also debated female labour *versus* machines, such as for milking cows on the asylum farm, a task previously undertaken by men.[85] No-one appeared to advocate for fair-play for the cheapest option: patient labour. Patients replaced female staff on Claybury's farm when seven out of the eight staff left, dissatisfied with their wages. The patients who took over were allowed "extra cheese and jam for lunch and oatmeal water during the afternoon" but received no salary.[86]

Regarding education and training, a better trained workforce was assumed to be more productive and effective.[87] The MPA accepted that ward staff needed training, although Vicky Long argued that this was associated with a degree of self-interest, psychiatrists recognising that their own image was inexorably bound up with that of other staff.[88] Even if psychiatrists' image was a major concern of the MPA, it is admirable that it established a mental nursing syllabus, examinations and the "Certificate of Proficiency in Nursing the Insane", in the context of the general nursing profession keeping itself at arm's length from the asylums and there being no comparable established system of asylum ward staff leadership to develop the training themselves.[89] Introducing formal training to a workforce which had had little opportunity for study after leaving school, typically at age 12 years,[90] was an achievement. It was also a challenge for some asylum doctors who were expected to train their staff, having had little formal psychiatric training themselves. They might perceive that giving staff a recognised specialist qualification, when they had none, was a threat to their own status.[91]

The MPA's *Handbook for Attendants on the Insane*, was updated regularly and reached its sixth edition in 1911.[92] Asylums purchased the *Handbook* by the dozen.[93] The doctors gave lectures, which in some asylums received sufficient priority to be continued during the war.[94] The subject matter of the course was mostly theoretical, a watered-down version of the medical curriculum, lacking creativity to take into account the different practical tasks undertaken by doctors and ward staff. Not everyone regarded formal training as important: one doctor cited a staff representative who said that formal training was un-necessary, because "to be boxed up with the insane means becoming a qualified nurse."[95] Some medical officers questioned whether it was necessary for "ordinary attendants" to know about scientific subjects, such as physiology, to help them care for patients.[96] Others hoped that it would improve practice and recruitment and "eradicate faults of character".[97] "Faults of character" appeared to be a euphemism for unkind behaviour.

Anecdotal evidence suggested limited effects of the training. A former patient reported that he asked an attendant "Don't they give you talks on psychology?" and the attendant replied "What is that, something to eat?"[98] The attendant may have intended to be witty, but his comment suggested that his training lacked relevant content. Psychological skills might have been learnt on the wards, but it is less clear that there were enough knowledgeable senior ward staff with time and ability to demonstrate or encourage relevant therapeutic approaches.

Staff interest in training varied, even though the certificate was key to promotion within the asylum system[99] and to a salary bonus, usually £2 a year.[100] At some asylums, such as Claybury almost one-third of ward staff held the certificate in 1914.[101] Elsewhere, none possessed it.[102] Pre-war, more attendants than nurses passed the exam,[103] probably because attendants were more likely to consider their work as a life time job, compared to nurses who were less motivated to study because of the marriage bar. However, during the war, exam successes reversed: temporary attendants probably had less incentive than nurses on permanent contracts.[104]

The MPA considered that the work of asylum nurses and attendants was equivalent to that of general nurses and should be recognised as such. Consequently, it wanted the Royal British Nursing Association (RBNA) register to include asylum staff who held the MPA certificate. The RBNA rejected their request as it did not consider asylum staff trained nurses. The RNBA would have provided some trade union representation for the asylum ward staff, similar to the way the British Medical Association acted for doctors.[105] Their rejection was associated with the establishment of a separate organisation the Asylum Worker's Association which became the National Asylum Worker's Union (NAWU) in 1910.[106] It represented a disheartened and under-trained body of staff, and it focussed primarily on the well-being of the workforce rather than directly on the patients. In contrast to the NAWU, the College of Nursing (later, Royal College), established in 1916, had educational objectives. Its nurses were beginning to take a greater role in teaching their own profession. However, general nursing textbooks, similar to general textbooks for training doctors, hardly mentioned psychiatric symptoms, further reinforcing the compartmentalisation of mental and physical nursing.[107] The College of Nursing and the NAWU indicated workers' needs: for general nurses, better education; for asylum workers, improved wages and employment conditions. Contrasting priorities indicated a self-confident general nursing profession, and an unsettled asylum workforce. In 1919 the establishment of the General Nursing Council, a regulatory body for the nursing profession in England and Wales, was heavily influenced by the RNBA leadership. It too did not recognise the MPA qualification, and in 1921 introduced its own. Soberingly, Kathleen Jones argued that "there were many mental nurses with neither the will nor the apparent ability to take either."[108]

MEDICAL STAFF: DOCTORS AND DILEMMAS

Medical students were taught a fairly standardised curriculum in "psychological medicine". Tracy Loughran analysed their education in psychological and psychiatric subjects in the context of her research on shell shock, arguing that medical students would have found it difficult to avoid acquiring some psychological knowledge in the course of their studies.[109] However, clinical work was (and is) a practical art backed up by science, and art requires practice, not just knowledge. Medical students received practical training in medicine, surgery, pathology, obstetrics and gynaecology, but rarely in psychiatry. Without practice, lectures were unlikely to give them a secure grounding in the subject for their future careers. In addition, senior asylum doctors usually taught their courses, focussing on mental disorders encountered in daily asylum work, rather than those which most doctors would face in their general hospital or community practice. Standard textbooks were also often inadequate concerning psychiatry. Whereas they contained descriptions of physical symptoms (e.g. coughs) and indicated the characteristics and clinical significance of each type, they were likely only to define a psychiatric term (e.g. delusion) but neither explain its significance nor indicate its subtypes.[110] Bernard Hollander, a psychiatrist, and Edward Younger, a physician with some psychiatric training, both questioned the relevance of the medical school curriculum.[111] Younger worked at London's Finsbury Dispensary, providing out-patient services for working-class people. His textbook in 1914 contrasted with usual teaching, particularly by emphasising early stages of mental disorder, clinical assessment and legal matters relevant to the work of general practitioners.[112]

Pre-war, with little psychiatric training in medical schools, doctors working in asylums needed, but received, little in-service training to supplement their clinical experiences. A few spent time away from psychiatry, working in general hospitals, and sat the examination for Membership of the Royal College of Physicians. The MPA, as it had done for asylum nurses and attendants, set the ball rolling in asylum doctors' education. However, the MPA's "Certificate of Efficiency in Psychological Medicine" had neither a published curriculum nor official recognition. Several universities began to provide teaching for asylum doctors,[113] giving them the opportunity to gain a Diploma in Psychological Medicine. That too was problematic. Although it went some way towards indicating a doctor's suitability to become a specialist, the diploma lacked the rigour and status of the examinations of the medical Royal Colleges.[114] It thus did not increase the esteem of asylum doctors in the eyes of their physician and surgeon colleagues, for whom Royal College memberships and fellowships, and work in teaching hospitals, private clinics and charity-funded ("voluntary") general hospitals, comprised the pinnacle of professional clinical practice.

As with many other asylum staff, the doctors were dissatisfied with their terms and conditions of service. An anonymous asylum medical officer wrote to the *British Medical Journal* (*BMJ*) shortly before the war, drawing attention to medical staff vacancies: the recent pay rise was welcome but insufficient, and "Until some action is taken to improve existing conditions, the asylum medical officer will remain a professional pariah, whose life, like the policeman's, is 'not a happy one'." He ascribed some of the blame to medical superintendents who made little effort to improve matters.[115] Around the same time, the *BMJ* also cited an MPA report that medical work in asylums, "leads to the stunting of ambition and a gradual loss of interest in scientific medicine, and it tends to produce a deteriorating effect upon those who remain long in the service." It also commented that the problem "demands the earnest attention of public authorities and all interested in the welfare of the insane"[116]; asylum medical posts needed improving to attract and keep good staff. The MPA dedicated a half-day session to this at its annual meeting in July 1914, two weeks before war broke out. It recommended a greater variety of clinical responsibilities including investigating and treating new patients, better clinical supervision from senior medical officers, more training and study leave and some experience working in a general hospital. Medical officers should also be allowed to marry after 5 years' service and have house in the grounds; promotion should depend upon qualifications and personal qualities; and lay committees which lacked expertise to evaluate the clinical knowledge or skills of the applicant were unsuitable for appointing medical staff.[117] Implementing the changes would need collaboration between various bodies such as local authorities to fund locums to cover study leave; general hospitals to facilitate placements; and VCs to build more staff accommodation.

With numerous vacancies for asylum doctors, some took jobs in asylums when they were unable to find work elsewhere. This may have given Herbert Ellis, a magistrate and VC member, the impression that assistant medical officers lacked ability, interest and enthusiasm, contrasting with often impressive medical superintendents who had high standards and knew their patients well.[118] Former patient, Charles McCarthy, a retired civil servant, was less charitable, describing one asylum doctor as "after the type of a low English navvy", and the medical superintendent as "an English snob with an imitation University accent."[119] Standards of asylum clinical work could be dismal. Medical assessments might not be entered in the patients' notes and a batch of mandatory clinical reviews might be added just before a Board inspection.[120] The Board nudged: "instead of making so many on one day (sometimes we observe over 100)" it would be better if "an endeavour were made to distribute them over the year, so that only a few fall due each day."[121] Neglectful, rushed and superficial clinical assessments may have been due to doctors' laziness or lack of skills or interest, but could also have been an effect of the asylum system, its values and economic restrictions, with unsuitable recruitment processes, medical understaffing and excessive workloads. As with the relationship between VCs and the asylum workforce generally, that between a medical superintendent and his junior staff could be equally fraught. The medical superintendent at Prestwich Asylum showed little respect for his junior doctors. He described them as "the flotsam and jetsam and scum of the earth", with the second part of the sentence deleted in the transcript of the Cobb Inquiry.[122] The comments from the superintendent about his medical staff seem excessive, even if some of them were second-rate.

Many doctors endeavoured to practice high standards of medicine, but things could still go wrong. In those circumstances, doctors appear to have been punished more leniently than their non-medical colleagues, probably because their professional status unfairly accorded them some immunity. Five women patients died one night in 1914 at the Bethlem Hospital, all by poisoning from amylene hydrate, a sedative. A seriously depleted staff at the beginning of the war resulted in the on-call doctor, Henry Jones, being called on to dispense medications from stock bottles. He poured amylene from the bottle containing the concentrated, rather than the diluted, solution, giving each woman eight times the usual dose. The *Times* reported the coroner's jury's verdicts of "death by misadventure".[123] The coroner recommended that medical officers should not have to undertake dispensing and a "qualified paid dispenser" should be employed. The Bethlem adopted this proposal and arranged for concentrated and diluted medications to be stored separately.[124] There is no evidence that Jones was punished for his error. Indeed, his career progressed, despite the disaster. Jones became medical superintendent at

Fulbourn Hospital, Cambridge, where his eccentricities and personal style received greater acclaim than his clinical leadership.[125]

In summary, poor standards of medical practice, scarcity of doctors willing to enter asylum work, plus many medical officers enlisting early in the war, were likely to prejudice patient care.[126]

SERVING THE COLOURS

Medical officers, alongside attendants and some staff who fulfilled unique roles in the asylum, enlisted or transferred to war work. When Hanwell's tin smith went to work in a munitions factory, colleagues at other LCC asylums covered for him.[127] From Colney Hatch, the "last permanent hand in the tailor's shop" and the upholsterer, whose jobs included furniture renovation and repairing blinds and mattresses,[128] left to join the army in the same week.[129] That was especially tricky when repair rather than replacement had become the norm. The Board complied with instructions, in line with national propaganda and public opinion, to release the maximum numbers of staff to achieve the overriding goal of bringing hostilities to a satisfactory close and return to a "proper standard" as soon as possible thereafter.[130] With many men serving the Colours, women, and men over military recruitment age, took over their duties.[131] Much leave was curtailed at the beginning of the war, with promises that annual leave would accrue and that overtime would be paid.[132]

Nationally, over one million volunteers were recruited into military service by the end of 1914, but more were needed. The LCC encouraged asylum staff to enlist.[133] By March 1915, over 500 men, about a quarter of the total male staff across all the LCC asylums, were serving with the military forces. At the end of 1915, the LCC resolved that any asylum employee who wanted to join the army under the scheme established by Lord Derby, Director General of Recruiting, should be permitted to do so. If he could not be spared immediately, his name would be transferred to the army reserve list, to provide time to find a substitute.[134] The LCC based its strategy on the premise that difficulties in the asylums could be overcome with careful financial management and a "helpful fluidity of staff". The latter implied that staff would move from asylum to asylum as required, although the LCC did not state how it might find enough adequately trained staff for this. The Board encouraged the LCC scheme with a little flattery, that "the London Asylums, the pioneers in the Asylum world" would set an example to others.[135]

In March 1916 the Military Service Act introduced conscription except for those in essential occupations. Very few asylum jobs fell into this category. Of 6500 attendants in the asylum service in England and Wales before the war, a skeleton of 1500 were deemed indispensable.[136] Doctors were in demand to serve the nation, and almost half those working in asylums undertook military service. Many of those who replaced them had less asylum experience, were physically unfit, or had retired from clinical practice.[137] (Lomax was an older, retired doctor, working in this capacity at Prestwich Asylum.[138]) By mid-1916, the ratio of doctors to patients in the asylums deteriorated from an average of 1 to 250, to 1 to 390.[139] Medical staffing was so inadequate that some asylum doctors spent their leave from the army working in the asylum which had agreed to their military service and to which they expected to return. More clinical work fell on the shoulders of the medical superintendents. One asylum reported a "large amount of illness in the institution" which needed a "reliable permanent assistant who could relive him [the medical superintendent] of some of the very heavy responsibilities which he is now called upon to bear."[140]

The LCC offered financial support to military recruits, topping up military pay where necessary to its usual asylum level, including emoluments and increments.[141] The principle was that those undertaking military service should not be financially disadvantaged compared to those remaining behind. To ensure this, asylums also caped the salaries of existing staff, such as when "acting up" into more senior roles. However, as the war lengthened some asylums had to ignore the salary caps to allay staff unrest and to stem the tide of pay-related resignations.[142] Elsewhere, VCs deferred payment of additional wages, promising that the matter would be considered at some later date.[143] VCs were also prohibited from appointing new permanent staff. This was well intentioned, aiming to ensure that eligible staff on military service would have equal opportunity to apply for permanent posts on their return, but the consequences of temporary appointments, or rapid promotion into acting roles, risked sub-standard leadership and destabilising asylum function.[144]

In 1916, the MPA approached the Board, concerned about falling staff levels. It feared the consequences of lower standards of care, such as "extensive resort to seclusion and mechanical and chemical restraint which prevailed in the days when attendants were few and inefficient."

It asked the Board to help secure exemptions from military service "To save the already dangerously depleted asylums from the almost complete denudation of a skilled and physically fit staff of male attendants."[145] The Board appeared keener to follow the national priorities rather than more patient focussed advocacy of the MPA. In 1917, on behalf of the War Office, the Board appealed for more medical men from the asylums.[146] The LCC, which until then had encouraged military recruitment, uncompromising refused.[147] The Board reiterated the recruitment request early in 1918, continuing to comply with the War Office, "that every fit man of military age should be available for military service".[148] The Board rejected pleas from the LCC and MPA about falling standards of care.

At the end of the war, asylums were desperate for their staff to return, but there was no plan to demob asylum employees any earlier than anyone else.[149] By April 1919, most LCC asylum staff had returned to their peace-time work. However, despite concern by the asylum authorities about medical staffing levels, 26 of 28 medical officers from LCC asylums remained absent from their civilian posts, still not demobbed.[150] The asylums were not alone in their dissatisfaction about the slow rate of demobilisation and the inequities of its application. Demobilisation aimed to be in accordance with the strategic importance of an individual's civilian occupation: a coal miner, for example, was high priority.[151] Regarding asylum doctors, there seemed to be little official awareness of their civilian roles. This fitted with national understanding and priorities concerning civilian mental and physical health.[152] However, the return of doctors was probably also delayed because physical and mental war wounds did not disappear with the signing of the Armistice. Thus, in the established hierarchies of military needs and civilian mental health needs, it is hardly surprising that asylum doctors experienced late demobilisation. Nationally, one million men were still in uniform in September 1919 and 125,000 awaited return to civilian life in early 1920. The delays caused much distress,[153] not solely to asylums.

Through the war, the Board and VCs regularly reported on asylum personnel serving the Colours. News of their deaths, injuries, promotions and gallantry[154] may have motivated remaining staff to work harder, in line with propaganda and despite the challenges they faced. From the LCC asylums, 952 men (about half of the male workforce) served in the forces. Ninety-seven were killed, dead or missing, 160 wounded, and 31 gained military distinctions including three with the Military Cross.[155]

Others suffered physical illnesses and shell shock.[156] Some, such as attendant Thomas Wells received support when back at his asylum. Employed at Claybury since 1907, he served in the army for two years. On his return, he had difficulty undertaking some tasks. When he refused to bathe a patient, his seniors reported him to the medical superintendent. The superintendent recognised that he was suffering from shell shock and negotiated alternative, less distressing work for him on the farm.[157] Not all traumatised returning staff received sympathy. Attendant Franklin Graimes from Hanwell enlisted in 1914 age 26, and served for three years, and was invalided out of the army suffering from shell shock.[158] Back at Hanwell, he was too unwell to resume his duties. The VC showed little tolerance of his symptoms or willingness to modify his duties. Instead they encouraged him to resign, which he did.[159] Lack of sympathy towards people with mental disorders existed, including within the mental health service leadership, and even towards former soldiers who public mandate demanded were to be treated with respect.

The Board unswervingly followed the patriotic party line, despite intermittent opposition from the MPA and the LCC who were concerned about the risks to asylum patients. It was rare for the Board to advocate for patients in the face of competing national pressures, despite the image they sought to present of themselves as working in their best interests.[160] Rather, they seemed to prioritise their organisational and personal reputations: Marriott Cooke, chairman of the Board during the war, was knighted for his war services, not for his commitment to the asylums and their staff and patients.[161]

Towards the End of the War

Despite simmering staff discontent, the NAWU kept a fairly low profile until 1918.[162] By then, some ward staff were working 100 hours a week and there was a nadir of morale. At the same time, trade unions were becoming more influential across many occupational groups[163] and strikes by public service workers, including the police, took place before the war ended. The NAWU placed before the Lancashire Asylums Board (LAB) a list of nine requests, varying from permission to post their union notices in the staff mess rooms to improving pay and conditions for attendants and nurses. The LAB rejected them all. On 4 September 1918, 200 asylum staff came out on strike at Prestwich. The following day 449 attendants stopped work at Whittingham. At Winwick there was a go slow and a suggestion that the strike would spread to asylums outside Lancashire. The LAB agreed to submit the items under dispute to arbitration by the Ministry of Labour (established in 1916) and promised that no employee on strike would be penalized. In the light of having organised this protest, despite the claims eventually being rejected at arbitration, the NAWU's prestige rose and its membership increased. Capitalizing on their success, at the end of September 1918 the NAWU adopted a national programme for the future. It included plans to implement a 48-hour week; a minimum weekly wage of £2 for the most junior nurses; equal pay for equal work for men and women; registration for the profession of mental nursing; and universal recognition by the asylum authorities of the union as a negotiating body.[164] The Board's fifth annual report for 1918 acknowledged the NAWU for the first time. The Board situated asylum changes in the context of a general "movement of the working classes" to secure better pay and employment conditions. It stated that it was already aware of the need to do this, but counter-balanced its argument by repeating the problem of economic hurdles concerning "the burden imposed on the nation by the mass of mental defect and disorder".[165] The Board, having done little to advocate for patients or staff over the previous 4 years, said that it knew what to do and paid short shrift to the NAWU.

Conclusions

Strict rules and attitudes of asylum leaders towards their staff echoed military discipline as a means of controlling lower ranks. This style may have been appropriate to soldiers on the front line in battle, but it was unsuited to the asylum front line where the aim was to improve the health and wellbeing of patients through "care and treatment". The "systematic petty tyranny" detected in Scottish asylums was also present in their English counterparts, a culture of excessively harsh and rigid attitudes and behaviours which passed through the asylums as far as the patients whose treatment often fell short of ideal. Insufficiently trained lower levels of staff were likely to perpetuate the tyranny, modelling their own behaviours and attitudes on their experiences of those in authority who demonstrated how seniors behaved towards subordinates.

Organisational rigidity imposed by the Lunacy Act and the leadership discouraged changes in asylum practices and inhibited creativity to deal proactively with new eventualities. Lay management committees running the asylums, despite working closely with senior asylum officers, particularly the medical superintendent, may have contributed to this. Their lack of expertise may have made them uncertain in their decision making and more dependent on rules and regulations. Concerning staff, the management showed little interest in their wellbeing, although some helpful flexibility appeared regarding rules about marriage and about giving staff options to live beyond the perimeter wall, although that commenced pre-war. The motivation for these changes may have been the limited amount of married accommodation available, the cost and inconvenience of building more, and fear of further workforce depletion, rather than staff wellbeing as such. Albeit small, the changes were in line with staff needs, and did not precipitate disaster.

Goffman wrote about a two-way staff-inmate split in institutions:

> Each group tends to conceive of the other in terms of narrow hostile stereotypes, staff often seeing inmates as bitter, secretive, and untrustworthy, while inmates often see staff as condescending, high handed and mean. Staff tends to feel superior and righteous; inmates tend, in some way at least, to feel inferior, weak, blameworthy and guilty.[166]

The wartime asylums appeared to have a three-way split: seniors including the VC; subordinate staff; and patients. The relationship between seniors and subordinate staff and that between subordinate staff and patients both fitted with Goffman's staff-inmate pattern. Neither facilitated a happy working relationship.

Although some staff worked long-term in the asylums and appeared settled within an institutional regime, many others were discontent, morale was low, and staff had a high turnover both before and during the war. The establishment of the NAWU indicated staff concerns—pay, hours, accommodation and other conditions of employment—in contrast to the education and professionalisation priorities in general nursing. By the end of the war, with increased staff unrest and higher union membership, the NAWU was a greater force for change. A similar shift occurred in other employment sectors.[167] The NAWU appeared to listen to staff feedback about their needs in contrast to the asylum leadership which was out of touch with its workforce.

Official status or rank carried significant weight in the asylums, affecting who listened to whom, and to whom punishment—or sometimes praise—was directed. Praise and punishment were doled out inequitably, such as punishing doctors more leniently than ward staff for breaching rules or making errors. Responses to staff deemed unsuitable varied in other ways, such as how to support former soldiers who returned to their asylum employment while suffering from shell shock, or what to do when nurses were unhappy about working on male wards. Although we do not have details, such as about individual staff members' past work record, decisions on their employment status appear unfair, and sometimes lacking compassion.

The asylum leadership prioritised conforming to rules and expected everyone to do likewise. A conformist system could contribute to a sense of place and security for the leadership and belief that they behaved in the correct manner. This would reinforce existing practices, but would not encourage lateral thinking about alternatives, or querying whether some of the asylum's staffing difficulties were due to the system which they led. It is likely that the asylum leadership contributed to a dysfunctional system in which lower ranks of staff were undervalued and unappreciated.

NOTES

1. Select Committee on the Asylum Officers (Employment, Pensions and Superannuation) Bill, *Report and Special Report Together with the Proceedings of the Committee* (London: HMSO, 1911), iv.
2. Dr. Pasmore in discussion about "Asylum Administration as Affected by Present Events," *Journal of Mental Science* (*JMS*) 65 (1919): 124–29, 127.
3. *First Annual Report of the Board of Control, for the Year 1914* (London: HMSO, 1916) (*BoC AR 1914*), Part 2, 154; Anon. *The LCC Hospitals: A Retrospect* (London: LCC, 1949), 108; LCC LCC/MIN/00754 Minutes of miscellaneous sub-committees 1915–1919: Summary of staff numbers required for a 48-hour week, LMA.
4. LCC LCC/MIN/00759 Presented papers of sub-committee 1909–1923: tradesmen in asylums 1910, LMA.
5. Colney Hatch LCC/MIN/01005 Meeting, 19 May 1916, 162; H12/CH/C/04/003 Male attendants' wages book 1915–1916, LMA.
6. Asylums Officers (Employment, Pensions, and Superannuation) Bill. *Hansard* HC Deb, 21 May 1914, vol. 62, c2132.
7. E. Marriott Cooke and C. Hubert Bond, *History of the Asylum War Hospitals in England and Wales* (London: HMSO, 1920), 2.
8. "Asylum Worker's Association, Extract from Sir James Crichton-Browne's Address," *JMS* 61 (1915): 479–80.

9. Colney Hatch LCC/MIN/01006 Meeting, 7 September 1917, 234–36 LMA.

10. Erving Goffman, *Asylums: Essays on the Social Situation of Mental Patients and Other Inmates* (1961; Harmondsworth: Penguin, 1980).

11. Colney Hatch LCC/MIN/01003 Meeting, 31 July 1914, 57 LMA.

12. Hanwell H11/HLL/C/06/006 Male attendants' fine book 1914–1935, 18 June 1917 LMA.

13. Colney Hatch LCC/MIN/01006 Meeting, 1 December 1916, 37 LMA; *BoC AR 1914*, Part 2, Salop Asylum 8 July 1914, 298; Peter Nolan, *A History of Mental Nursing* (London: Chapman and Hall, 1993), 57, 74.

14. Hanwell H11/HLL/C/06/006 Male attendants' fine book 1914–1935, 22 May 1916 LMA.

15. LCC LCC/MIN/00579 Meeting, 26 May 1914, 463 LMA; Colney Hatch LCC/MIN/01003 Meeting, 18 December 1914, 215–16 LMA.

16. Claybury LCC/MIN/00948 Meeting, 8 November 1917, 244 LMA.

17. Hanwell H11/HLL/C/06/006 Male attendants' fine book 1914–1935; 18 June 1917; 16 February 1914; 15 November 1920; 21 July 1913 LMA.

18. Bedford Pierce, "Some Present Day Problems Connected with the Administration of Asylums," *JMS* 65 (1919): 198–201, 198.

19. Colney Hatch LCC/MIN/01001 Meeting, 25 April 1913, 42 LMA.

20. Nolan, *History*, 74.

21. Colney Hatch LCC/MIN/01007 Meeting, 17 May 1918, 75 LMA; sometimes 10.30 p.m. in summer.

22. Napsbury H50/A/01/024 Meeting, 6 August 1915, 117 LMA.

23. Colney Hatch LCC/MIN/01002 Meeting, 27 March 1914, 183 LMA.

24. England Census 1891, 1901, 1911, https://www.ancestry.co.uk/search/categories/ukicen/.

25. Colney Hatch LCC/MIN/01005 Meeting, 7 April 1916, 122 LMA.

26. Colney Hatch LCC/MIN/01002 Meeting, 13 February 1914, 125 LMA.

27. LCC LCC/MIN/00583 Meeting, 24 July 1917, 35 LMA.

28. LCC LCC/MIN/00582 Meeting, 30 January 1917, 408–9 LMA.

29. Colney Hatch LCC/MIN/01006 Meeting, 17 November 1916, 57 LMA.

30. LCC LCC/MIN/00583 Meeting, 26 March 1918, 429 LMA.

31. Colney Hatch LCC/MIN/01005 Meeting, 19 May 1916, 165 LMA.

32. LCC LCC/MIN/00580 Meeting, 27 April 1915, 392 LMA.

33. *BoC AR 1914*, Part 2, Isle of Wight Asylum 21 April 1914, 319.

34. Montagu Lomax, *The Experiences of an Asylum Doctor* (London: Allen and Unwin, 1921), 117–18.

35. Colney Hatch LCC/MIN/01002 Meeting, 13 March 1914, 163–64 LMA.
36. Hanwell LCC/MIN/01093 Meeting, 22 December 1913, 27 LMA.
37. Hanwell LCC/MIN/01095 Meeting, 7 June 1915, 66 LMA.
38. Select Committee on the Asylum Officers Bill, *Report*, iv; Neil Brimblecombe, "Asylum Nursing as a Career in the United Kingdom, 1890–1910," *Journal of Advanced Nursing* 55 (2006): 770–77, 770.
39. Nolan, *History*, 75; *BoC AR 1914*, Part 2, Cumberland and Westmorland Asylum 23 July 1914, 212; Oxford Asylum 4 August 1914, 296.
40. *BoC AR 1914*, Part 2, Winwick Asylum 24 February 1914, 257.
41. Select Committee on the Asylum Officers Bill, *Report*, iii–v, vii.
42. *BoC AR 1914*, Part 2, Winwick Asylum 24 February 1914, 257.
43. LCC LCC/MIN/00579 Meetings: 16 December 1913, 94; 27 January 1914, 135 LMA; Department of Employment and Productivity, *British Labour Statistics: Historical Abstract 1886–1968* (London: HMSO, 1971), 28, 30, 39.
44. Select Committee on the Asylum Officers Bill, *Report*, iv.
45. Nolan, *History*, 75, 77.
46. Select Committee on the Asylum Officers Bill, *Report*, v.
47. *BoC AR 1914*, Part 2, Oxford Asylum 4 August 1914, 295.
48. Colney Hatch LCC/MIN/01004 Meeting, 2 July 1915, 155 LMA.
49. Hanwell LCC/MIN/01097 Meeting, 24 September 1917, 181–83 LMA.
50. Committee on the Administration of Public Mental Hospitals (Chairman: Sir Cyril Cobb) (Cobb Inquiry), 15 March 1922 AM Donaldson Q:576, MH 58/219 TNA.
51. Colney Hatch H12/CH/C/03/004 Officers' salaries book 1910–1917, LMA.
52. Lunacy Act 1890 section 276 (1) (b) (c).
53. Claybury LCC/MIN/00946 Meeting, 24 March 1915, 81 and between pp. 71–72 LMA.
54. Colney Hatch H12/CH/C/04/004 Male attendants' wages book 1917–1918 LMA.
55. Colney Hatch H12/CH/C/03/004 Officers' salaries book 1910–1917 LMA; Hanwell LCC/MIN/01096 Meeting, 5 June 1916, 83 LMA.
56. Department of Employment and Productivity, *British Labour Statistics*, 38–39; Brimblecombe, "Asylum Nursing": 770.
57. Leonard Smith, "Behind Closed Doors: Lunatic Asylum Keepers, 1800–1860," *Social History of Medicine* 1 (1988): 301–27, 327.
58. Ministry of Health, *Report of the Committee on Administration of Public Mental Hospitals* Cmd. 1730 (Chairman: Sir Cyril Cobb) (London: HMSO, 1922); Lomax, *Experiences*, 51.

59. BoC, "Memorandum for the Minister of Health on Mr. Montagu Lomax's Book *The Experiences of an Asylum Doctor,*" 21 September 1921, MH 52/222 TNA.
60. Colney Hatch LCC/MIN/01002 Meeting, 30 January 1914, 113 LMA.
61. *BoC AR 1914*, Part 2, Dorset Asylum 12 May 1914, 222.
62. Cobb Inquiry, 15 March 1922 Mr. Cox Q:401, MH 58/219 TNA.
63. Cobb Inquiry, 30 March 1922 Edward Mason Q:2112, MH 58/220 TNA.
64. Lomax, *Experiences*, 84; Nolan, *History*, 83.
65. Charles Mercier, *The Attendant's Companion: A Manual of the Duties of Attendants in Lunatic Asylums* (London: J and A Churchill, 1898), 2.
66. Lunacy Act 1890, section 53.
67. Napsbury H50/A/01/026 Meeting, 22 July 1916, 37 LMA.
68. George Robertson, "The Employment of Female Nurses in the Male Wards of Mental Hospitals in Scotland," *JMS* 62 (1916): 351–62, 361.
69. Robertson, "Employment of Female Nurses": 362.
70. Nolan, *History*, 70.
71. Tom Walmsley, "Psychiatry in Scotland," 294–305, in *150 Years of British Psychiatry 1841–1991*, ed. German Berrios and Hugh Freeman (London: Gaskell, 1991), 303.
72. Hanwell H11/HLL/A/06/05 Draft annual report 1917 LMA.
73. *BoC AR 1914*, Part 2, Northumberland Asylum 4 May 1914, 292.
74. Claybury LCC/MIN/00946 Meeting, 14 October 1915, 241 LMA; *BoC AR 1914*, Part 2, Severalls Asylum 27 October 1914, 227.
75. Claybury LCC/MIN/00946 Meeting, 14 October 1915, 241 LMA; Hanwell LCC/MIN/01097 Meeting, 2 July 1917, 118–19 LMA.
76. Brimblecombe, "Asylum Nursing": 770.
77. Hanwell H11/HLL/C/03/001 Letters of recommendation and testimonials of female asylum staff 1903–1923, using sample from 1910 to 1919 LMA.
78. LCC LCC/MIN/00580 Meeting, 29 June 1915, 638–39; Colney Hatch LCC/MIN/01004 Meeting, 2 July 1915, 152: LCC/MIN/01005 Meeting, 22 September 1916, 270 LMA.
79. LCC LCC/MIN/00582 Meeting, 30 January 1917, 402 LMA.
80. Claybury LCC/MIN/00949 Meeting, 5 December 1918, 250 LMA; Napsbury H50/A/01/026 Meeting, 6 October 1916, 115 LMA; Louise Hide, *Gender and Class in English Asylums, 1890–1914* (London: Palgrave Macmillan, 2014), 45–46.
81. *BoC AR 1914*, Part 1, vi; LCC LCC/MIN/00581 Meeting, 14 March 1916, 424; LCC/MIN/00584 Meeting, 8 October 1918, 2–4 LMA.
82. Colney Hatch LCC/MIN/01004 Meeting, 27 August 1915, 197 LMA.
83. Claybury LCC/MIN/00948 Meeting, 15 March 1917, 57 LMA.

84. LCC: LCC/MIN/00581 Meeting, 30 November 1915, 178; LCC/MIN/00584 Meeting, 8 October 1918, 3 LMA.
85. LCC LCC/MIN/00581 Meeting, 18 April 1916, 484 LMA.
86. Claybury LCC/MIN/00949 Meeting, 20 June 1918, 130 LMA.
87. Nolan, *History*, 62.
88. Vicky Long, *Destigmatising Mental Illness? Professional Politics and Public Education in Britain, 1870–1970* (Manchester, UK: Manchester University Press, 2014), 67.
89. Thomas Bewley, *Madness to Mental Illness: A History of the Royal College of Psychiatrists* (London: RCPsych Publications, 2008), 115.
90. Age 14 after Education Act 1918.
91. Nolan, *History*, 62.
92. MPA, *Handbook for the Instruction of Attendants on the Insane* (London: Baillière, Tindall and Cox, 1885); MPA, *Handbook for Attendants on the Insane* (6th Edition) (London: Baillière, Tindall and Cox, 1911); Bewley, *Madness to Mental Illness*, 114.
93. Napsbury H50/A/01/024 Meeting, 16 October 1915, 220 LMA.
94. Colney Hatch LCC/MIN/01007 Meeting, 22 February 1918, 39 LMA.
95. Dr. Turner in discussion about "Asylum Administration as Affected by Present Events," *JMS* 65 (1919): 124–29, 129.
96. Bewley, *Madness to Mental Illness*, 114.
97. Nolan, *History*, 82.
98. Cobb Inquiry, 30 March 1922 Edward Mason Q:2138, MH 58/220 TNA.
99. Colney Hatch LCC/MIN/01007 Meeting, 22 February 1918, 39 LMA.
100. LCC LCC/MIN/00579 Meeting, 4 November 1913, 19 LMA.
101. *BoC AR 1914*, Part 2, 1914 Claybury Asylum 27 June 1914, 270.
102. *BoC AR 1914*, Part 2, Berks Asylum 6 May 1914, 198.
103. *BoC AR 1914*, Part 2, Brecon and Radnor Asylum 6 May 1914, 199.
104. Claybury LCC/MIN/00946 Meeting, 22 July 1915, 190 LMA; Colney Hatch LCC/MIN/01005 Meeting, 2 June 1916, 192 LMA.
105. Royal British Nursing Association, https://www.rbna.org.uk/.
106. Francis Adams, "From Association to Union: Professional Organization of Asylum Attendants, 1869–1919," *British Journal of Sociology* 20 (1969): 11–26, 12.
107. Georgiana Sanders, *Modern Methods in Nursing* (Philadelphia and London: WB Saunders, 1912), 703–9.
108. Kathleen Jones, *Mental Health and Social Policy, 1845–1959* (London: Routledge and Kegan Paul, 1960), 102.
109. Tracy Loughran, *Shell Shock and Medical Culture in First World War Britain* (Cambridge: Cambridge University Press, 2017), 23, 33.

110. G Elliott Smith and Tom Pear, *Shell Shock and Its Lessons* (Manchester: University Press, 1917), 111, 118–19.
111. Edward Younger, *Insanity in Everyday Practice* (London: Baillière, Tindall and Cox, 1914), 1; Bernard Hollander, *The First Signs of Insanity: Their Prevention and Treatment* (London: Stanley Paul and Co, 1912), 21.
112. Younger, *Insanity*, vii, 16–22.
113. Anon. "Facilities Provided for the Teaching of Psychiatry," *JMS* 59 (1913): 159–60.
114. Hugh Freeman, "Psychiatry in Britain c. 1900," *History of Psychiatry* 21 (2010): 312–24, 320.
115. An AMO, "Assistant Medical Officers in Asylums," *BMJ* 9 August 1913, 349.
116. Anon. "The Asylum Service," *BMJ* 29 November 1913, 1447–1448, 1448.
117. Anon. "The Medico-Psychological Association of Great Britain and Ireland," *JMS* 60 (1914): 644–95, 669–73.
118. Cobb Inquiry, 16 March 1922 Herbert Ellis Q:862, 872, MH 58/219 TNA.
119. Cobb Inquiry, 16 March 1922 Charles McCarthy Q:819, 823, MH 58/219 TNA.
120. *BoC AR 1914*, Part 2, Kesteven Asylum 27 January 1914, 263.
121. *BoC AR 1914*, Part 2, Hants Asylum 6 November 1914, 234.
122. Cobb Inquiry, 24 February 1922 Dr. Perceval Q:410, MH 58/219 TNA.
123. BoC W/FM, 11 November 1914, 236 MH 50/43 TNA; Anon. "News in Brief," *Times*, 13 November 1914.
124. *BoC AR 1914*, Part 1, 37.
125. David Clark, *The Story of a Mental Hospital: Fulbourn 1858–1983* (London: Process Press, 1996), 54, 192.
126. *BoC AR 1914*, Part 1, 15–16.
127. Hanwell LCC/MIN/01095 Meeting, 7 June 1915, 96 LMA.
128. Cobb Inquiry, 30 March 1922 Dr. Ogilvy Q:1806–7, MH 58/220 TNA.
129. Colney Hatch LCC/MIN/01006 Meeting, 17 November 1916, 12 LMA.
130. *Third Annual Report of the Board of Control, for the Year 1916* (London: HMSO, 1917) (*BoC AR 1916*), 10; BoC to MPA, untitled letter 17 May 1916, *JMS* 62 (1916): 637–38.
131. Initially 19–30 years, then 18–41. From April 1918, 18–51.
132. LCC LCC/MIN/00579 Meeting, 29 September 1914, 649 LMA.
133. LCC LCC/MIN/00580 Meeting, 22 December 1914, 131 LMA.

134. LCC LCC/MIN/00581 Meeting, 9 November 1915, 111, 128 LMA; *BoC AR 1916*, 9–10.
135. LCC LCC/MIN/00581 Meeting, 30 May 1916, 604–5 LMA.
136. *BoC AR 1916*, 9–10.
137. Kathleen Jones, *Asylums and After* (London: Athlone Press, 1993), 124.
138. Anon. "Montagu Lomax MRCS Eng, LRCP Edin," *Lancet* 25 March 1933, 668.
139. Anon. "Asylum accommodation," *JMS* 62 (1916): 827–28.
140. Colney Hatch LCC/MIN/01007 Meeting, 11 January 1918, 5–6 LMA.
141. LCC LCC/MIN/00579 Meeting, 29 September 1914, 646 LMA.
142. Colney Hatch LCC/MIN/01007 Meeting, 11 January 1918, 4 LMA; LCC/MIN/01005 Meeting, 2 June 1916, 173; LCC LCC/MIN/00584 Meeting, 8 October 1918, 2–4 LMA; Hanwell LCC/MIN/01094 Meeting, 15 March 1915, 284–85 LMA.
143. LCC LCC/MIN/00581 Meeting, 26 October 1915, 56 LMA.
144. Claybury LCC/MIN/00948 Meeting, 5 July 1917, 134–35 LMA.
145. MPA to BoC, untitled letter, 17 May 1916, *JMS* 62 (1916): 636–37.
146. BoC W/FM, 21 March 1917, 97 MH 50/45 TNA.
147. LCC LCC/MIN/00582 Meeting, 27 March 1917, 568–69; 3 April 1917, 589 LMA.
148. LCC LCC/MIN/00583 Meeting, 29 January 1918, 319 LMA.
149. BoC, circular to superintendents, 23 December 1918, MH 51/239 TNA.
150. LCC LCC/MIN/00584 Meeting, 1 April 1919, 432 LMA.
151. Richard van Emden and Steve Humphries, *All Quiet on the Home Front: An Oral History of Life in Britain During the First World War* (London: Headline, 2003), 297.
152. Pat Thane, *Divided Kingdom: A History of Britain, 1900 to the Present* (Cambridge: Cambridge University Press, 2018), 56–57; JM Winter, "Military Fitness and Civilian Health in Britain During the First World War," *Journal of Contemporary History* 15 (1980): 211–44, 211.
153. Van Emden and Humphries, *All Quiet*, 300.
154. Hanwell LCC/MIN/01097 Meeting, 17 December 1917, 251 LMA.
155. LCC LCC/MIN/00584 Meeting, 1 April 1919, 432 LMA.
156. Colney Hatch LCC/MIN/01006 Meeting, 30 November 1917, 301; Claybury LCC/MIN/00946 Meeting, 23 December 1915, 318 LMA.
157. Claybury LCC/MIN/00948 Meeting, 19 July 1917, 176–77 LMA.
158. British Army WW1 Pension Records 1914–1920, https://www.ancestry.co.uk/search/collections/britisharmy/; UK, Silver War Badge Records 1914–1920, https://www.ancestry.co.uk/search/collections/silverwarbadgemedals/.
159. Hanwell LCC/MIN/01097 Meetings: 22 October 1917, 19; 17 December 1917, 252–54 LMA.

160. Robert Armstrong-Jones, "The Eighth Annual Report of the Board of Control for the Year 1921," *Eugenics Review* 15 (1923): 426–32, 432.
161. HB, "Sir Marriott Cooke KBE MB," *BMJ* 31 October 1931, 829–30.
162. Nolan, *History*, 79.
163. Trades Union Congress, *A Short History of British Trade Unionism: A TUC Study Pamphlet* (London: Trades Union Congress, 1947), 21.
164. Adams, "From Association to Union": 19–20.
165. *Fifth Annual Report of the Board of Control, for the Year 1918* (London: HMSO, 1919), 4.
166. Goffman, *Asylums*, 18.
167. Trades Union Congress, *A Short History*, 21.

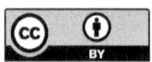

CHAPTER 5

Food, Farm and Fuel: An Inequitable Supply Chain

Introduction

Within days of war breaking out the country faced a torrent of problems including "extraordinary chaos in the Food Market". At Napsbury Asylum, the grain and flour supplier backed out of his contract because imports failed to arrive, and Nestlé stopped deliveries because the government required its stocks. The standard of bread fell because much yeast was imported and consequently unobtainable. Fish was suddenly unavailable because "as the Steamers return they are being laid up pending events."[1] Foods such as meat, and other items considered healthy by early twentieth century nutritional scientists, were prioritised for the soldiers.[2] The large contracts for food required by the asylums became particularly vulnerable. There were many challenges in addition to obtaining supplies, including coping with a capped budget, concerns about cooking to avoid exhausting limited fuel supplies, and resident staff voicing discontent about the food provided for them. Limited understanding of nutrition, and patterns of inequitable food distribution within the asylums according to rank rather than health need, also contributed to an unsatisfactory diet for patients.

In order to contextualise and explain the situation in the asylums, this chapter begins by outlining the national position with regard to food, then, in the context of nutritional understanding, explores asylum supply and demand issues, patients' communal meals, and food distribution.

© The Author(s) 2021   147
C. Hilton, *Civilian Lunatic Asylums During the First World War*,
Mental Health in Historical Perspective,
https://doi.org/10.1007/978-3-030-54871-1_5

Some of the challenges faced by asylum farms, and the use of fuel, another precious commodity, are also discussed.

THE NATIONAL FOOD CONTEXT

Until the war, Britain imported about 60 per cent of its food. As in the lyrics of *Rule, Britannia!*, "Britannia rule the waves",[3] it could not conceive of any way in which its sea routes could be disrupted, neither had it envisaged the possibility of a prolonged conflict nor interruption of trade by submarines.[4] The country produced one fifth of its wheat, two fifths of its butter and cheese, three-fifths of its meat and bacon, and none of its sugar. Only in respect of fish, milk and potatoes was it self-sufficient.

A few days after war was declared, the government passed the Defence of the Realm Act (DORA) which gave it authority to control many aspects of civilian life, including food supplies. This system of national government-led welfare was new: earlier, providing and controlling resources would have been in the hands of voluntary bodies.[5] It was a change with potential to influence future welfare policy. At the same time, Walter Runciman was appointed president of the Board of Trade. Consistent with Runciman's free-trade principles and the Liberal government's general philosophy, his lack of intervention inhibited the development of a coherent food policy.[6] Nevertheless, behind the scenes, the government amassed emergency supplies of essential food stuffs such as wheat,[7] and took control of the sugar supply, two-thirds of which was usually imported from Austria-Hungary.[8] Inclement weather and the reduced availability of ammonia, which was used to produce both fertilisers and explosives, affected home-grown crops.[9] Despite threats to the food supply, in the view of William Beveridge (later, draftsman of the welfare state), until late 1916 "there was no general food problem in Britain".[10]

Administrative errors caused local shortages, such as sugar supplies to retailers being based on pre-war sales patterns, due to failing to take into account large scale civilian population movement for munitions and other work.[11] War inflation, higher costs of freight, and panic buying, all contributed to higher food prices and caused public discontent, but according to an analysis by Gerd Hardach, most food stuffs remained within reach of poorer people.[12] An independent committee, appointed by the government, which investigated wartime life for working class people found that dietary energy levels for community dwellers were

generally maintained, although intakes of some key nutrients deteriorated.[13] For some households, with a father in the forces and a mother
with young children relying on the meagre "separation allowance", life
was a struggle.[14] Some oral histories recalled experiences of persistent
hunger among working class children, and families who attributed deaths
of younger siblings to malnutrition.[15] Two years into the war, food prices
had almost doubled.[16] For many in the community, high rates of employment and some increase in salary partly compensated for the steep price
rises.[17] An asylum, of course, was an employer, so was responsible for
paying the "war bonus" increases to its non-resident staff to cover their
higher daily living costs. Within a framework of a budget capped by the
Lunacy Act 1890 which stipulated a maximum outlay of 14s (shillings,
70p) per patient per week to cover all asylum running expenses, including
staff salaries,[18] the outcome was less money to spend on food for patients
and staff who were resident in the asylum.

The government aimed to avoid compulsory rationing and invited
the public to participate in voluntary dietary restrictions, much as it
initially encouraged voluntary military recruitment rather than introduce conscription.[19] However, from 1916, German "U-boat" submarines
specifically targeted merchant ships with great loss of life and cargo, and
food supplies were again in crisis. The government feared that if families
sent letters to soldiers describing their daily problems, or if soldiers experienced the difficulties when home on leave, this would undermine military
morale.[20] To deal with this, to "maintain war production and prevent
unrest at home" the government established a Ministry of Food.[21] It was
headed by a "Food Controller", rather than a Minister, and was empow-
ered to regulate supply and consumption and to take steps to encourage
food production.[22] Beveridge was appointed Permanent Secretary to the
Ministry.[23]

The first Food Controller, Lord Devonport, a grocery stores magnate,
continued to promote voluntary dietary adaptations, aiming to reduce the
consumption of foods in short supply and to avoid waste when cooking.
Some commentators have proposed that his *laissez faire* approach was
founded on a financial conflict of interest.[24] The Ministry of Food
proposed dietary guidelines in February 1917 (Table 5.1) which applied
to domestic environments where each household member was assumed
to have different nutritional requirements: food needs of a labourer and
young child in the same household would probably balance out so that
neither went hungry. Some households could supplement diets with

Table 5.1   Weekly food allowances under various rationing schemes

Recommended intake, general population, Feb. 1917	Compulsory rationing, general population, Nov. 1917	LCC asylum patients, Nov. 1917	Compulsory rationing, general population, early 1918
Sugar 12 oz	Sugar 8 oz Fats 10 oz	Sugar 7¼ oz Fats 7¼ oz	Sugar (adult or child) 8 oz Fats (adult or child) 8 oz
Bread 4 lb	Bread (age/gender/occupation) 3½ lb ("sedentary/unoccupied woman")–8 lb	Bread (average) 4¾ lb	Bread (age/gender/occupation) 3–7 lb
Meat 2½ lb	Meat 2 lb	Meat 1¾ lb	Meat 2 lb Use carefully: Cheese, milk, oatmeal, rice, tea, jam Unrestricted: Potatoes, fruit, vegetables, eggs, fish

Sources LCC LCC/MIN/00582 Meeting, 27 February 1917, 434 LMA; LCC LCC/MIN/00583, 27 November 1917, 175–76 LMA; BBC, "World War One: What Shops Were on the High Street? Rationing," http://www.bbc.co.uk/schools/0/ww1/25235371

home-grown produce, and a cook "in an ordinary household" could make many "small economies". Regarding institutions, those which solely housed adults lost the benefits of juggling supplies on the basis of individual nutritional requirements across the lifespan, and a handful of cooks feeding 2000 resident patients and staff seven days a week were unlikely to be able to replicate economies made in a household kitchen.

The second Food Controller, Lord Rhondda, an industrialist and politician, introduced compulsory rationing at the end of 1917, beginning with butter, margarine and sugar (Table 5.1).[25] Food queues in London, which had reached one and a half million people a week, diminished with compulsory rationing.[26] Rationing was intended to provide a state determined allocation of food to all, with flexibility for age, health, religious and other needs.[27] The entire country, including King George and Queen Mary had ration books, with their allowances calculated on the same ration scale as their subjects.[28] Everyone had their rations derived from a scale roughly tailored to their needs, but this would only be achieved if those rations were distributed equitably. In asylums, the hierarchical culture, difficulties in economising in ways which might be possible in a household setting, together with escalating food prices and other higher expenses within a limited budget, contributed to a precarious food situation.

ASYLUM DIETS: SUPPLY AND DEMAND

The asylums contended with unpredictable food supplies pre-war,[29] in contrast to the relatively stable situation for the rest of the country. They procured enormous quantities, had little access to refrigeration, and kept only minimal stocks. Suppliers knew this, and its implications, that asylums had to accept deliveries even if substandard.[30] Food might be "stale and unfit for consumption" at the time of delivery,[31] and even when fit, it was often best cooked the same day to prevent deterioration, serving it the following day.[32] Some asylums spent as little as 4s (20p) per patient per week on food, a sum independent of the amount of food provided by the asylum farm.[33]

Benjamin Seebohm Rowntree's study of poverty in *fin de siècle* York provides useful dietary comparators for the asylums in 1914. These comparisons are possible because there was almost no inflation or change in eating habits during this period. Rowntree found weekly food expenditure to be approximately 3s6d (18½p) per adult male in households of the lowest wage earners and 3s9½d (19p) in the workhouse. He incorporated into his analysis the most up-to-date estimates of the nutritional value of these people's diets. Analyses were generally limited to calorie and protein content, standardised to the bodily needs of a person at rest in a warm room.[34] Not only was the situation of being at rest in a warm room likely to be unusual for the poorest of the working classes in York, but even when based on these calculations, their diet was deficient in calories and protein by around 25 per cent.[35] Similar deficiencies were likely for patients living in asylums with poor quality clothes and inadequate heating and with high levels of bodily energy usage due to restlessness, co-existing physical illness, much manual work and having long distances to walk such as to the lavatories and dining hall.

In contrast to Rowntree's analysis, Diane Carpenter, in her study of two Hampshire asylums pre-war, concluded that asylum food was better than in workhouses and often better balanced than that available to most poor people.[36] Her conclusions suggest variation between asylums, but for those functioning at Rowntree's level, diet would have been insufficient to promote health and wellbeing, or to help the recovery of patients who required more calories due to their mental and physical disorders. Keeping to the Lunacy Act's budget of 14s per week per patient, was a constant challenge for the asylums. Barely feasible in the low inflation period pre-1914, the London County Council (LCC) found it unachievable during the war.[37] The financial target contributed to a culture of minimising expenditure, accompanied by the temptation to divert savings made by cutting food costs to benefit other, more outwardly visible, asylum needs. The 14s compared unrealistically with the average weekly general hospital cost of 28s per patient, or 45s in one Red Cross Hospital, even allowing for the different disorders being treated.[38] With wartime inflation, expenditure on asylum food did not increase: there were other priorities, including paying the staff to keep the asylums functioning. Psychiatrist William Stoddart cautioned in 1916: "It is false economy on the part of the authorities of many county asylums to keep down the maintenance rate by economising food."[39] His message fell on deaf ears.

In contrast to the situation for the general public, wartime food rationing began early for people in the asylums. We hear little from patients about the food, although one patient later alleged: "My wife brought in food. Else I should have been starved",[40] and another volunteered for kitchen work, and "got better food because I really stole it".[41] We hear more from the resident staff who were also subject to early rationing. With compulsory deductions from their already low wages for board and lodging, they had little option but to eat the food provided. They resented the dietary restrictions and food monotony which those outside did not have to endure.[42] At Hanwell, one nurse left, alleging that she was being starved. Others complained about rancid margarine, poor quality bacon, only one potato at dinner, small meat allowances and bread inferior to what was on sale outside.[43] The LCC attempted to improve staff food,[44] occasional seeking expert external advice to try to make it more palatable.[45] It justified allocating more and better quality food to staff to keep them well enough to care for the patients, to alleviate employee discontent, and to prevent them taking the patients' food.[46] However, since food supplies within the asylum were pooled,[47] a strategy of providing more for staff, automatically diminished quantities available for patients. One asylum management "visiting" committee (VC), pleased with its ingenuity in issuing bread directly to wards, reported that it reduced expenditure and waste and "every patient or member of the staff has what he requires". Other evidence throws this open to dispute, because only staff held keys to the store cupboards, and when they were hungry, they took the patients' bread.[48] Visiting committee members lived in the un-rationed community outside the asylum, and sometimes appeared to lack a detailed appreciation of asylum life.[49]

The asylum economy and the external supply chain were major considerations throughout the war for the VCs and the national asylums' Board of Control ("the Board"). Regarding the main dietary staple of bread, shortage of wheat flour necessitated substitutions of un-rationed ingredients such as barley, oatmeal, rice, sago, tapioca, maize or potatoes.[50] Twenty pounds (20 lb, 9 kg) of potatoes could be mixed with 1 sack (280 lb, 127 kg) of flour.[51] Kitchen staff disliked the additional labour it required without a potato mashing machine.[52] Bread made with potatoes also tasted different and was unpopular with consumers.[53] Bran or wheatgerm could be added, a financially sound alternative,[54] but not always acceptable in a culinary culture which considered white bread best and wholemeal inferior.[55] The Board welcomed the news of a glut of cheap pickled and smoked herring on the market. It distributed to the asylums the Ministry of Food's recipe guide: herrings could be boiled, steamed, fried, grilled, baked, poached, stuffed, soused or curried, served with lemon sauce, in a pie or salad, or potted in vinegar.[56] The recipes were generally for household quantities, and whether they would translate effectively into mass-catering was uncertain.

Asylum Diets and Nutritional Understanding

The VCs' track record of prioritising lowest possible expenditure, plus little grasp of emerging nutritional science,[57] was a potentially disastrous combination. Although the Board made recommendations in line with nutritional knowledge, for example suggesting high protein substitutes such as cheese, beans, lentils or peas when meat was in short supply, VCs, with one eye on the books, proposed puddings, fruit pies and rice, cheaper but hardly equivalent nutritionally.[58] Tenna Jensen's study of nutritional science and early twentieth-century institutional diets (in Denmark) indicated that, in spite of societal awareness of nutrition, incorporating that knowledge into institutional diets was far from universal. Instead, institutional diets focussed more on the need for food to be filling.[59] Knowledge could have a time lag of several years before filtering through to institutional implementation, with the result that war time asylum diets tended to follow obsolete guidelines.

Regarding vitamins, discovered around 1912, their mode of action was still "immature views and guesses"[60] and their presence in food unquantifiable,[61] but the medical profession acknowledged their "astonishing properties" which could "profoundly affect" physical and mental health.[62] Regarding vitamin C just before the war, patients at Colney Hatch received "½lb fruit weekly per head in the summer" (0.25 kg).[63] When combined with plenty of potatoes and other root vegetables, vitamin C intake was probably adequate: none of the medical records examined in the course of researching this book referred to scurvy. Although more fruit may not have been considered essential to the diet, sugar, because of its calorie content was regarded as a vital nutrient. Prewar, the nine LCC lunatic asylums consumed 10 tons of sugar between them each week, about 1 lb (0.5 kg) per person.[64] It was standard asylum practice to sweeten hot drinks. Typically, a gallon size pot contained 1 oz (28 g) tea, 4 oz sugar and 12 oz milk, with similar proportions for a gallon of coffee or cocoa.[65] In 1916, the LCC asked medical superintendents to suggest "dietary substitutes...to take the place of necessary food for patients caused by the great reduction of sugar allowance".[66] It also asked the Royal Commission on the Sugar Supply for more sugar for asylums "having regard to the fact that the issues of sugar at the asylums have already been reduced to the lowest limit which is believed to be compatible with good health". Nevertheless, the LCC oversaw inequitable distribution of sugar: ½ lb per patient and 1 lb per resident member of staff per week in 1916,[67] pointing to the nutrition of staff being prioritised over that of patients.

Nutritional understanding by VCs also contributed to how they interpreted government dietary recommendations which were often formulated in terms of maximum amounts which were not to be exceeded.[68] The general understanding was that if individuals did not need the maximum, it was fine if they ate less of their own volition.[69] Maximum quantities, however, in the asylums, were interpreted on behalf of the patients who had little individual choice or agency. Claybury's VC wanted to provide patients with "less than the maximum scale" of bread, cake, potatoes, meat, pudding, fish, coffee, tea, sugar, margarine, flour, dripping, jam and cheese.[70] Two weeks later, at the VC's next meeting, medical superintendent Robert Armstrong-Jones argued against their proposal: "The standards in use are the result of many years of thought and experience and a lowering of standard does not necessarily lead to a saving", echoing Stoddart's message.[71] If any reductions were made, Armstrong-Jones continued, they should be on the basis of careful study of the entire food contract, not just chosen arbitrarily or to make financial savings.[72] Armstrong-Jones was aware of his VC's tendency to make decisions based on finance rather than on patients' wellbeing. Claybury did not introduce this across-the-board food reduction, but less dramatic dietary reductions followed. By contrast, interventions to increase patients' food intake were miniscule and half-hearted: when a medical officer at Hanwell suggested that each patient should receive an extra pound of potatoes a week, the VC reduced it to half-a-pound.[73] Asylums neglected to provide food according to the patient's needs. The simple and recommended act of weighing asylum patients regularly to detect malnutrition or disease was implemented inconsistently, suggesting a lack of concern or interest.[74] Patient Mary Riggall reported in her memoir of asylum life that her weight declined from 9 to 6 stones (57–38 kg) during her 18-month admission,[75] supporting the notion that balancing diet with energy expenditure, whether due to illness or occupation, was ignored.

The emphasis on balancing-the-books rather than patients' wellbeing fitted with the practice of allocating additional food to "working" patients, that is, to those whose work the asylum considered economically useful.[76] In contrast, a patient undertaking physical activities for their therapeutic benefit alone did not receive extra, regardless of energy expenditure. This valued a patients' economic contribution above stated ideals of considering activities as intrinsically therapeutic and important to wellbeing and self-esteem, regardless of whether they benefited the institution financially. When one considers the meagre lunch provided to female patients employed on Hanwell's farm—3 oz (90 g) bread with either ½ oz cheese or ½ oz treacle depending on availability—probably under 300 calories,[77] it is hard to identify what might have been considered "additional".

In 1917, the medical superintendents discussed weight loss and high asylum death rates side by side and drew the Board's attention to the effects of food restrictions.[78] At Hanwell acting medical superintendent Alfred Daniel informed the VC that the rising death rate was "partly due to shortage of food", noting the introduction of dry bread for supper instead of bread and dripping,[79] and that "pudding" had only one-fifth the calories of the same item produced earlier in the war. Food preparation advice to asylums included to boil food rather than roasting or frying it, to conform with government demands to economise on gas consumption,[80] but this reduced both calorie and nutritional content. In July 1918, with rising death rates at Hanwell—26 people in one month—Daniel sought advice from the local authority medical officer of health.[81] The same month, the Board reiterated that all patients should be weighed every 3 months "If not already done as a matter of routine" to monitor dietary adequacy, and that patients and resident staff should be allocated food to provide 2600 calories a day.[82] However, Hanwell did not even provide that amount to its shell-shocked patients, those deemed worthy of the best care. They received 2200 calories daily; the VC minutes did not state what was provided for the civilian patients. Diets at Hanwell for the shell shocked patients compared unfavourably to the 3350 calories daily provided at the Maudsley Military Hospital, dedicated entirely to soldier's mental health.[83] Rations in asylums were also inequitable when compared to those provided in the war hospitals which were created by vacating asylums. When Napsbury became a war hospital, about eighty male asylum patients and some asylum staff remained on site to tend the farm and gardens. The Board's circulated guidance on maximum dietary allowances only applied to these patients and staff. It was "not intended to apply to Military patients or any of the staff" looking after them.[84] Many of the soldier-patients recovering from injuries would have needed more calories than physically healthy individuals, but farm work was no less strenuous and demanding of an adequate diet than nursing the soldier-patients. The Board's action was nonsensical based on recognised nutritional criteria. Apart from desiring to minimise financial expenditure, or wanting to comply with Whitehall's directives, it is hard to see the rationale or humanity of making this distinction.

When the distinguished psychiatrist and researcher Frederick Mott, probably the most knowledgeable authority about the health of asylum patients in England, communicated his concerns about food restrictions directly to the Board, it minuted its intention to enquire from asylums to what extent there were grounds for his anxiety.[85] No answers appear in subsequent minutes. The asylum leadership sometimes tried to avoid discussing awkward issues, including about diet, and evaded questions when asked directly. The Cobb Inquiry about asylum standards demonstrated this: when the panel asked the chairman of one VC: "You must have been badly off during the war for potatoes?" he replied: "We gave them an excellent quality of margarine".[86] It was hardly an adequate response.

The Board's preoccupation with doing as the Ministry of Food asked and maintaining its reputation as a compliant authority, may have contributed to its lack of action to ensure adequate food for patients. Throughout the war, its rigid advice to asylums contrasted with the government's strategy of encouraging voluntary initiative before compulsion. The Board emphasised compliance with dietary restrictions, even when uncertain whether the rules were applicable to institutions entirely for adults.[87] In contrast to the Board's inactivity, the prison authorities interpreted the Ministry's recommendations less stringently. They negotiated with the Ministry, so that in their institutions with all adult prisoners, bread was provided at the standard rate plus 2 lb (1 kg), giving each person an extra 2000 calories a week. Although directly comparing asylum and prison dietary regimes is complex, because different categories of prisoner received different diets, overall, calorie intake of prisoners exceeded that of patients in asylums.[88] Notably, prisoners did not suffer the high rate of infectious diseases, such as tuberculosis, compared to asylum patients. In addition, unlike most prisoners who had a release date, asylum patients could be detained indefinitely, so for many of them, poor nutrition could be of prolonged and indeterminate duration. The Board's minutes available at the National Archives provide no evidence that it knew about, asked about, or acted on, the prison diet experience.

COMMUNAL EATING FOR PATIENTS AND STAFF

"The healthfulness of a variety of food is allowed by the best authorities; but beyond its healthfulness, its desirability is beyond doubt" wrote Charles Mercier in his book on asylum management.[89] Not only nutrition, but also palatability and presentation of food were important in Mercier's eyes. For patients, the food which arrived on their plates could be unappetising. Mott regarded oatmeal porridge with treacle four days a week for tea at Hanwell as particularly uninviting.[90] Too often food was poor quality and could be "abominably cooked".[91]

On the first day of a Board inspection at one asylum in November 1914, the stew was unpopular, but the following day there was "roast beef and mutton with bread and two vegetables, the enjoyment of which was obvious".[92] Two meats in one meal was rare on asylum menus. It is likely that, having made an unfavourable initial impression, the asylum then laid on a culinary treat. Food often improved on Board inspection days or when the VC made its rounds. Staff at Claybury described "Committee-day soup", which was far better than the usual "flour with the water", and vegetables which were "stalks, dead leaves and slugs" and "When one man picks up a caterpillar with his fork the others are done."[93] In one asylum, the main meal of the day consisted of rhubarb pudding with bread and cheese: the Board reported that the "change from a meat diet on one day in the week is looked upon with favour by the patients".[94] This may have been the Board's genuine understanding, but at a time when meat or fish was an expected constituent of a main meal, patients may have expressed their appreciation as they felt obliged to do so. Unlike when the inspectors received criticism from patients, they warmly accepted their praise, without attributing it to mental disorder. If the inspectors observed patients and staff enjoying a good meal they were unlikely to take food-related complaints seriously. They appeared unaware that a display might be created for their benefit.

Inspectors also evaluated routines of communal eating. Meals were often rushed: "Toothless old men had sometimes to wrestle with chunks of fat or gristle; they swallowed their food somehow or other, but had no time to masticate it properly".[95] Stoddart criticised nurses who rushed patients with their food due to their own working demands. He used military metaphor: "just as the velocity of a fleet is that of its slowest vessel, the duration of a meal must be that of the slowest eater."[96] Some patients who ate with great haste were labelled as greedy, but some were probably extremely hungry or worried that other patients would snatch their food.[97] So-called greediness also occurred in some brain diseases, such as general paralysis of the insane (GPI, syphilis), which could predispose patients to disinhibited table manners and to bolt their food. GPI could also impair swallowing which could result in choking.[98] A soft diet eaten with a teaspoon could reduce that risk, but if the need was not recognised, a patient could choke to death. That happened to Louis L, a prisoner of war at Colney Hatch, a horrible ending of life for the patient, and very disturbing to those around.[99]

The Board noted other aspects of mealtimes, which they thought could help make them as pleasant as possible. It was keen on communal recitation or singing of grace when patients were all seated, as a prelude to an orderly meal.[100] Inspectors advised one asylum that chipped and broken mugs should be replaced "at once", but did not state whether this was for safety, hygiene, or aesthetics.[101] They praised another where "crockery plates and glass tumblers are gradually being substituted for the enamelled iron plates and mugs".[102] Some patients must have been considered sufficiently trustworthy for the change, but it is unclear for how long others continued to use the enamelled implements, or whether inspection routines influenced the changeover. Every meal, whether on a ward, in the dining hall, or in the staff mess room, concluded with the routine of counting in the cutlery, for fear it could be used to injure self or others.[103]

Food Distribution in the Asylums

The bureaucratic web embedded in the asylum's hierarchical culture, determined food distribution, and the quality and quantity of food served. It often failed to produce an equitable share for all. The medical officers, matron and assistant matrons usually received the best, and patients the worst.[104] Inequalities were enshrined in official guidance, such as the LCC's instruction: "Instead of Officers' Fish at 7d. and patients' at 2½d., take a contract for mixed fish and pick out the best for the officers",[105] or their recommended Christmas spending of 6d for each patient and 2s3d for each resident member of staff.[106] Dietary plans for patients and lower tiers of staff included serving them preserved beef, when the same asylums aimed to provide senior staff with "joints of English killed mutton".[107] When charge nurses, from the middle ranks of Claybury's work force, complained that the kitchen staff reserved the best flour for bread for the most senior staff, the VC ended the practice with haste.[108] Neither the reason for the VC's rapid response nor the motivation behind the kitchen staff action were recorded, although obsequiousness to seniors was replayed throughout the asylum system in multiple ways. Montagu Lomax recalled that during the war at Prestwich Asylum, cream for medical officers was provided by skimming the patients' milk.[109] Also, according to Lomax (with his italics), the following contributed to impairing patients' vitality[110]:

> unjust and unequal distribution of the *sufficient and available food*, the combination of official lavishness and waste, the incompetent management, the careless and unscientific cooking,…the neglect of opportunities for increasing the supply of asylum-grown vegetables—in a word, all the evils of the administrative system.[111]

As well as externally sourced food, produce home-grown on the asylum farm was also distributed unevenly. At Claybury, when 400 lb of strawberries were harvested just over half was shared between the 2000 patients, and the rest between 200 staff.[112] When VC minutes mentioned that their farm provided staff with fruit for desert or lettuce with their tea, they failed to indicate any similar provision for patients.[113] In view of asylums' lack of attention to vitamins in food, distribution was probably based on a desire to add interest to the diet. There could be little justification, however, for the inequity demonstrated at Colney Hatch, where, in stark contrast to the low allowance of fresh fruit for patients, the most senior asylum personnel were permitted to purchase up to 7 lbs of fruit a week and unlimited quantities of milk and vegetables.[114] There were other inequitable purchases: in spring 1915, Armstrong-Jones purchased goods to the value of £25 from Claybury's stores, three times that of the next highest spender in the same period. The VC scrutinised the list of staff spending without further comment.[115] Armstrong-Jones might have had a legitimate reason for doing this, or he might have exploited his privilege of rank. Backdoor shopping by higher social classes occurred in the community where it caused fury among those less privileged.[116] When it occurred in the asylums, the patients would have suffered most as a result. Even if patients knew about it, if they complained, there is little evidence that their voices were heard.

Asylum Farms

Asylum farms were integral to the institutions. They produced milk, eggs, fruit and vegetables to supplement asylum diets, provided employment for many patients and generated income from sales to staff, to other asylums and on the open market.[117] Shortly before the war, some asylums produced large quantities of food. In one fortnight in 1913, Colney Hatch farm produced 2300 eggs and farrowed 28 pigs, and slaughtered 20 pigs and 2 cows for use in the asylum. Later that year it harvested 22,000 lb onions, most of which were used in asylum food.[118] Crop success stories are harder to find during the war. In autumn 1914, Hanwell's farm had poor vegetable and root crops due to drought. The following month blight destroyed all the Brussels sprouts. In discussion with the farm bailiff, in early 1915 the VC approved the proposal to grow wheat under the special circumstance of the war. This was controversial in an urban area where house sparrows were known to "exact a very heavy

toll" on grain crops. Inexplicably, it was "left to the medical superintendent to decide as to the acreage to be sown".[119] Whether he had the
agricultural expertise to take this decision, or if it was delegated to him
on the basis of his overall leadership of the asylum, was not stated.

The weather over successive war years was deleterious to farming. At
Hanwell, drought affected the farm early in 1915, upsetting sewing and
transplanting.[120] The protracted and harsh winter of 1915–1916 particularly affected early crops and poultry, with only 3000 eggs laid compared
to 5000 in the same period the previous year.[121] Heavy rain and hail
after sowing late wheat in 1917 battered down the soil which became
"so hard that the young shoots could not break through".[122] In 1918,
incessant rain followed the worst drought for 12 years.[123] Some senior
farm staff, such as the bailiff, ploughman and head cowman, were exempt
from military service,[124] but many others enlisted or moved into munitions work. Adverse weather conditions, reduced availability of synthetic
fertilisers, bureaucratic asylum management, and less experienced farm
staff,[125] probably all contributed to lower yield.

Land usually used for recreation in asylums (Fig. 5.1) was ploughed

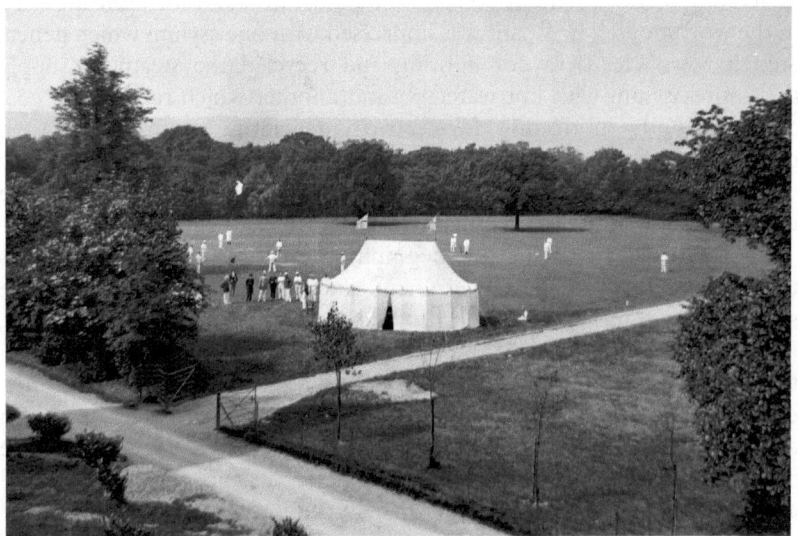

Fig. 5.1 Cricket pitch at Claybury, before 1917 (Armstrong-Jones collection,
Royal College of Psychiatrists' Archives)

and cultivated,[126] as elsewhere, such as in the nine LCC parks which together produced 3½ tons of tomatoes in 1917 and the vegetable patches which replaced flowerbeds at Buckingham Palace.[127] Occasionally farms undertook new projects, such as bee keeping at Colney Hatch. Shortages of materials and staff affected the farms. Hanwell's VC declined the chance to purchase a motorised tractor, which could have compensated for fewer farm staff, sped-up farm work and replaced the fittest horses which had been enlisted alongside the men.[128] The decision not to purchase the tractor may have been one of finance: in the farm bailiff's view, the asylum had the philosophy of doing everything atleast expense, which probably adversely affected "the returns from the stock and the present condition of all the herds".[129] Relentless economising and understaffing may also have been associated with lack of attention to the environment, probably linked to the death of one cow, found to have nails, wire, tin, stones and ashes in her stomach at post mortem.[130]

FUEL

Before the war, in most asylums, coal provided heating and was used to generate gas and electricity for domestic amenities and for light industry in the workshops. The Board was impressed with one asylum which generated its own electricity for lighting and recycled the steam to supply the entire asylum with hot water,[131] and another which reduced its coal consumption by lubricating the electricity-generating steam-engines with graphite rather than oil, which allowed vast quantities of water, previously wasted due to oil contamination, to be re-used in the boilers.[132] Praise for these innovations was aligned with achieving budgetary targets.[133]

Coal shortages started at the beginning of the war, "with the Railways under the control of the Government, and the first necessity being the safety of the Nation",[134] leading to additional reasons for fuel economy, both for private households and public institutions.[135] One way in which the authorities tried to prevent "fuel fraud" and inequity, was to allow each household to register with only one coal merchant.[136] However, in asylums, as with food, the coal was pooled which facilitated inequitable distribution. One medical superintendent, for example, received a coal allowance for his "motor garage".[137] By contrast, the VC at Hanwell reprimanded a nurse for unnecessary use of gas when she was caught frying onions late at night over the gas in her bedroom. She justified her cooking as not wasting gas, because after dark she needed a light anyway and the gas served both purposes simultaneously. The same asylum used gas to make tea for working women patients when they returned to the ward in the afternoon. The VC wanted to discontinue this practice, but the medical superintendent refused to allow them to do so, since "it would do away with perhaps the last pleasure and privilege" left to those patients, which could only be "justified in case of grave necessity".[138]

Fuel supplies became dangerously depleted, but not quite "grave". Six months into the war, in mid-winter, the LCC asylums at Banstead and Long Grove had only 4 days' coal in stock. Claybury had sufficient for one week, and the others had marginally more. Military demands for coal, plus reduced labour and flooding in the mines, hindered collieries from filling the LCC's coal order. Lack of equipment to unload coal from boats on the Thames, plus "congestion on the railways" delayed deliveries.[139] Hanwell had a slight advantage over the other asylums: its coal was delivered by barge as it had its own dock on the Grand Union Canal which ran along its southern perimeter. To monitor coal deliveries, each asylum had a weighbridge. Sometimes asylums received under-deliveries, and very occasionally, slight excess.[140] The variability might have been due to deliberate under-supply or genuine error, due to faulty weighbridges at collieries or trucks being filled with wet coal which then dried.[141] Large deficits in the region of 2 tons were harder to explain and asylums sought answers or refunds from their suppliers.[142] With rising fuel prices, careful tendering was needed for contracts on huge purchases for institutions, such as for an order of over 6000 tons of "house coal" to provide ward heating for six months in the LCC asylums.[143]

Late in 1915, the LCC advised its asylums that infirmary wards could be heated at night, but other wards should be heated only if temperatures fell below freezing,[144] hardly likely to promote a good night's sleep for patients or provide a healthy work environment for night staff. When the Board inspected Claybury in 1916, and patients complained about intense cold, it advised more heating,[145] but conflicting advice from higher authorities hardly helped VCs steer a safe course. The Household Coal Distribution Order 1917 prompted the LCC to state that:

> consumption of coal and coke at the London County Asylums has always been closely studied, and that the quantities consumed have been brought to what is believed to be the lowest level which is compatible with the efficiency of the administration of the asylums and the health of the inmates.[146]

It is unclear who, if anyone, defined "compatible…with health" or what it meant in practice. Using the outdated derogatory term "inmates", rather than the more respectful "patients" which was usually found in official asylum documents at this time, suggested negativity towards those in their care, which may have reflected on decisions regarding distribution of precious resources.

In autumn 1918, because of the cold, Claybury's VC predicted increasing death rates, which were already well above those in the community and in most other asylums. The LCC could envisage no way to prevent them.[147] By closing some wards for the winter to help economise on fuel,[148] other wards became unhealthily overcrowded, creating environments ripe for spreading infectious diseases. The authorities were under pressure to conform to fuel economy targets, and compared to the other LCC asylums, Claybury used more than its expected share, attributed to its damp location on London clay soil.[149] However, both the LCC and Claybury's VC were complacent about the risks of their austerity measures. As with food, the authorities tended to accept their allocations of fuel without demanding more, even when human tragedy was predicted.

CONCLUSIONS

John Walton wrote in his book on fish and chips that, in 1910, the eminent Scottish psychiatrist Sir James Crichton Brown praised the warming, sustaining and nourishing benefits of fish and chips, which might also be "a useful auxiliary in the fight against tuberculosis".[150] Walton commented that "Perceptions of living standards were as important as actual nutritional levels", and that the warmth, tastiness and timesaving qualities of fish and chips for the general population was an argument for eating it during the war.[151] Fish and chips would have had value against tuberculosis in the general sense of being nutritious, high in calories and protein, but no asylum menus have come to light which included it, despite the country being self-sufficient for fish and potatoes.

Aiming to feed the patients and resident staff and keep them warm was an enormous juggling act with moving goal posts to conform to restrictions and to ensure best use of erratic supplies with lowest expenditure. The asylum leadership obeyed directives, enforced national guidelines, and accepted negative outcomes—including a high death rate—as inevitable. Strictly obeying orders given by superiors effectively displaced responsibility and accountability for adverse consequences from any one level of staff or leadership onto someone higher in the chain. The authoritarian management system may have inhibited lateral thinking, innovation and communication to find solutions, such as by consulting or working collaboratively with the prison service to overcome shared challenges. The rigidity of management was compatible with Erving Goffman's administrative structure of a "total institution",[152] but it contrasted with government tactics at the time, demonstrated in its initial attempts to involve the public in the war effort voluntarily rather than through compulsion.

Whether due to lack of scientific and nutritional knowledge, or deliberately disregarding it, the leadership demonstrated little awareness of potential interactions between diet, cold and illness. Some doctors opposed the decisions of VCs, or at least warned of the consequences, regarding reducing patients' food intake. Occasionally the doctors requested more food for patients, but most remedial action concerning food and warmth was minimal and sluggish at best. Potential adverse consequences were rarely used as a basis for arguing for more by VCs or the Board, but the supposition that no more would be provided was hardly an ethical reason for not asking for it. It is also hard to justify why ward staff were allowed to neglect the simple, cheap and valuable practice of weighing patients to detect malnutrition and chronic disease. Overall, these findings suggest a lack of care rather than just a lack of resources.

Frugality towards patients and obsequiousness to seniors were parts of asylum culture, and institutional culture was (and is) notoriously hard to change. The culture of an acceptable way to care for patients established before the war did not adapt in a humane manner to the extreme challenges of wartime. The hierarchical structure of the asylums created a discriminatory scenario when considering basic needs such as food and warmth. Senior staff, particularly medical superintendents, received excessive life-style privileges. This demonstrated to other staff that it was acceptable for those with greater authority to consume more than those lower in the pecking order. It may therefore have encouraged and perpetuated staff taking food intended for patients. Social class inequality was not unique to asylums, but hierarchical food provision, which was detrimental to patients, was a potentially avoidable situation.[153] The authorities, however, could justify prioritising the needs of staff by arguing that the fragile asylum care system risked disintegration if they did not. They had no such incentive for patients.

The war time supply chain and distribution of food and fuel in the asylums is a study of the effects of austerity, rigid rules and questionable management methods by the authorities, concerning the lives of mentally unwell people. A *Times* leader in 1919 about the asylums asked: "Have we been sending some of our lunatics into the Army and starving the others?" It called the Board to account.[154]

Notes

1. Napsbury H50/A/01/022 Meeting, 6 August 1914, 167–72 LMA.
2. Tenna Jensen, "The Importance of Age Perceptions and Nutritional Science to Early Twentieth-Century Institutional Diets," *Social History of Medicine* 30 (2017): 158–174, 171; LCC LCC/MIN/00581 Meeting, 21 December 1915, 260–62 LMA.
3. James Thomson, *The Works of James Thomson: With His Last Corrections and Improvements … To Which Is Prefixed, the Life of the Author, by Patrick Murdoch* (London: J Rivington, 1788).
4. Gerd Hardach, *The First World War, 1914–1918* (tr. Peter and Betty Ross) (London: Allen Lane, 1977), 112; Derek Oddy, *From Plain Fare to Fusion Food: British Diet from the 1890s to the 1990s* (Suffolk: Boydell Press, 2003), 71.
5. Ian Beckett, *Home Front 1914–18: How Britain Survived the Great War* (Richmond: The National Archives, 2006), 107–8.
6. Oddy, *From Plain Fare*, 71.
7. William Beveridge, *British Food Control* (London: Oxford University Press, 1928), 1.
8. Beveridge, *Food Control*, 6.
9. Hardach, *First World War*, 127.
10. Beveridge, *Food Control*, 1.
11. Hardach, *First World War*, 124.
12. Hardach, *First World War*, 130.
13. Working Class Cost of Living Committee, *Report of the Committee Appointed to Enquire Into and Report Upon (i) The Actual Increase Since June 1914, in the Cost of Living to the Working Classes and (ii) Any Counterbalancing Factors (Apart from Increases in Wages) Which May Have Arisen Under War Conditions* Cd. 8980 (Sumner Committee) (London: HMSO, 1918); Ian Gazeley and Andrew Newell, "The First World War and Working-Class Food Consumption in Britain," *European Review of Economic History* 17 (2013): 71–94.
14. Beckett, *Home Front*, 110.

15. Richard van Emden and Steve Humphries, *All Quiet on the Home Front: An Oral History of Life in Britain During the First World War* (London: Headline, 2003), 199.
16. Beveridge, *Food Control*, 19.
17. Beveridge, *Food Control*, 20.
18. Lunacy Act 1890 section 283.
19. Beveridge, *Food Control*, 2.
20. Oddy, *From Plain Fare*, 78.
21. Oddy, *From Plain Fare*, 72.
22. Director of the Horticultural Section of the Food Production Department of the Board of Agriculture, BoC W/FM, 21 March 1917, 98 MH 50/45 TNA.
23. Beveridge, *Food Control*, 1.
24. Jeremy Paxman, *Great Britain's Great War* (London: Penguin, 2013), 216.
25. Beveridge, *Food Control*, 217.
26. Beveridge, *Food Control*, 206–7.
27. Beveridge, *Food Control*, 221.
28. Beveridge, *Food Control*, 233.
29. LCC LCC/MIN/00580 Meeting, 6 January 1915, 163–64; Claybury LCC/MIN/00947 Meeting, 2 March 1916, 172; Claybury LCC/MIN/00948 Meeting, 15 March 1917, 54 LMA.
30. Rules made by the Commissioners in Lunacy 1907–1929, MH 51/682 TNA.
31. Claybury LCC/MIN/00948 Meeting, 21 June 1917, 201 LMA.
32. Claybury LCC/MIN/00949 Meeting, 23 May 1918, 78 LMA.
33. Committee on the Administration of Public Mental Hospitals (Chairman: Sir Cyril Cobb) (Cobb Inquiry), 24 February 1922 Dr. Perceval Q:426–32, MH 58/219 TNA; Ministry of Health (MoH), *Report of the Departmental Committee on the Administration of Public Mental Hospitals* Cmd. 1730 (London: HMSO, 1922).
34. Beveridge, *Food Control*, 329; Major Greenwood and Cecily Thompson, "An Epidemiological Study of the Food Problem," *Proceedings of the Royal Society of Medicine* 11 (1918) (Section on Epidemiology and State Medicine): 61–84, 65.
35. Benjamin Seebohm Rowntree, *Poverty: A Study of Town Life* (London: Macmillan, 1902), 234, 235, 239.
36. Diane Carpenter, "'Above All a Patient Should Never Be Terrified': An Examination of Mental Health Care and Treatment in Hampshire 1845–1914" (PhD thesis, University of Portsmouth, 2010), https://researchportal.port.ac.uk/portal/files/5877161/Diane_Carpenter_PhD_Thesis_2010.pdf, 166.
37. LCC LCC/MIN/00583 Meeting, 30 April 1918, 534 LMA.

38. Robert Armstrong-Jones, "Mortality Among Lunatics," *Times*, 10 September 1919.
39. William Stoddart, *Mental Nursing* (London: Scientific Press, 1916), 72.
40. Cobb Inquiry, 15 March 1922 Mr. Sale Q:700, MH 58/219 TNA.
41. Cobb Inquiry, 30 March 1922 Edward Mason Q:2130, MH 58/220 TNA.
42. LCC LCC/MIN/00583 Meeting, 24 July 1917, 14 LMA.
43. Hanwell LCC/MIN/01097 Meeting, 24 September 1917, 181–83 LMA.
44. LCC LCC/MIN/00580 Meeting, 27 July 1915, 695 LMA.
45. Claybury LCC/MIN/00949 Meeting, 23 May 1918, 66 LMA.
46. LCC LCC/MIN/00582 Meeting, 27 February 1917, 441 LMA.
47. Beveridge, *Food Control*, 222.
48. LCC LCC/MIN/00580 Meeting, 27 July 1915, 694 LMA.
49. Cobb Inquiry, 11 April 1922 Rev WD Yoward (VC chairman) Q:3092–98, 3048–50, MH 58/220 TNA.
50. BoC, letter to MSs, 2 March 1917 MH 51/239 TNA; LCC LCC/MIN/00583 Meeting, 29 January 1918, 283 LMA.
51. BoC, letter to MSs, 19 January 1918 MH 51/239 TNA.
52. LCC LCC/MIN/00583 Meeting, 26 March 1918, 436 LMA.
53. Van Emden and Humphries, *All Quiet*, 196.
54. LCC/MIN/00759 Presented papers of sub-committee 1909–1923, Summaries of replies from asylums, 2 November 1915 LMA.
55. Van Emden and Humphries, *All Quiet*, 196.
56. Ministry of Food (Fish Section), "Pickled Herrings," September 1917, MH 51/239 TNA.
57. Montagu Lomax, *The Experiences of an Asylum Doctor* (London: Allen and Unwin, 1921), 127; John Crammer, "Extraordinary Deaths of Asylum Inpatients During the 1914–1918 War," *Medical History* 36 (1992): 430–41, 439, citing Annual Reports of the Commissioners in Lunacy, 1908, 1911.
58. BoC, letter to MSs, 2 March 1917 MH 51/239 TNA; LCC/MIN/00759 Presented papers of sub-committee 1909–1923 Suggested further economies 4 August 1915; Claybury LCC/MIN/00947 Meeting, 2 March 1916, 62; Hanwell LCC/MIN/01094 Meeting, 17 August 1914, 40 LMA.
59. Jensen, "Early Twentieth-Century Institutional Diets": 164, 166.
60. WD Halliburton, "Cooking and Vitamins," *Lancet* 28 March 1914, 931–32.
61. Robert Branthwaite, *Some Observations on the Prevalence of Tuberculosis, Dysentery, and "Severe Diarrhoea" in Mental Hospitals* (London: HMSO, 1923), 8.

62. Charles Mercier, "Diet as a Factor in the Causation of Mental Disease," *Journal of Mental Science* (*JMS*) 62 (1916): 505–29, 507.
63. Colney Hatch LCC/MIN/01001 Meeting, 6 June 1913, 111 LMA.
64. LCC LCC/MIN/00581 Meeting, 30 May 1916, 590 LMA.
65. Cobb Inquiry, "Reports of Visits to Mental Institutions: Dietary at Powick," 1922, MH 58/221 TNA.
66. LCC LCC/MIN/00582 Meeting, 25 July 1916, 33 LMA.
67. LCC LCC/MIN/00582 Meeting, 1 August 1916, 76–77 LMA.
68. BoC, letter to MSs, 13 February 1917, MH 51/239 TNA.
69. Oddy, *From Plain Fare*, 84.
70. Claybury LCC/MIN/00946 Meeting, 8 July 1915, 180 LMA.
71. Stoddart, *Mental Nursing*, 72.
72. LCC LCC/MIN/00580 Meeting, 27 July 1915, 699 LMA.
73. Hanwell LCC/MIN/01097 Meetings: 30 July 1917; 27 August 1917, 165 LMA.
74. Hanwell H11/HLL/B/35/006 Patients' records: male deaths 1936–1937 LMA.
75. Mary Riggall, *Reminiscences of a Stay in a Mental Hospital* (London: Arthur Stockwell, 1929), 5.
76. LCC LCC/MIN/00581 Meeting, 30 November 1915, 160 LMA.
77. Hanwell LCC/MIN/01098 Meeting, 23 September 1918, 140 LMA.
78. Claybury LCC/MIN/00949 Meeting, 23 May 1918, 71–72 LMA; *Fourth Annual Report of the Board of Control, for the Year 1917* (London: HMSO, 1918), 23.
79. Hanwell LCC/MIN/01097 Meeting, 11 March 1918, 323 LMA.
80. Hanwell LCC/MIN/01098 Meeting, 6 May 1918, 40; 3 June 1918, 61 LMA.
81. Hanwell LCC/MIN/01098 Meeting, 1 July 1918, 77, 86 LMA.
82. BoC, circular to superintendents, "Food Allowances," 23 July 1918 MH 51/239 TNA.
83. LCC LCC/MIN/00584 Meeting, 25 February 1919, 305–6 LMA.
84. Napsbury H50/A/01/026 Meeting, 17 February 1916, 262 LMA.
85. BoC W/FM 3 October 1917, 279 MH 50/45 TNA.
86. Cobb Inquiry, 23 March 1922 JR Smith Q:1286, MH 58/219 TNA; MoH, *Committee on Administration*.
87. BoC W/FM, 14 February 1917, 53 MH 50/45 TNA; Napsbury H50/A/01/026 Meeting, 13 February 1917, 261 LMA; LCC LCC/MIN/00582 Meeting, 27 February 1917, 438–39 LMA.
88. Prison dietary scales, Present and proposed diets, 9 March 1917 HO 45/14152 TNA.
89. Charles Mercier, *Lunatic Asylums, Their Organisation and Management* (London: Griffin, 1894), 63.

90. Hanwell H11/HLL/A/14/003/012/001 Letter book, including in-letters and copies of out-letters, statistics and other information 1915–1927, 25 February 1919, 61 LMA.

91. Colney Hatch LCC/MIN/01005 Meeting, 20 October 1916, 297–98 (*Islington Daily Gazette*, 15 October 1916) LMA.

92. *First Annual Report of the Board of Control, for the Year 1914* (London: HMSO, 1916) (*BoC AR 1914*), Part 2, Glamorgan Asylum 4 November 1914, 229.

93. Claybury LCC/MIN/00948 Meeting, 8 November 1917. Between pp. 231–32, notes of conference on staff food, LMA.

94. *BoC AR 1914*, Part 2, Derbyshire Asylum 8 July 1914, 216.

95. Cobb Inquiry, 15 March 1922 AM Donaldson Q:619–21, MH 58/219 TNA.

96. Stoddart, *Mental Nursing*, 88.

97. Cobb Inquiry: 15 March 1922 Mr. Sale Q:700, MH 58/219; 30 March 1922 Edward Mason Q:2130, MH 58/220 TNA; Charles Mercier, *The Attendant's Companion: A Manual of the Duties of Attendants in Lunatic Asylums* (London: J and A Churchill, 1898), 41; Stoddart, *Mental Nursing*, 88.

98. William Julius Mickle, *General Paralysis of the Insane* (London: HK Lewis, 1886), 84.

99. Mercier, *Attendant's Companion*, 41; Colney Hatch H12/CH/A/08/001 Reports to sub-committee, 25 January 1918, 12 LMA.

100. *BoC AR 1914*, Part 2, Brighton Asylum 27 March 1914, 345.

101. *BoC AR 1914*, Part 2, Nottingham City Asylum 29 January 1914, 370.

102. *BoC AR 1914*, Part 2, Cambridge and Isle of Ely Asylum 21 October 1914, 202.

103. Colney Hatch LCC/MIN/01001 Meeting, 23 May 1913, 93 LMA.

104. LCC LCC/MIN/00583 Meeting, 24 July 1917, 26 LMA.

105. LCC/MIN/00759 Presented papers of sub-committee 1909–1923 Suggested further economies, 4 August 1915 LMA.

106. LCC LCC/MIN/00581 Meeting, 30 November 1915, 166 LMA; and LCC LCC/MIN/00584 Meeting, 26 November 1918, 109: for Christmas; patients, 9d per head; staff 2s9d per head.

107. LCC LCC/MIN/00581 Meeting, 25 January 1916, 300–1 LMA.

108. Claybury LCC/MIN/00948 Meeting, 21 June 1917, 158–59 LMA.

109. Lomax, *Experiences*, 131.

110. Lomax, *Experiences*, 18.

111. Lomax, *Experiences*, 123.

112. Claybury LCC/MIN/00949 Meeting, 18 July 1918, 129 LMA.

113. Colney Hatch LCC/MIN/01007 Meeting, 11 January 1918, 16 LMA; Hanwell LCC/MIN/01095 Meeting, 7 June 1915, 97 LMA.

114. LCC LCC/MIN/00583 Meeting, 18 December 1917, 237 LMA.
115. Claybury LCC/MIN/00946 Meeting, 22 July 1915, 94 LMA.
116. van Emden and Humphries, *All Quiet*, 218.
117. Hanwell LCC/MIN/01096 Meeting, 5 June 1916, 85, 95–96 LMA.
118. Colney Hatch LCC/MIN/01001 Meetings: 25 April 1913, 53; 6 June 1913, 123 LMA.
119. Hanwell LCC/MIN/01094 Meetings, 26 October 1914, 113, 23 November 1914, 142, 1 February 1915, 219 LMA.
120. Hanwell LCC/MIN/01095 Meeting, 5 July 1915, 115 LMA.
121. Hanwell LCC/MIN/01096 Meeting, 27 March 1916, 19 LMA.
122. Hanwell LCC/MIN/01097 Meeting, 7 May 1917, 67 LMA.
123. Hanwell LCC/MIN/01098 Meeting, 29 July 1918, 107 LMA.
124. Bonnie White, "Feeding the War Effort: Agricultural Experiences in First World War Devon, 1914–17," *Agricultural History Review* 58 (2010): 95–112, 99; LCC LCC/MIN/00581 Meeting, 30 May 1916, 602 LMA.
125. White, "Feeding the War Effort".
126. Hanwell LCC/MIN/01096 Meeting, 20 November 1916, 241 LMA.
127. Anon. "Happenings," *United Methodist*, 7 February 1918, 62; Beckett, *Home Front*, 113.
128. Eric Pryor, *Claybury 1893–1993: A Century of Caring* (London: Forest Healthcare, 1993), 62.
129. Hanwell LCC/MIN/01096 Meeting, 27 March 1916, 20 LMA.
130. Hanwell LCC/MIN/01094 Meeting, 1 February 1915, 230 LMA.
131. *BoC AR 1914*, Part 2, 309–10.
132. Anon. "Asylum Reports: *London County Council, 1914*," *JMS* 62 (1916): 627–34, 631.
133. Lomax, *Experiences*, 123.
134. Napsbury H50/A/01/022 Meeting, 6 August 1914, 167–72 LMA.
135. LCC LCC/MIN/00581 Meeting, 18 April 1916, 523 LMA.
136. Beveridge, *Food Control*, 228.
137. LCC LCC/MIN/00583 Meeting, 27 November 1917, 181 LMA.
138. Hanwell LCC/MIN/01098 Meeting, 3 June 1918, 60; 26 August 1918, 127 LMA.
139. LCC LCC/MIN/00580 Meetings: 26 January 1915, 182, 23 February 1915, 263; 23 March 1915, 369 LMA.
140. Hanwell LCC/MIN/01094 Meeting, 15 February 1915, 250 LMA.
141. Colney Hatch LCC/MIN/01005 Meeting, 28 January 1916, 61 LMA.
142. Colney Hatch LCC/MIN/01003 Meeting, 25 September 1914, 105 LMA.
143. LCC LCC/MIN/00580 Meeting, 23 March 1915, 369 LMA; LCC LCC/MIN/00581 Meeting, 26 October 1915, 23–24 LMA.

144. LCC/MIN/00759 Presented papers of sub-committee 1909–1923, letter LCC to MSs, 5 November 1915 LMA.
145. Claybury LCC/MIN/00947 Meeting, 23 November 1916, between pp. 273–74 report on BoC visit, 17 November 1916 LMA.
146. LCC LCC/MIN/00583 Meeting, 30 October 1917, 143 LMA.
147. Claybury LCC/MIN/00949 Meeting, 12 September 1918, 169 LMA; LCC LCC/MIN/00584 Meeting, 29 October 1918, 25 LMA.
148. Colney Hatch H12/CH/A/08/001 Reports to sub-committee, 1 November 1918, 107 LMA.
149. Claybury LCC/MIN/00947 Meeting, 11 May 1916, 104 LMA.
150. John Walton, *Fish and Chips, and the British Working Class, 1870–1940* (London: Leicester University Press, 2000), 13.
151. Walton, *Fish and Chips*, 18.
152. Erving Goffman, *Asylums: Essays on the Social Situation of Mental Patients and other Inmates* (1961; Harmondsworth: Penguin, 1980).
153. Carpenter, "Above All," 144: meat ration per week: male patients, 30 oz (0.85 kg, uncooked); female staff 5¼ lbs (2.4 kg); male staff 7 lbs (3.2 kg).
154. Anon. "Lunacy During the War," *Times*, 6 September 1919.

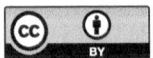

CHAPTER 6

Patients and Their Daily Life

INTRODUCTION

When asylums were converted to war hospitals, scenes of departure of their civilian patients captured some sense of the asylum as a community.[1] Many patients lost their "home", and staff and other patients with whom they had supportive relationships. Dr. Thompson, a medical superintendent, wrote:

> The scenes on departure aroused varying emotions in myself, my medical colleagues, and the nurses. It was all interesting, some of it most amusing, and much sadly pathetic....[T]he whole gamut of emotion was exhibited by the patients on leaving, ranging from acute distress and misery, through gay indifference, to maniacal fury and indignation....I did not realise the strong mutual attachment till it was severed.[2]

Marriott Cooke and Hubert Bond, in their *History of the Asylum War Hospitals*, also acknowledged the distress of departures, for both patients and staff.[3] The asylums were by no means ideal, and the dependence which asylums created for their patients probably contributed to their sense of loss, but meaningful human relationships still existed within them.

The day Britain declared war against Germany, the Board of Control ("the Board") was inspecting Oxford Asylum. Patients were restless on

© The Author(s) 2021   173
C. Hilton, *Civilian Lunatic Asylums During the First World War*,
Mental Health in Historical Perspective,
https://doi.org/10.1007/978-3-030-54871-1_6

one overcrowded and understaffed ward, but the inspectors complimented the asylum because most patients were calm and the wards
peaceful.[4] The inspectors interpreted their observations as indicating
that patients were "evidently very well treated" and their insanities well
managed.[5] The Board recognised that personal dignity and providing
appropriate employment, social diversions and as much freedom as
possible could alleviate patients' distress, lessen untoward behaviours and
enhance wellbeing.[6] However, it appeared less aware of the damaging
effects of institutional living or that a bullying or oppressive regime
could produce apathetic and subdued patients. These only became widely
acknowledged several decades later. In the 1950s, psychiatrist Russell
Barton, working in England, regarded the quiet and submissive state of
many mental hospital patients almost as an illness in its own right. He
termed it "institutional neurosis". Others used the terms "prison stupor",
"prison psychosis", "institutionalism" or "institutionalisation".[7] Erving
Goffman in his ethnographic study of an asylum in the United States of
America (USA), also in the 1950s, identified many of the mechanisms by
which patients were institutionalised, beginning with admission processes
which forced "role dispossession" and "curtailment of self" relative to life
outside.[8]

The Board did not have recourse to uniform criteria to set and monitor
healthcare standards of the sort which began to emerge in the USA in the
1930s.[9] The Board set its own standards, based on experience of what it
knew could be achieved and ideals expressed by colleagues, such as those
which psychiatrist Charles Mercier incorporated into his textbooks.[10]
Disconcertingly, Mercier's books were published almost 20 years before
the war, and two decades of relative prosperity failed to achieve many
of the recommendations. In addition to comparing asylum standards
to ideals stated by psychiatrists or to workhouse and domestic norms,
wartime comparators included care considered acceptable for soldiers. In
contrast to the minimal public attention paid to care for civilian "pauper
lunatics", there was widespread concern about the necessity to provide
dignified care for shell shocked men who had served their country.

When the Board recognised conditions which it deemed detrimental
to patients, it encouraged the asylum management "visiting" committee
(VC) to remedy them.[11] Despite this, and the asylums running according
to tight rules, different standards of care were experienced from patient to
patient, ward to ward and asylum to asylum. There was no such thing as
an average ward, but we can still attempt to understand something of the

daily life of patients who spent days, or years, in them. In earlier chapters we discussed how the asylum system worked, the nature of the patients' mental disorders and their treatments, and issues around staffing and the provision and distribution of food and fuel, all of which underpinned and influenced daily life. In this chapter exploring facets of daily life, we begin by considering sources which reveal something of the patients' perspectives. We then move onto some specific aspects of their lives: clothing; cleanliness and provision of basic amenities; night times; links with the outside world; and the asylum work which they undertook.

SEEKING THE PATIENTS' VIEW

To understand patients' experiences, it is best to use sources which they created. Some wrote memoirs about their admissions. Mary Riggall, Rachel Grant-Smith and James Scott described their experiences in England; D Davidson wrote about his experience in England and Australia; and Clifford Beers about his in the USA.[12] They wrote their reminiscences months or years after discharge. Time for reflection, and their intention to inform the public about mental illness and to encourage improvements in prevention, care and treatment could have influenced their content and style.[13] Despite being situated on several continents before, during and after the war, their asylum experiences suggest that institutional psychiatric treatment and care across the English-speaking Western world had many commonalities. Their descriptions, when combined with those from more patients, such as in committee minutes and the Cobb Inquiry triggered by Montagu Lomax's book,[14] give a range of bottom-up, personal perspectives. All need careful interpretation: official minutes, for example, may be biased against a patient's testimony.

The value of patient-derived written sources is particularly important as senior asylum personnel and the institutions' inspectors largely ignored the patients' words. The Lunacy Act 1890 stipulated that asylum inspectors must "see" every patient, and "give everyone, as far as possible, full opportunity of complaint".[15] The Board interpreted this literally, probably a necessity during a typical two-day inspection of a large asylum. If inspectors entered a ward with patients and staff gathered, they could "see" everyone, and could then ask the group if anyone wanted to speak to them, thus giving them the "opportunity". It would be a brave patient to indicate that he or she wanted to make a complaint. If staff accompanied inspectors on their rounds, a patient might not be permitted to speak with one in confidence. Also, if a staff member offered an alternative perspective, staff words usually had primacy over those of patients.[16]

The Board inspectors handed their written report to the asylum leadership at the end of their inspection and intended to publish it in their own annual report. The published narratives informed the public of standards expected, what was found, and the advice given to make improvements. Inspection reports for 1914 mentioned complaints from patients, but they were often trivialised: "We had but few complaints, and none of a serious character", or they were "evidently based on a delusional condition of mind", or were not "worthy of mention", or "we did not receive any complaints...which had any foundation of fact".[17] The rapidly written reports would have allowed little time for anything other than cursory discussion of complaints with senior asylum staff who tended to offer reassuring explanations, with the Board concluding that complaints required no further attention. Generalisations about patients' complaints were compatible with psychiatric opinion which regarded insanity as all-encompassing: patients needed guidance and supervision in all matters and their interpretation of events was distorted by their mental state.[18] Inconsistently, however, these assumptions disappeared if a patient complimented the leadership or made comments with which they agreed.[19] Positive comments were acknowledged at face value, despite the illogicality of accepting one sort of comment while automatically rejecting another. Allegations from patients of ephemeral, unprovable occurrences, such as dietary inadequacies or staff rough handling them, were particularly likely not to be believed by a self-assured, defensive leadership which assumed that staff behaved kindly and appropriately and patients were untrustworthy.

Neglecting complaints on the basis of a patient's mental disorder was a recurring grievance expressed in memoirs. Grant-Smith reflected: "Once tainted with a certificate of madness, every statement made by the so-called lunatic can be characterised as a further sign of his or her unsoundness of mind."[20] When she complained, the authorities transferred her to another asylum[21]: it was easier to move a so-called troublemaker than to deal with their concerns.[22] When she wrote to the Lord Chancellor (her right under the Lunacy Act), he replied two days later, stating that he had made inquiries into her complaints and "sees no reason for thinking they are well founded". No one had discussed her complaints with her during that time and she found it hard to believe that such speedy inquiries were meaningful.[23] The impression given was that she was fobbed off.

Despite questioning the validity of patients' opinions, the Board expected VCs to listen to their patients, although VCs tended to follow the Board's example rather than its advice.[24] The Cobb Inquiry took evidence from patients but rationalised that they would only want to speak if they were aggrieved at their experience, about which their memories would inevitably be distorted because of their mental state. Otherwise, if happy with the treatment they received, they would want to avoid the risk of inquiry-related publicity about them ever having suffered from a mental disorder which required certification.[25] Thus, preconceived ideas affected the analysis of the inquiry's evidence, with negative accounts from patients documented in the transcript, but overlooked in writing the inquiry report. Similar happened at the Royal Commission on Lunacy (1924–1926) which followed the Cobb Inquiry.[26]

Patients continued to complain, despite their words being rejected. One woman, Elizabeth T, an in-patient for over 20 years, transferred to Claybury from Horton when it became a war hospital in 1915, alleged that staff stole some of her money and belongings. Her doctor explained away the allegations, saying that she was "subject to frequent lapses and loses her property, and as it is necessary to prevent her from collecting rubbish, she imagines her money is taken". His analysis meant that allegations of theft could be overlooked, protecting his colleagues, but if Elizabeth was correct, in effect he was condoning criminal activity. The doctor also did not acknowledge that his perception of rubbish might have included objects meaningful to Elizabeth.[27] As Goffman explained, in an institution where everyone was stripped of their possessions on admission, they were also stripped of their personal identity, so that when a patient

> fills his pockets with bits of string and rolled up paper, and when he fights to keep these possessions in spite of the consequent inconvenience to those who must regularly go through his pockets, he is usually seen as engaging in symptomatic behaviour befitting a very sick patient, not as someone who is attempting to stand apart from the place accorded him.[28]

Rather than talking to patients, inspectors focussed on the asylum environment, activities they witnessed, ledgers of standardised forms, and reports from VC members and a few senior staff. This was less taxing, time consuming and conflict-laden than speaking to patients. Similarly, in the absence of the patient's voice, Diane Carpenter, historian of asylums in Hampshire before 1914, based her study on objectively quantifiable material commodities as proxy indicators of standards.[29] When she compared them to domestic dwellings and workhouses, she found that the asylums' basic provision was relatively satisfactory. Asylum cleanliness and personal hygiene, for example, usually compared favourably with other living environments, and clothes, though institutional, provided warmth and were of good quality. Carpenter concluded that "In every respect improvements occurred as time progressed."[30] As we shall see in this chapter, standards varied, and when wartime priorities engulfed the country, with resources diverted away from civilian needs, especially from people considered a burden on public funds, any pre-war improvements did not continue.

In-Patient Life

Mary Riggall expressed her feelings about being admitted to an asylum in 1918 and being confined there for 18 months: "It seems to me that Liberty is one of the best things in the world – Liberty in the truest sense of the word, I mean, and not licence."[31] As with other aspects of asylum life, the Lunacy Act underpinned decisions about freedom for patients, but it did not define if "asylum" meant the ward, the buildings or the entire estate within the perimeter wall. The VCs tended to interpret it narrowly, but the Board regarded confining patients to the wards and their adjacent "airing courts" as unacceptable, unless they were physically unwell.[32] Psychiatrist Bernard Hollander, took a stronger line: he described locked doors as "a torture", and deprivation of liberty for less ill patients as "cruel and uncalled for."[33] Mercier cautioned staff to be ever vigilant about their patients to avoid catastrophe,[34] but also considered the blanket restrictions on patient's liberty as overly stringent and devoid of attention to individual need.[35] It was particularly difficult to achieve a balance of freedoms based on individual need with reduced staff levels and expertise during wartime.

The Board advocated for patients to have as "normal" a life as possible. Wards needed to be pleasant and homely, with "plants, birds and flowers" and pictures on the walls, with their frames made in the asylum workshops.[36] Wards with the most disturbed patients needed the same recreational facilities as those with calmer patients, even if items might be damaged.[37] The Board emphasised that equipment such as pianos, billiard tables and bagatelle boards should be well maintained, and that staff should "be ready to start a game, such as skittles, quoits, bowls or badminton, and when it is started, to yield his place in it to a patient, and go on with some other duty".[38] The Board expected wards to be "well supplied with books and bound periodicals", including some suitable for "demented patients" and for patients of lower intellectual ability, so all can "be improved and ameliorated".[39] Books on the wards required changing regularly and were never to be kept in locked book cases.[40] One asylum subscribed to a braille lending library for a blind patient.[41] Asylums purchased newspapers and magazines to suit diverse interests, although good intentions fell foul to war time austerity and rising prices when many "half-penny dailies" became "penny dailies".[42] Staff were directed to read newspapers to patients, if required, and ensure that papers were neither monopolised by a few nor destroyed by those with destructive tendencies.[43]

Life was influenced by rules and expectations about gender segregation. Separate gender spheres reflected societal attitudes that women were best equipped for private or domestic realms, while men were naturally suited to active, aggressive and intellectual domains of public life.[44] Lives of most women were constrained by reproduction and domestic duties, gendered educational opportunities, workplaces and types of employment. Outside asylums, respectable young unmarried women were chaperoned during social encounters with men. As middle-class Vera Brittain wrote in her wartime autobiography, it was "considered correct and inevitable that my aunt should cling to me like a limpet throughout the precious hours" that she spent with her special male friend.[45] In asylums, the Lunacy Act forbade male staff having responsibility for female patients,[46] and the architecture reinforced gender segregation, typically separating men from women, both staff and patients, on either side of a central administration block.

Both inside and outside the asylums, a perceived vulnerability of women imposed greater restrictions on their activities compared to those of men. Riggall envied the male patients their cricket matches and long walks.[47] Trustworthy male patients might be accorded parole within or outside the grounds, a privilege usually beneficial and seldom abused.[48] Male and female patients were not usually allowed to be together in the asylum's designated patients' gardens (Fig. 6.1) as trees and well-matured shrubs created "risk in the opportunities afforded for the mixing

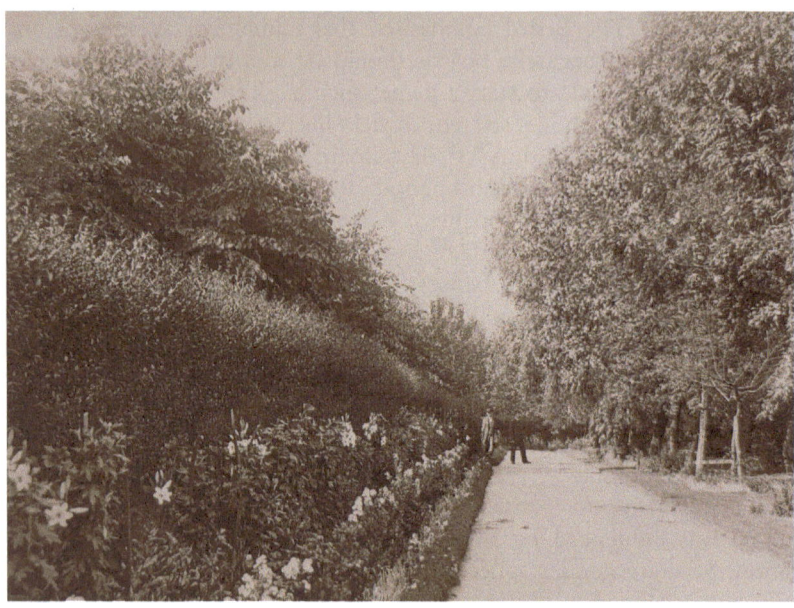

Fig. 6.1   Patients' garden at Claybury, before 1917 (Armstrong-Jones collection, Royal College of Psychiatrists' Archives)

of the sexes".[49] Occasionally a sexual assault occurred, but those reported in minutes identified staff as perpetrators, not patients. One male staff member was sentenced to six months hard labour for a sexual assault on a woman patient.[50] This sort of offence reinforced the asylum authorities' determination to "prevent the association of the sexes" except under "complete and careful supervision".[51]

As Riggall found, options for physical exercise differed for male and female patients. Some gender segregated outdoor exercise was feasible in each ward's airing court. An ideal airing court was about one acre (¾ of a football pitch) for a ward of 50 patients, properly laid out as a garden, not asphalted or paved, and not like a "bear pit", as one low lying airing court at Hanwell was known.[52] Wire fences with evergreen shrubs were attractive and therefore preferable to a high wall.[53] Elsewhere on the estate, accompanied walks for the men provided fresh air and were convenient for staff, with just a few of them required to observe many patients. After a patient escaped from a group of 90 accompanied by five staff on a "boundary walk" at Claybury, the VC grudgingly listened to the patients who disliked these large group walks, and proposed a maximum of 50 patients accompanied by five staff.[54] We are not privy to know whether that satisfied the patients or achieved the VC's goals of preventing escapes, but 50 was still an enormous group for a walk. Such groups may have provided physical exercise, but hardly contributed to a therapeutic staff–patient relationship.

Since asylum activities were part of treatment, Mercier cautioned against punishing patients by preventing them from joining in, as participant, performer or spectator.[55] On the other hand, activities were used as rewards, such as tram outings to Uxbridge for working patients at Hanwell (Fig. 6.2).[56] Entertainment programmes continued as usual in the early months of the war, including the annual patients' fancy dress ball at Claybury and a Vaudeville show at Colney Hatch. By Christmas 1914, celebrations faced disruption because of night-time lighting restrictions and risk of cancelation at short notice in the event of an air raid

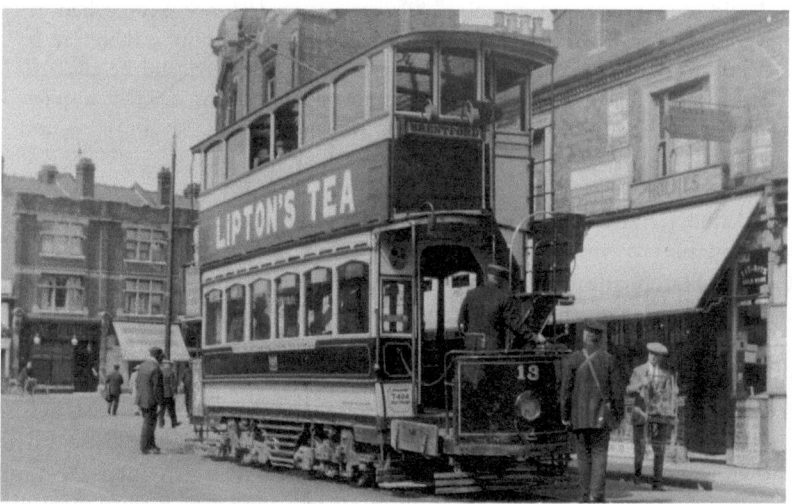

Fig. 6.2 Tram, a few minutes' walk from Hanwell Asylum c.1910 (Public domain), https://en.wikipedia.org/wiki/Hanwell#/media/File:Tram_in_hanw ell_boston_road.JPG

warning.[57] Social events declined further as the war progressed. Cricket matches were curtailed at asylums where pitches were ploughed or used for billeting troops.[58] If a pitch was available, a diminished workforce precluded staff from working with patients to prepare it and to provide a team, and match refreshments were considered an unnecessary luxury.[59] Other out-door events, which allowed staff, patients, their relatives and local people to mix and glimpse a display of positive features of asylum life, such as the annual fete, were curtailed by austerity: Claybury budgeted £80 for a fete pre-war and £10 during it.[60] At Colney Hatch, special grants for events and entertainments ceased for the duration of the war.[61]

Spiritual as well as social needs needed to be attended to. The Lunacy Act stipulated that each asylum employ a Church of England chaplain.[62] Riggall described that she did not go to the laundry to iron on Sundays.[63] Instead, she went twice to the church in the asylum grounds, where she enjoyed the organ, the singing and "orderly services". Male patients sat on the right with the attendants, and women on the left with the nurses. She compared patients to St. Peter in prison:

> I said, one day, to a companion, "Prayer was made for St Peter when he was in prison, and God sent an angel and delivered him – therefore it seems to me that we had better pray that we may recover and be allowed to go home." So two other women and myself used to meet in a quiet corner of the grounds for prayer. And who will dare to say we were not helped and blessed by doing so.[64]

The Lunacy Act also advised that appropriate ministers of religion should be available to visit patients of different denominations and faiths.[65] Colney Hatch admitted many patients from the East End of London which had a large immigrant Jewish community and for whom it made suitable arrangements. The asylum had a supply of skull caps for the men.[66] There was a kosher kitchen.[67] Special arrangements were made for fasts such as the Day of Atonement[68] and for festivals. Just before the war, 241 patients attended a Passover "seder" service and meal with the visiting chaplain, Reverend Solomon Lipson, who provided the additional, special foods for the ceremony.[69] During the war, kosher meat was prohibitively expensive[70] so Lipson advised on dietary changes, with the asylum eventually substituting fish and haricot beans for meat.[71] If Jewish patients had limited knowledge of English, they were placed on wards with other Yiddish speakers.[72] The asylum also organised interpreters for these patients and for others, through the relevant community, or by a staff member who received a salary supplement for his services, or on an *ad hoc* basis.[73]

The London County Council (LCC) encouraged admission to Colney Hatch of people belonging to various minority groups, as, based on their experience of catering for the Jewish community, it deemed the asylum's arrangements for "foreigners" better than elsewhere.[74] Thus, alongside civilian patients who normally resided in the London area and "service" patients, Belgian refugees, prisoners of war and interned enemy aliens were admitted, sometimes transferred from as far afield as Scotland or the Isle of Man.[75]

Over 200,000 Belgian refugees who had fled "the rape of Belgium", the German army advance through their country, arrived in England in the first months of the war. Many were initially taken to one of the British government's largest refugee reception centres, Alexandra Palace, in Hornsey,[76] two miles from Colney Hatch, before being dispersed throughout the country. Some required asylum admission, either directly from the reception centre or after being housed further afield. If refugee lunatics or their families wished, they could opt to be admitted directly to, or transferred to, Colney Hatch where they had access to an interpreter and they "could be amongst patients who would be able to converse with them and also be visited by their country people".[77] The asylum authorities worked closely with voluntary committees to support the refugees.[78] Occasionally, "foreigners" caused concern to civilian patients, such as one who believed he would be harmed by "Germans". It is unclear whether that was part of his psychiatric disorder, but the VC approved his wife's request to transfer him to another asylum.[79] Colney Hatch minutes recorded little about how the new groups of patients were distributed within the asylum, or how they interacted, suggesting that the social diversity was harmonious. The Board's annual reports raised no concerns.[80]

CLOTHING

Exchange of a patient's own clothes for institutional garments, alongside relinquishing most personal possessions, was part of the asylum admission process. This was problematic as clothing and grooming tools, in Goffman's words, are part of an individual's "'identity kit' for the management of his personal front".[81] Removing personal identity was convenient for the institution as it could help ensure patients' compliance with the regime and simplify the organisation of batch-living. In addition, uniformity meant that the leadership could achieve a neat and tidy appearance of their patients as a whole, propagating an image of enlightened care.[82] This contrasted with the patients' view about asylum clothes. According to Lomax:

> Few things are more deeply resented by the ordinary pauper lunatic and his friends than the depriving him of his own clothes, and the compulsory wearing of what he and they regard as "prison" attire.[83]

Asylum clothes differed from both prison attire and workhouse uniforms, but they were institutional, rarely met recommendations about variety, and had little "regard to appearance".[84] Lomax concurred with the patients and explained that asylum clothing destroyed self-respect, intensified stigma, and gave the impression that admission to an asylum was a crime and disgrace, contributing to patients and their families trying to avoid seeking treatment until late stages of illness.[85] Jane Hamlett and Lesley Hoskins, in their study of asylum clothing, agreed with Lomax's understanding, but they also argued that despite uniformity or standardization within each asylum, there was no "uniform" as such, and although the clothes identified those who wore them as institutionalized pauper lunatics, clothing was not deliberately used to shame or punish patients or to represent or develop identification with the institution.[86] Hamlett and Hoskins also argued that by the early twentieth-century the provision of standardized apparel was increasingly criticized and representations were made (though not generally adopted) that patients should be allowed to wear their own clothes.[87]

The Board preferred some variety in attire for both for men and women, such as men's caps being provided in various shapes and colours.[88] Asylum clothing appeared more uniform if a particular style, fabric or colour became identified with a specific ward. This was convenient and practical, particularly for laundry staff, and ease for staff carried greater weight than choice for patients.[89] Similarly, for staff convenience, women patients in some asylums had uniform short haircuts, even though in the community women tended to wear their hair long, often plaited or pinned in place. Although Mercier advised only to cut women's hair short "for medical reasons", and the Board criticised asylums where short hair for women was commonplace, staff priorities overruled patient choice.[90] Shared hairbrushes and combs, sometimes less than three of each for over 30 patients[91] were unlikely to inspire Stoddart's standard that "the hair should be neatly dressed."[92]

As well as having some variety, asylum clothes were meant to be durable, washable and suitable for summer and winter. For women, clothes were often old fashioned. Sufficient supplies were needed for them to have a change of dress once a fortnight and clean underwear twice a week, with more underwear allowed for patients of "faulty" or "dirty" habits (incontinence).[93] In contrast to Carpenter's findings on quality of asylum clothing, the LCC admitted that women's clothes were often "very bad quality", and replacements were low on the agenda, even post-war.[94] Male patients were allocated two clean shirts a week and a weekly change of undershirt and drawers.[95] Their clothing could be threadbare or otherwise inadequate, and in some wet and windy locations, overcoats were not distributed, even to men working outdoors.[96] Men's asylum garb resembled workmen's clothes so they might be indistinguishable from any other workman beyond the asylum walls.[97] However, there was still a risk of being identified as a patient if attempting to escape, so some men devised ingenious ways to change their clothes: Frederick S probably hid in the grounds for one night, returning the following night to deposit his hospital garb and take workshop clothes belonging to a paid worker.[98]

Asylum clothes were often crumpled, baggy, and fitted poorly. Admission photographs of women patients at Colney Hatch reveal much about their clothes, indicating ways in which they tried to convey their individuality and exert a degree of choice. They also provide clues to their physical health and state of mind.[99] Regarding clothing, Jenny K's and Rachel K's clothes were identical, apart from some mismatched, probably replaced buttons, and a blouse under Jenny's dress (Fig. 6.3). Jenny's blouse may have been her way of projecting some individuality, despite expected uniformity, while others tucked in their collars to make v-necks, or added detachable lace collars or bows (Fig. 6.4). Importantly, staff respected these individual choices of clothing adjustments. Photographs of most male patients at Colney Hatch show greater uniformity in the design of their clothes, although variation in colour cannot be assessed in the images. Slightly built 15-year-old Harold H looked nonplussed in his

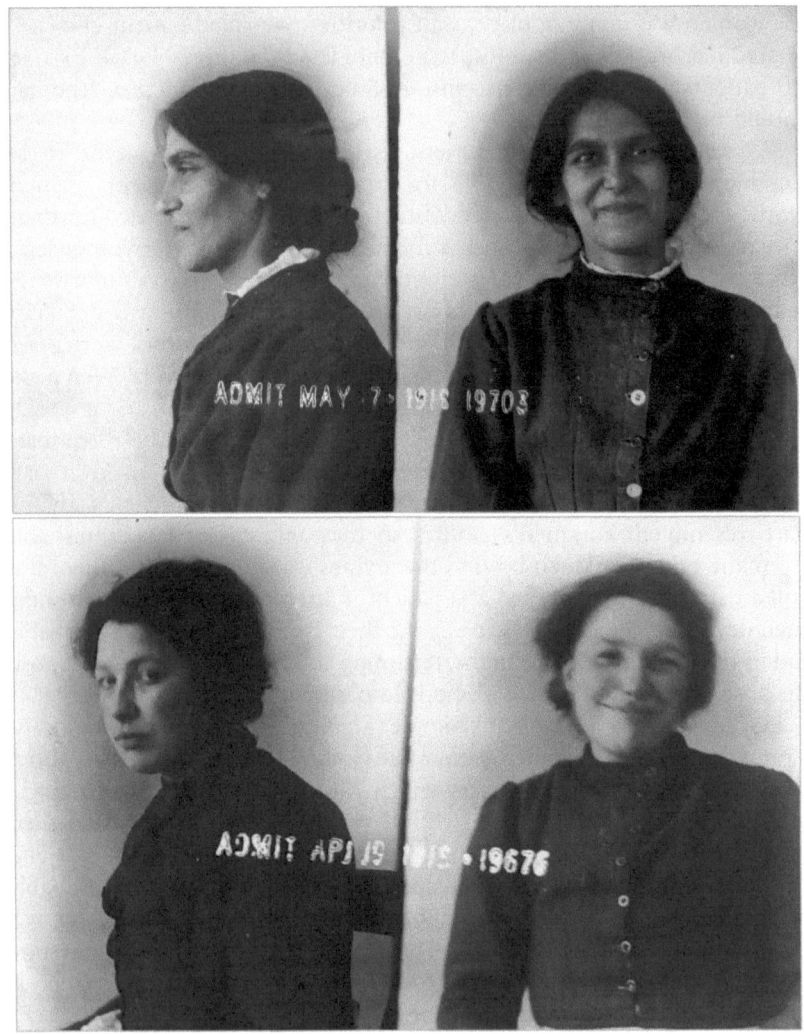

Fig. 6.3 Jenny K and Rachel K: uniform asylum clothes (Photographs of female patients at Colney Hatch 1918–1920 H12/CH/B/18/004 LMA)

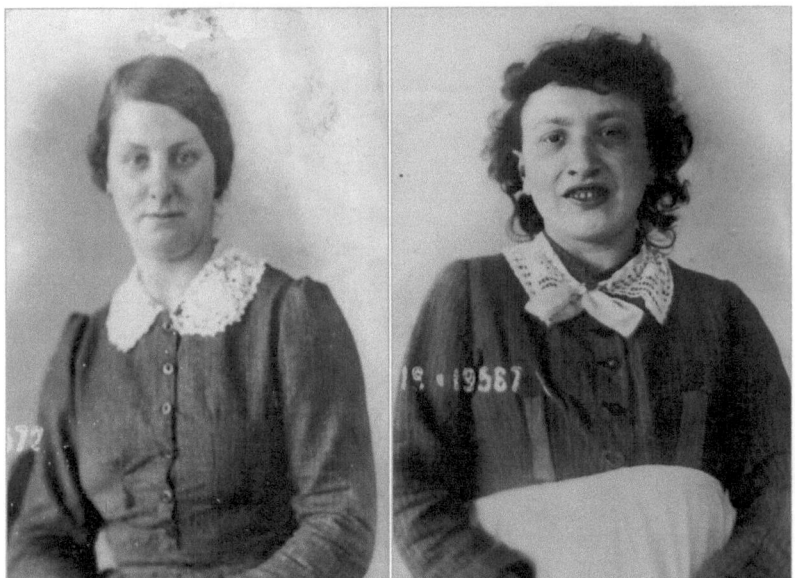

Fig. 6.4 Annie L and Annie S: detachable lace collars (Photographs of female patients at Colney Hatch 1918–1920 H12/CH/B/18/004 LMA)

over-sized asylum-issue of shirt, tie, waistcoat and jacket. Unusually, Max G, was photographed in his shirt sleeves, failing to make eye contact and in a defiant pose (Fig. 6.5).[100]

One patient, Margarita K (Fig. 6.6), had a tear in her sleeve and a steadying hand on her shoulder, and a dress with no buttons on the front, unlike most of the other women's clothes. We do not know how the sleeve was torn, but the hand on Margarita's shoulder suggests a staff member trying to settle her, and the lack of buttons may have been to prevent her from removing her clothes. The pose suggests genuine care of the staff member attending to her.

Other aspects of clothing management could be undignified and detrimental to well-being and recovery, such as staff searching patients' clothes every night, in case they had concealed a home-made weapon in them.[101] However, a new dimension was added to discussion on dignity and patients' clothing with the arrival of service patients. Initially, the Board

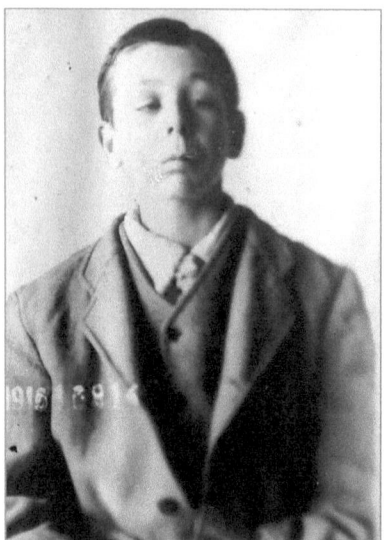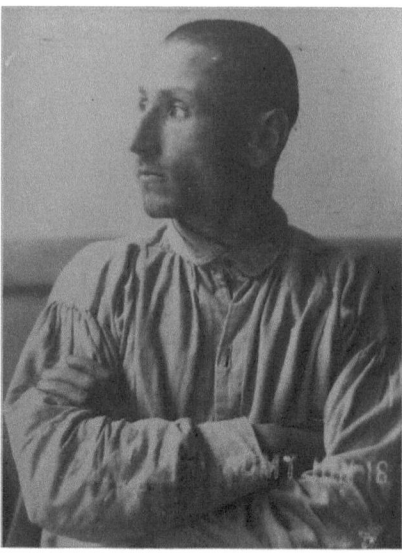

Fig. 6.5   Harold H and Max G: bewildered and defiant (Photographs of male patients at Colney Hatch 1908–1920 H12/CH/B/19/003 LMA)

agreed with the military authorities that they would have a distinctive uniform, to avoid the stigma of pauper lunatics' asylum clothes and distinguish them as war-traumatised.[102] The uniform was abandoned when many refused to wear it, as it triggered memories of their army uniforms and their traumatic experiences, and it had a detrimental effect on recovery.[103] As an alternative, service patients wore tweed suits, "to distinguish them from the others, and to mark the appreciation of a grateful county for their war services".[104] By providing better and less workman-like clothes for service patients and commenting that their clothing could affect recovery, the authorities tacitly acknowledged the drawbacks of the garments provided to pauper lunatics.

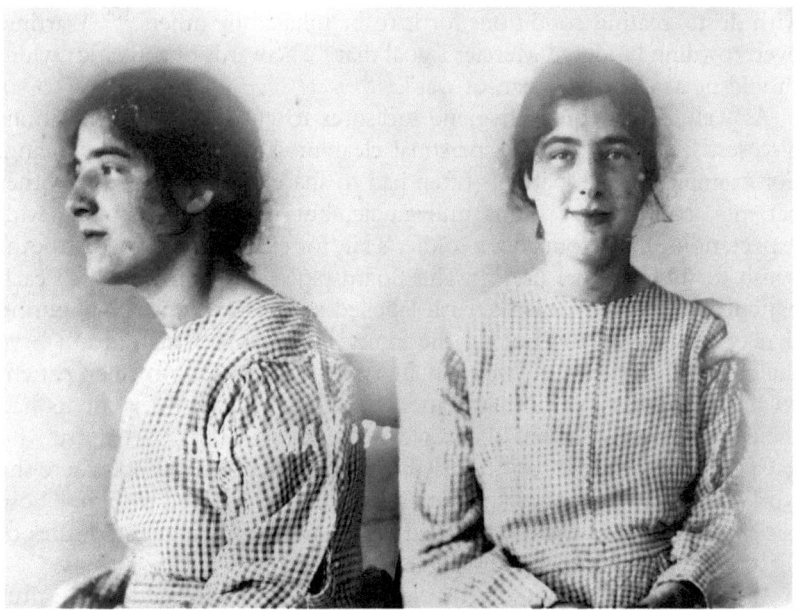

Fig. 6.6 Margarita K, with a steadying hand on her shoulder (Photographs of female patients at Colney Hatch 1918–1920 H12/CH/B/18/004 LMA)

CLEANLINESS

From time to time, asylums sought assistance to help rid their buildings of beetles and cockroaches which occasionally appeared in the food.[105] Some asylums employed rat catchers,[106] and at Hanwell, rats bred in the asylum tip and escaped along the railway bank if the rat catcher disturbed them. To use rat poison, also a risk to humans, required special permission, and in this instance, it was granted.[107] In the pre-war decades, discoveries in microbiology increased understanding of disease prevention and the need for hygiene and public health measures. The Board was aware of these developments, but this knowledge was a far cry from the conditions on asylum wards, where practices were often unhygienic and neither met recommended standards nor those described by Carpenter.[108] Poor hygiene contributed to spread of infection in asylums, such as tuberculosis (discussed further in the next chapter). Some patients with that disease coughed up sputum, spat it on the floor where it dried and mixed with dust, creating conditions for it to be inhaled by others.[109] Wartime overcrowding hindered Mercier's goal that "The wards of a lunatic asylum should be as clean as a man-of-war".[110]

As well as inadequate hygiene measures to curb spread of infectious diseases, facilities to ensure personal cleanliness were far from enticing. For example, asylum patients often had to share toothbrushes with other patients. Not only was this unhygienic, but it was incompatible with expectations on the outside: a soldier's kit, for example, included a tooth-brush for his personal use.[111] The Board praised asylums in which each patient had their own toothbrush labelled with their name, highlighting that other asylums did not do the same.[112] Some patients did not have their own hand towels, even on infirmary wards. One former patient recalled 3 towels for over 30 patients.[113] At Long Grove, patients had their own towels, but only had cold water for washing.[114] A nurse who gave evidence at the Cobb Inquiry mentioned that some wards where she worked lacked washbasins and patients washed in a shared trough. Those patients also lacked towels, so dried themselves on their night clothes or on a soiled sheet from the dirty linen cupboard.[115]

In Goffman's analysis, "territories of the self are violated" in institutions, with removal of the boundaries which a person would put between himself and the next person if living in the community: contamination could be physical and psychological.[116] Alongside shared toothbrushes and towels, undignified asylum bathing routines fit this model. Despite acknowledgement that bathing could be beneficial for more than just ensuring cleanliness, its therapeutic potential was frequently neglected. An asylum chaplain, giving evidence to the Cobb Inquiry, described it as "positive indecency" with patients "treated more like animals" than human beings.[117] His report was incompatible with Mercier's stipulation that staff should never allow a "crowd of naked patients [to] accumulate".[118] Mercier also criticised the lack of privacy due to an absence of curtains between baths and "spray baths" (showers),[119] and Stoddart criticised the rigid weekly bathing regime as punitive and "unnecessary tyranny" and requested flexibility for patients accustomed to bathing daily.[120]

The mechanistic rules for safe bathing which were displayed in the bathrooms had to be followed even though they disregarded the psycho-logical wellbeing of patients.[121] They included directions on how to fill the bath to avoid scalding (although that still occurred), the need to change the bath water between patients, never to put a patient's head under water, and only to give cold baths on medical advice.[122] The rules also required staff to supervise patients when bathing even though they did not all require it, and to inspect patients' bodies for bruises.[123] In reality, bruises told the staff little, as examination would not disclose their causes. The weekly mass bathing ritual in accordance with the bathing rules was convenient for staff. Checking for bruises legitimised it as a pseudo-medical routine, but the process undermined dignity, individuality, autonomy and rehabilitation, and the rules probably protected staff more than patients.

Carpenter noted that, pre-war, sanitary facilities in the Hampshire asylums compared favourably to those which Benjamin Seebohm Rowntree found in working-class York around 1900.[124] However, judging by the Board repeatedly cajoling asylums to improve sanitary facilities,[125] this was not the asylum picture nationally. In some asylums, water closets (WCs) merely required decorating.[126] In others, more were needed, ideally one for 12 patients, because "insufficiency leads to constant squabbling and contention among the patients".[127] Elsewhere, WCs had no doors.[128] Fearful of being negligent in their duty to observe patients to keep them safe, VCs repeatedly argued for toilets without doors, although the Board recommended "dwarf doors" as a minimum.[129] Mercier stipulated that the top of closet doors should be at least 5 ft 6 inches (1.7 m) from the floor, to ensure that the occupant was "decently concealed". There could be a gap at floor level up to 1 ft (30 cm) so it was obvious if it was occupied,[130] which would also allow staff to monitor patients who "Must not get the opportunity of loitering and spending their time in the closets – a time which is frequently occupied in evil practices."[131] Perhaps the greatest fear for staff was to be blamed if a patient took their own life by hanging on exposed pipework. That risk, however, was remediable as pipes could be enclosed. Nevertheless, some VCs ignored the Board's instructions to do that, even after a suicide by hanging in their own asylum. Reasons given included that it "would involve too great a cost".[132] Even the Board naming-and-shaming to indicate its disapproval of negligent VCs,[133] did not ensure action, raising questions about the principles upon which those running the asylums made their decisions.

Another upgrade required for lavatories in some asylums was to replace earth closets (ECs) by WCs. Public health experts had recommended this since the turn of the century, particularly in population-dense towns and cities, where, by 1914, ECs were rare.[134] Asylums, despite their rural locations were mini-population dense areas and required similar facilities.

Mercier did not mention ECs in his book of asylum management in 1898, appearing unaware of their continued asylum use.[135] The Board criticised their on-going use pre-war, such as at Prestwich, where patients used ECs while the medical superintendent and senior staff had WCs. Lomax drew attention to the ECs and the "closet-barrow gang" of patients who emptied them.[136] Prestwich's VC made no changes between the time of publication of Lomax's book and the Cobb Inquiry nine months later, despite the asylum being under scrutiny of the Board and of the Ministry of Health. When the inquiry panel asked the chairman of Prestwich VC what he was doing about the ECs, he answered: "I have made a note of it. We are getting the contract in now."[137] The inquiry indicated the VC's apathy towards improving sanitation, hygiene and personal dignity of patients and eliminating the need for the closet-barrow gang, in stark contrast to it providing modern facilities for those at the top of the asylum hierarchy. The inquiry risked creating adverse publicity for Prestwich concerning their standards of care in a way that Lomax's book (where the asylum was unnamed) had not.

Night Times

In overcrowded asylums, mattresses were placed on floors and beds made up in washing areas and store-rooms.[138] Straw paillasses on old fashioned wooden bedsteads without springs, a shortage of sheets and blankets, and sometimes two patients in one bed with a pillow at each end was hardly conducive to a good night's sleep.[139] Some wards lacked blinds, so light could disrupt patients' sleep in summer time.[140] Some asylums allocated night-wear to individual patients, a practice which the Board wanted more widely adopted.[141] Elsewhere, the patients' nightwear was bundled-up in the morning and re-distributed randomly the following night.[142] Even just numbering garments could have ensured more hygienic and dignified redistribution.[143] Patients might also be moved from one bed to another, but when sheets were only changed once a week, they could be sleeping in a stranger's bed linen.[144] Mercier and the Board made other practical suggestions to overcome some sleep-disturbing environmental factors, such as providing individual chamber pots for night use since toilets were often at a distance, and instructing attendants to wear "noiseless slippers", not to flash their lanterns in patients' faces and not to wake sleeping patients to give them medication.[145]

Typical asylum bed time for patients was about 8 p.m., when the night shift came on duty, but Board inspectors were "more than pleased" when they saw patients socialising until 10 p.m.[146] At Horton, before it became a war hospital, the Board wrote: "We might from all appearances have been in the rooms of a working men's club, where the amusements and recreations of an ordinary social evening were in progress." The patients were reading, playing billiards, cards or dominoes, and singing songs round a piano.[147] Smoking was encouraged as a social pass-time.[148] Some women also had evening privileges, with gender suitable activities such as needlework.[149] The Board praised asylums which instigated evening socialising. It encouraged others to follow suit, but by 1922, the practice was still not widespread.[150] Implementation of Board suggestions was neither promptly nor consistently followed, much to their chagrin at subsequent inspections.

Despite the Board's encouragement for evening socialising, most patients spent over eleven hours in bed each night. Patients considered this regime "monstrous".[151] The theory that acutely mentally unwell patients needed to rest their brain was extrapolated from the common practice of resting a diseased part of the body to aid recovery, linked to the understanding that mental and physical disorders were caused by similar biological mechanisms. Mercier explained that in acute mental disorders, "the demand upon the energy of the brain is greater than it can supply; it becomes so depleted that it cannot carry on its current function, and the depletion manifests itself in some form of insanity."[152] Although Mercier's explanation was for acute mental disorders, the regime frequently extended to the whole asylum. This was irreconcilable with the Board's objective that patients should have as normal a life as possible and with their praise for asylums which allowed patients to stay up late.[153] Time in bed, like other aspects of asylum culture, was justified by theories, rather than evidence, and dovetailed with asylum organisation and staff convenience. In this instance, it was easier to supervise patients if they were expected to stay in bed, and eleven hours aligned with the seven-times fewer staff on night shift compared to day shift. As with shared bed linen and nightwear, practices convenient for staff and economical for VCs became accepted and therefore unquestioned as part of asylum life even when not in the patients' best interests.

PATIENTS' LINKS WITH PEOPLE OUTSIDE

Riggall described "those unfortunate folk, who, through no fault of their own, are doomed to live [in an asylum], cut off from their friends and the outside world. No one could possibly explain the monotony of such a life. It has to be experienced to be believed."[154] Having visitors was important, Riggall said, "one can form no idea what these visits mean to people"; and for those without visitors, "I have seen them cry with disappointment on visiting days as they heard the more fortunate ones called out to go down to the visiting-room."[155]

Visiting hours were restricted, typically a couple of hours on a handful of days each month, unless a patient was dangerously ill, when relatives might be invited to stay day and night.[156] At Hanwell, patients could have up to 2 visitors at a time, but no infants, and caution was advised about bringing in "children of tender years". Visitors were instructed that conversation with the patient should be comforting and reassuring. They had to obey rules: they must not post patients' letters nor give them money, nor give gratuities to staff who could be dismissed for accepting them.[157] At Hanwell, visitors were permitted to bring fruit and cake for patients, but that was sometimes prohibited, such as during an outbreak of typhoid when the authorities could not identify a source for it inside the asylum.[158] Through much of the war, visitors could purchase cake at Claybury, or tea for 1½d (0.6p) and "two small dry biscuits" for ½d at Colney Hatch.[159] When flour and tea were in short supply, these refreshments indicated recognition of the visitors' often arduous journeys on public transport, and were significant gestures of welcome.

Despite infrequent visiting times, the Board recognised the importance of maintaining contact with family and friends. For patients transferred from their usual asylum to one further away in the process of creating war hospitals, the Board negotiated for the War Office to cover the additional travel costs incurred by visitors, and by patients returning to their home area for trial leave pre-discharge.[160] The Treasury initially opposed the subsidy, only agreeing after the Board gave them an ultimatum that it would otherwise cease to cooperate to provide accommodation for wounded men.[161] This was a rare example of timely advocacy by the Board for its asylum patients and their families. The Board also issued instructions to VCs to be lenient when judging if reimbursement should be made: assessment should be based on whether visitors were "reasonably able to afford" the additional cost, not on whether they could "scrape together a sufficient amount of money" to do so.[162] Admirably humanely based, it is less clear how the VCs interpreted the directive or if they informed relatives about the scheme.

Another means of communication with the outside world was by post. The Board criticised wards which failed to provide writing materials, envelopes and stamps. In some asylums, paper was available, but not envelopes, so the patient would write the address on the foot of page and the letter would be taken to the office to be put in an envelope. This was hardly compatible with the Lunacy Act which permitted patients to communicate in confidence with the asylum authorities in charge of their detention, treatment and care.[163] Sometimes a medical superintendent authorised staff to read all letters so that they knew as much as possible about their patients.[164] Elsewhere, attendants read them unauthorised.[165] Staff also opened in-coming letters and parcels, fearing that patients might receive plans for escape or money which might help them do so. It was a pointless intrusion into the patients' privacy in that patients could receive the same from determined visitors. It also contributed to distrust between staff and patients. Practices of staff reading incoming mail seemingly functioned more to protect staff in the event of an escape or other breach in the Lunacy Act rules, by proving that they had done everything in their power to prevent it.

The *Journal of Mental Science* cited an opinion that letter writing was "highly dangerous" during acute mental disturbance: it could make the patients' condition worse due to

> jangling intellects [being] taxed by futile efforts to co-ordinate thought....A patient should not be permitted to tax his diseased brain any more than a patient with pneumonia should be permitted to join in a game of football. This is in reality a question of medicine, and not one of legal ordinance.[166]

This was consistent with other biological hypotheses about resting the disordered brain.[167] Although it was less overtly compatible with minimising staff effort when compared to the argument about time in bed, it did create one less demand on staff, that of providing patients with writing materials.

PATIENTS AT WORK

In Edwardian times, in the community, working outside the house for men and household duties (or their organisation with tasks delegated to servants) for women, were regarded as civic obligations which could be empowering.[168] The asylums reflected these social norms in the work opportunities given to patients. In addition, it was recognised that suitable asylum work could help self-esteem, distract patients from introspective brooding and provide a barometer of a patient's mental state and recovery.[169] The laundry, for example, was "the stepping stone to liberty for more patients than any other workshop", according to Lomax, because only the most trustworthy could be placed there.[170]

Mercier regarded work for patients as therapeutic, whether or not useful to the asylum economy.[171] Likewise, Lomax acknowledged that work had intrinsic therapeutic benefits, although it also subsidised the asylum and could be exploitative, such as the most menial and dirty tasks often falling to patients, whether the closet barrow gang, or others carrying sacks of coal to the wards or distributing patients' chamber pots each evening.[172] The Board recognised the dual aspects of work, dividing it into categories "daily" and "useful", or work which was solely therapeutic and that which also subsidised the economy. In 1914, the Board praised asylums with work rates of around 90 per cent in daily employment or 75 per cent usefully employed.[173] Some work necessitated close interaction with staff, such as in the asylum fire brigade, which rapidly became depleted during the war, necessitating training patients and female staff.[174] Batch-living on overcrowded and understaffed wards contrasted with work-place supervision which provided staff attention to individuals or small groups which could be therapeutic even after decades in the asylum.[175] However, as Andrew Scull commented, and Kathleen Jones concurred, the purpose of employment in asylums shifted, away from the primary goal of benefit to the patients, to enabling the institution to run more smoothly and cheaply.[176]

For many working class patients, their asylum work mirrored their pre-admission daily activities.[177] However, this was less likely for patients from a growing middle-class population such as governesses, teachers, shop keepers, nurses and office workers.[178] Within the asylums, male patients had greater occupational diversity than female, although both helped on the wards. Male patients might work with the asylum's craftsmen and tradesmen, but employment for women was usually restricted to domestic tasks, mainly in the needlework room, laundry and kitchen. When male staff began to enlist, patients and existing staff took on new roles, and whole teams might change, in line with the principles of asylum gender segregation.[179] Women took over heavier work previously undertaken by men,[180] and when female staff began to work on the farms, they supervised female patients working alongside them.[181] Women patients, as women outside the asylums, took on new roles.

During the war, patients also contributed to the war effort, although sometimes, external policies, politics and opinions impinged on asylum activities, not necessarily in the patients' best interests. For example, the LCC decided that patients would not make garments for soldiers, even if they had the skills, as that risked putting women in the community out of work.[182] Asylums did, however, purchase wool which allowed patients to knit socks for men in the forces, and some patients helped on war hospital farms, as at Napsbury.[183] Patients at Colney Hatch collected about 30,000 horse chestnut "conkers" (about 240 kg) from the asylum grounds for the Ministry of Munitions to produce cordite, the smokeless powder used as a propellant in ammunition.[184] Late in the war, asylums collected fruit stones and hard nut shells which were burnt to produce charcoal for gas-mask filters, more effective than standard wood-charcoal.[185]

In addition to these contributions, some asylums undertook paid war work. Claybury took on munitions work, "roughing out" shells, as they had the correct size machinery or furnaces in the boiler room.[186] A photograph of the boiler room from the medical superintendent's personal collection was labelled "Claybury – making shells, 1915" (Fig. 6.7). Claybury produced 4000 shell bodies which generated £450 for the asylum.[187] At another asylum, trustworthy male patients worked with local farmers, who escorted them to the farm and back each day, and who paid a "small charge" to the asylum. A report about the scheme did not mention whether the patients received a share of the fee paid, although we hear that they, and the farmers, found the experience gratifying and neither party abused the system. The Board encouraged other asylums to do the same, but Board archives do not indicate whether that happened.[188]

As with making shells or keeping the boiler furnaces alight, asylum work on an industrial scale could be hazardous. Asylum premises were subject to the Factory and Workshops Act 1907 which aimed to promote health and safety.[189] Nevertheless, accidents happened. One patient

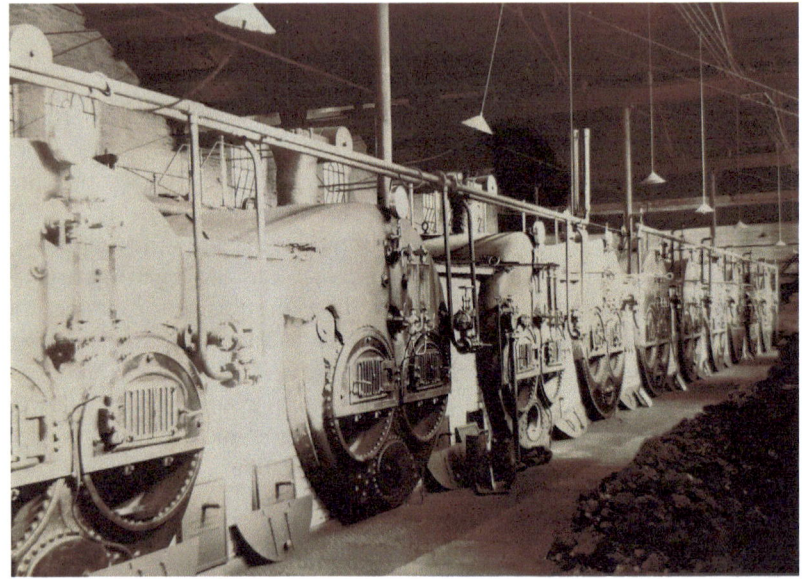

Fig. 6.7 "Claybury – making shells, 1915" (Armstrong-Jones collection, Royal College of Psychiatrists' Archives)

sustained a fracture when his arm caught in the hair-picking machine,[190] the device used to separate out different sorts of horsehair for stuffing mattresses. Laundry work was also dangerous: inadequate training before using the machinery, unhygienic processing of soiled linen, and lack of opportunity or encouragement for hand washing after handling it, all contributed.[191] Following Henrietta S's death in the laundry at Wakefield Asylum by scalding, the Board criticised the "persistent disregard" of laundry safety regulations.[192]

The VCs were concerned less about patients being injured at work and more that they might escape, the latter indicating that the asylum had failed in its duty under the Lunacy Act. Louis Z escaped from a party of four patients working with a farm labourer in the cow sheds, and Eugene T, working in the grounds at Colney Hatch, asked the attendant if he could go to the WC then scaled the boundary wall. Eugene was probably not "recaptured", judging by the dates when the VC discussed his escape and his discharge a week later.[193] In neither case were staff blamed, but as a precaution, attendants were issued with whistles should they needed to summon help outdoors.[194]

Mercier justified patients receiving inducements to work, partly to overcome reluctance to work in a system which they did not like and did not want to support. He, like Lomax, disapproved of the widespread practice of giving rewards in kind which were demeaning rather than having the desired objective of promoting self-esteem.[195] Rewards in kind at Hanwell in 1918 were given to patients who washed the dishes on their ward for a week without any breakages: men received ½ oz (14 g) tobacco, and women, 1 oz tea or ½ oz sugar.[196] Since sugar was rationed, using it in this way suggests that it was removed from the pooled supplies and that others did not receive their full allocation.

Patients disliked being paid in kind, and preferred to receive money.[197] Regarding rewards for working patients, Lomax was among those who advocated for useful payment which patients could use to choose and purchase items in an asylum shop, helping to "increase self-respect and sense of personal value, which the present soulless and machine-made system of asylum administration seems specially designed to destroy."[198] Around this time, the idea of using tallies or tokens, rather than real money, was gaining ground. As well as spending tokens, they could be used as fines for wilful misdemeanours or saved and converted to real money at the time of discharge.[199] Half-a-crown (2s6d, 12½d) was a convenient reward or incentive for many people to undertake an activity. Patient Joseph P, who stayed up all night to assist with "re-adjusting the clocks in the Institution for 'summer time'" received half-a-crown.[200] It compared with the daily remuneration of a washer woman in Kensington, west London.[201] It was also the flat-rate reward which asylums gave to a member of the public who "recaptured" and returned an "escaped lunatic".[202] In the context of the asylum, probationer nurses were among the lowest paid, and in 1916, after deductions for living-in, they received 8s a week.[203] Patients did not work the long and anti-social hours of nurses, so although half-a-crown was low, it was a meaningful amount.

In contrast to the civilian patients, service patients automatically received half-a-crown a week pocket money, whether or not they contributed to the asylum economy. Jealousy and theft by patients without the allowance was reported, and some service patients used the money to gamble, which caused arguments.[204] Asylums were unsure how to deal with these problems: communal living without safe personal storage space was unconducive to a monetary or a token economy.

The Board gave no guidance.[205] Lomax challenged the conclusions of the authorities that patients were inevitably untrustworthy with money. In his view, the more you trust the patients, the better they respond, but "Asylum authorities, of course, are far from believing this; the principle they act upon is just the opposite."[206]

Conclusions

According to Kathleen Jones, the asylum regime suited some people.[207] For others, the standard of care was sufficient for them to live many years beyond the average life expectancy for their generation.[208] In the asylums, compassion existed, and patients could experience a sense of community. There are indicators that individual staff showed kindness to their patients despite the pressures under which they worked. Asylums also attended to aspects of the diverse religious, linguistic and cultural needs of their patients. Sometimes, following the death or discharge of a patient, relatives donated money or presented a gift to the asylum in gratitude for their care.[209]

Among those in authority, there was limited acknowledgement of the harm which institutions could cause to patients. However, critics mainly from outside the ranks of the public asylums, indicated dismay at practices which were undignified and disrespectful of patients and undermined their self-esteem. Their words often passed unheeded. The Board advocated for patients to have as near normal a life as possible and there were ample guidelines about what a modern asylum should provide. However, these were interpreted and achieved variably, balanced against other needs, particularly cost of provision, constraints of the Lunacy Act, and convenience for staff and leadership, all of which shaped the patients' daily life. Staff convenience also affected the application of practices derived from unproven theories about mechanisms of mental disorder which could hinder the wellbeing of patients.

The Lunacy Act set a financial cap and promoted rigid risk-avoidance. Innovation risked overstepping both of these: it was safer to maintain the *status quo* than to deviate from it. Thus, the Act encouraged a conservative and *laissez faire* culture and lethargy towards changing practices. The culture, as demonstrated at Prestwich regarding modernising the ECs was ongoing, rather than just specific to the war years. Some things could not be changed, such as the architecture and external societal pressures, but for many aspects of care, knowing what needed to be done but making little effort to do it, was negligence of a particularly distressing kind. Visiting committee minutes repeatedly convey an attitude that anything-would-do for the lunatics. Some staff and patients spoke up about the deficits, but usually after they had left the asylum.[210] Relatives and friends of patients rarely appeared to complain. Some had no concerns, but others feared repercussions against the patient if they made a fuss.[211] Lack of evidence about their concerns might also be due to the authorities destroying correspondence when satisfied that the problem had been dealt with.[212]

In contrast to improving the pauper lunatics' lives, for whom ideas were tardily implemented, or not at all, providing more dignified care, pocket money and better clothing for service patients reflected public concern and received speedy attention. Finding the will and the way was associated with outside interest and the leadership's concerns about adverse publicity. This was evident at Prestwich where the VC began to deal with the ECs only after the Cobb Inquiry. With regard to benefits from public exposure, it is unfortunate that the Board's annual reports were truncated during the war and during the period of post-war reconstruction.

With the Board's tools being persuasion and suggestion, its effectiveness was dubious for motivating unenthusiastic VCs to implement change. The methods were likely to be more successful with asylums whose VCs and medical superintendents were already motivated. Decisions on care were influenced by wider social demands which were not necessarily in the patients' best interests. In austerity, public authorities had to decide who to support, and pauper lunatics were low on the list, hardly helped by their stigmatising designation and by public fear of the disorders from which they suffered and of the asylums where they were confined. Practices introduced for service patients had the potential to underpin improvements for all patients, but they could also inhibit change by creating practical challenges which appeared insurmountable, such as the need to provide safe personal storage space to prevent theft of cash allowances. The war gave everyone additional worries and distractions, making it easy for the public and the authorities to neglect standards of care for pauper lunatics in a culture where minimal provision was accepted as the norm.

NOTES

1. Steven Cherry, *Mental Healthcare in Modern England: The Norfolk Asylum/St. Andrews Hospital 1810–1998* (Woodbridge, Suffolk: Boydell Press, 2003), 144.
2. D Thomson, "A Descriptive Record of the Conversion of a County Asylum into a War Hospital for Sick and Wounded Soldiers in 1915," *Journal of Mental Science (JMS)* 62 (1916): 109–35, 122–23, 114.
3. E Marriott Cooke and C Hubert Bond, *History of the Asylum War Hospitals* (London: HMSO, 1920), 7.
4. *First Annual Report of the Board of Control, for the Year 1914* (London: HMSO, 1916) (*BoC AR 1914*), Part 2, Oxford Asylum 4 August 1914, 295.
5. *BoC AR 1914*, Part 2, Cambridge and Isle of Ely Asylum 21 October 1914, 202.
6. *BoC AR 1914*, Part 2, Carmarthen Asylum 7 May 1914, 205.
7. Russell Barton, *Institutional Neurosis* (Bristol: John Wright and Sons, 1959), 11.
8. Erving Goffman, *Asylums: Essays on the Social Situation of Mental Patients and Other Inmates* (1961; Harmondsworth: Penguin, 1980), 23–24.
9. Roger Lee and Lewis Jones, *The Fundamentals of Good Medical Care* (Chicago: Chicago University Press, 1933).
10. Charles Mercier, *Lunatic Asylums, Their Organisation and Management* (London: Griffin, 1894); Charles Mercier, *The Attendant's Companion: A Manual of the Duties of Attendants in Lunatic Asylums* (London: J and A Churchill, 1898).
11. *BoC AR 1914*, Part 2, Oxford Asylum 4 August 1914, 296.
12. Mary Riggall, *Reminiscences of a Stay in a Mental Hospital* (London: AH Stockwell, 1929); Rachel Grant-Smith, *The Experiences of an Asylum Patient* (London: Allen and Unwin, 1922); James Scott, *Sane in Asylum Walls* (London: Fowler Wright, 1931); D Davidson, *Remembrances of a Religio-Maniac* (Stratford-on-Avon: Shakespeare, 1912); Clifford Beers, *A Mind That Found Itself* (London: Longmans Green, 1908).
13. Riggall, *Reminiscences*, 23.
14. Ministry of Health (MoH), *Report on of the Committee on Administration of Public Mental Hospitals* Cmd. 1730 (Chairman: Sir Cyril Cobb) (London: HMSO, 1922); Montagu Lomax, *The Experiences of an Asylum Doctor* (London: Allen and Unwin, 1921).
15. Lunacy Act 1890 section 188.
16. Committee on the Administration of Public Mental Hospitals (Chairman: Sir Cyril Cobb) (Cobb Inquiry), 30 March 1922 Edward Mason Q:2113, MH 58/220 TNA.

17. *BoC AR 1914*, Part 2: Durham Asylum 8 May 1914, 222; City of London Asylum 8 June 1914, 362; Dorset Asylum 12 May 1914, 220; Rainhill Asylum 21 February 1914, 250.
18. Mercier, *Attendant's Companion*, 2.
19. *BoC AR 1914*, Part 2, Kesteven Asylum 27 January 1914, 262; Bristol Asylum 9 May 1914, 347.
20. Grant-Smith, *Experiences*, 50.
21. Grant-Smith, *Experiences*, 82.
22. Claire Hilton, *Improving Psychiatric Care for Older People: Barbara Robb's Campaign 1965–1975* (London: Palgrave Macmillan, 2017), 119.
23. Grant-Smith, *Experiences*, 82.
24. *BoC AR 1914*, Part 2, Whittingham Asylum 28 February 1914, 253; Kesteven Asylum 27 January 1914, 262; Bristol Asylum 9 May 1914, 347.
25. MoH, *Committee on Administration*, 6.
26. Kathleen Jones, *Mental Health and Social Policy, 1845–1959* (London: Routledge and Kegan Paul, 1967), 107.
27. England Census, https://www.ancestry.co.uk/cs/us/uk-census-records. Patient at Coulsdon Asylum 1891 and Horton Asylum 1911; Claybury: Female patient case notes 1907, Redbridge Heritage Centre.
28. Goffman, *Asylums*, 270.
29. Diane Carpenter, "'Above All a Patient Should Never Be Terrified': An Examination of Mental Health Care and Treatment in Hampshire 1845–1914" (PhD thesis, University of Portsmouth, 2010), https://researchportal.port.ac.uk/portal/files/5877161/Diane_Carpenter_PhD_Thesis_2010.pdf, 25, 120.
30. Carpenter, "Above All": 166.
31. Riggall, *Reminiscences*, Preface, 17.
32. *BoC AR 1914*, Part 2, Brecon and Radnor Asylum 6 May 1914, 199; Kesteven Asylum 27 January 1914, 262.
33. Bernard Hollander, *The First Signs of Insanity: Their Prevention and Treatment* (London: Stanley Paul and Co, 1912), 19–20.
34. Mercier, *Attendant's Companion*, 1.
35. Mercier, *Organisation*, 120.
36. *BoC AR 1914*, Part 2, Glamorgan Asylum 4 November 1914, 228; Severalls Asylum 27 October 1914, 226.
37. *BoC AR 1914*, Part 2, Durham Asylum 8 May 1914, 222.
38. *BoC AR 1914*, Part 2, Cornwall Asylum 25 May 1914, 209–10; Rainhill Asylum 21 February 1914, 250; Mercier, *Attendant's Companion*, 72.
39. *BoC AR 1914*, Part 2, Berks Asylum 6 May 1914, 197; Derby Borough Asylum 31 January 1914, 352; Portsmouth Asylum 2 April 1914, 372.
40. *BoC AR 1914*, Part 2, Suffolk Asylum 5 June 1914, 308; Hereford Asylum 4 May 1914, 235.

41. Claybury LCC/MIN/00947 Meeting, 20 July 1916, 170 LMA.

42. LCC LCC/MIN/00580 Meeting, 27 July 1915, 698; LCC LCC/MIN/00583 Meetings: 29 January 1918, 281; 30 April 1918, 500 LMA.

43. Mercier, *Attendant's Companion*, 72.

44. Diana Cordea, "Two Approaches on the Philosophy of Separate Spheres in Mid Victorian England: John Ruskin and John Stuart Mill," *Procedia—Social and Behavioral Sciences* 71 (2013): 115–22, 115.

45. Vera Brittain, *Testament of Youth* (1933; London: Virago Press, 1982), 114.

46. Lunacy Act 1890, section 53.

47. Riggall, *Reminiscences*, 6.

48. *BoC AR 1914*, Part 2, Bexley Asylum 20 March 1914, 266.

49. *BoC AR 1914*, Part 2, Dorset Asylum 12 May 1914, 220.

50. BoC W/FM, 9 December 1914, 271 MH 50/43 TNA.

51. *BoC AR 1914*, Part 1, 57–58.

52. *BoC AR 1914*, Part 2, Cardiff Asylum 2 November 1914, 349; Cobb Inquiry, "Reports of Visits to Mental Institutions: Hanwell" 1922, MH 58/221 TNA.

53. Mercier, *Organisation*, 57; *BoC AR 1914*, Part 2, West Ham Asylum 6 February 1914, 377.

54. Claybury LCC/MIN/00949 Meeting, 18 July 1918, 120 LMA.

55. Mercier, *Organisation*, 88, 100.

56. Hanwell H11/HLL/A/06/05 draft annual report 1916 LMA.

57. Claybury LCC/MIN/00945 Meetings: 17 September 1914, 161; 15 October 1914, 198 LMA; Colney Hatch LCC/MIN/01003 Meeting, 6 November 1914, 154 LMA; Claybury LCC/MIN/00946 Meeting, 28 October 1914, 262 LMA.

58. Hanwell LCC/MIN/01096 Meeting, 20 November 1916, 241 LMA; Diana Gittins, *Madness in Its Place: Narratives of Severalls Hospital, 1913–1997* (London: Routledge, 1998), 170.

59. Hanwell LCC/MIN/01095 Meeting, 26 April 1915, 17–18 LMA.

60. Claybury LCC/MIN/00945 Meeting, 30 April 1914, 64 LMA; Claybury LCC/MIN/00946 Meeting, 13 May 1915, 125 LMA; LCC LCC/MIN/00581 Meeting, 6 June 1916, 637 LMA.

61. Colney Hatch H12/CH/D/02/005 Special grants for entertainments and sporting events for patients and staff 1918–1939 LMA.

62. Lunacy Act 1890 section 276 (1) (a).

63. Riggall, *Reminiscences*, 14.

64. Riggall, *Reminiscences*, 21–22.

65. Lunacy Act 1890 section 277 (3); *BoC AR 1914*, Part 2, North Wales Asylum 20 March 1914, 214.

66. Colney Hatch LCC/MIN/01001 Meeting, 10 October 1913, 255–56 LMA.
67. Colney Hatch LCC/MIN/01005 Meeting, 28 July 1916, 230 LMA.
68. Colney Hatch LCC/MIN/01001 Meeting, 10 October 1913, 255–56 LMA.
69. Colney Hatch LCC/MIN/01002 Meeting, 24 April 1914, 215 LMA.
70. Colney Hatch LCC/MIN/01005 Meetings: 30 June 1916, 203; 20 October 1916, 292–94; LCC/MIN/01007 Meetings: 11 January 1918, 88; 17 May 1918, 16 LMA.
71. Colney Hatch LCC/MIN/01005 Meeting, 20 October 1916, 292–94 LMA.
72. Colney Hatch LCC/MIN/01007 Meeting, 24 January 1919, 227 LMA.
73. LCC LCC/MIN/00584 Meeting, 29 October 1918, 30 LMA; Colney Hatch LCC/MIN/01007 Meeting, 19 April 1918, 64 LMA; Colney Hatch LCC/MIN/01005 Meeting, 7 April 1916, 120 LMA.
74. LCC LCC/MIN/00581 Meeting, 29 February 1916, 393 LMA.
75. Colney Hatch LCC/MIN/01005 Meeting, 14 January 1916, 26 LMA.
76. H Cuff, "The Belgian Refugees at Alexandra Palace," *Hospital* 26 (September 1914): 699–700.
77. Colney Hatch LCC/MIN/01005 Meeting, 14 January 1916, 252–56 LMA; BoC, circular to MSs, War Refugees, 3 January 1916, 440 MH 51/240 TNA.
78. LCC LCC/MIN/00580 Meeting, 24 November 1914, 9; LCC LCC/MIN/00584 Meeting, 25 February 1919, 301 LMA.
79. Colney Hatch LCC/MIN/01004 Meeting, 12 March 1915, 4 LMA.
80. Colney Hatch LCC/MIN/01005 Meeting, 19 May 1916, 157 LMA; *Fourth Annual Report of the Board of Control, for the Year 1917* (London: HMSO, 1918) (*BoC AR 1917*); *Fifth Annual Report of the Board of Control, for the Year 1918* (London: HMSO, 1919).
81. Goffman, *Asylums*, 28–30.
82. Rebecca Wynter, "'Good in All Respects': Appearance and Dress at Staffordshire County Lunatic Asylum, 1818–54," *History of Psychiatry* 22 (2011): 40–57.
83. Lomax, *Experiences*, 57–58.
84. Carpenter, "Above All": 154; *BoC AR 1914*, Part 2, Lancaster Asylum 22 July 1914, 247; Mercier, *Organisation*, 78.
85. Lomax, *Experiences*, 57–58.
86. Jane Hamlett and Lesley Hoskins, "Comfort in Small Things? Clothing, Control and Agency in County Lunatic Asylums in Nineteenth- and Early Twentieth-Century England," *Journal of Victorian Culture* 18 (2013): 93–114.
87. Hamlett and Hoskins, "Comfort in Small Things?": 98.

88. *BoC AR 1914*, Part 2, Prestwich Asylum 4 March 1914, 247.
89. *BoC AR 1914*, Part 2, Lancaster Asylum 22 July 1914, 247.
90. Mercier, *Attendant's Companion*, 65; *BoC AR 1914*, Part 2, Hull City Asylum 12 October 1914, 357.
91. *BoC AR 1914*, Part 2, Yorkshire (East Riding) Asylum 13 October 1914, 326; Cobb Inquiry, 15 March 1922 Mr. Sale Q:664, 723–24, MH 58/219 TNA.
92. William Stoddart, *Mental Nursing* (London: Scientific Press, 1916), 87.
93. Mercier, *Organisation*, 81.
94. Carpenter, "Above All": 166; LCC LCC/MIN/00754 Miscellaneous sub-committees, meeting, 19 November 1919, 148 LMA.
95. Mercier, *Organisation*, 82.
96. BoC, Memorandum for the Minister of Health on Mr. Montagu Lomax's book *The Experiences of an Asylum Doctor*, 21 September 1921 MH 58/222 TNA.
97. Lomax, *Experiences*, 59.
98. Colney Hatch LCC/MIN/01004 Meeting, 12 March 1915, 7 LMA.
99. Colney Hatch H12/CH/B/18/004 Photographs of female patients admitted and discharged 1918–1920 LMA.
100. Colney Hatch H12/CH/B/19/003 Photographs of male patients admitted and discharged 1908–1920 LMA.
101. Mercier, *Attendant's Companion*, 24; Hamlett and Hoskins, "Comfort in Small Things?": 105.
102. LCC LCC/MIN/00582 Meeting, 21 March 1917, 498 LMA.
103. BoC, letter to War Pensions etc. Statutory Committee, 4 June 1917 MH 51/692; Hanwell, H11/HLL/A/14/003/012/001 Letter book, including in-letters and copies of out-letters, statistics and other information, 1 April 1919, 110 LMA.
104. Lomax, *Experiences*, 57.
105. Hanwell LCC/MIN/01093 Meeting, 27 April 1914, 197 LMA.
106. LCC LCC/MIN/00584 Meeting, 17 December 1918, 158 LMA.
107. Hanwell LCC/MIN/01094, 9 November 1914, 131–32 LMA.
108. Carpenter, "Above All": 166; Stoddart, *Mental Nursing*, 87.
109. Hanwell LCC/MIN/01098, 8 April 1918, 6–7 LMA.
110. Mercier, *Attendant's Companion*, 69.
111. Anon. "Oxen Thigh Bones to Make Wartime Brushes," *British Dental Journal* 217 (2014): 61.
112. *BoC AR 1914*, Part 2, Cardiff Asylum 2 November 1914, 349; Whittingham Asylum 28 February 1914, 254. Cobb Inquiry, 11 April 1922 Miss Bartlett (Birmingham VC) Q:3197–98, MH 58/220 TNA.
113. Cobb Inquiry, 15 March 1922 Mr. Sale Q:664, 723–24, MH 58/219 TNA.

114. Cobb Inquiry, 30 March 1922 Dr. Ogilvy Q:1900, 1907, MH 58/220 TNA.
115. Cobb Inquiry, 16 March 1922 Nurse Jane Dagg Q:1003–23, MH 58/219 TNA.
116. Goffman, *Asylums*, 31–34.
117. Cobb Inquiry, 6 April 1922 Rev JJ Brownhill Q:2422–26, MH 58/220 TNA.
118. Mercier, *Attendant's Companion*, 63.
119. *BoC AR 1914*, Part 2, Claybury Asylum 27 June 1914, 269; Storthes Hall Asylum 19 May 1914, 334.
120. Stoddart, *Mental Nursing*, 77.
121. *BoC AR 1914*, Part 2, Kesteven Asylum 27 January 1914, 262.
122. Mercier, *Attendant's Companion*, 42; *BoC AR 1917*, 38–39; BoC, Bathing Rules (to be displayed) MH 51/239 TNA.
123. *BoC AR 1914*, Part 2, Kesteven Asylum 27 January 1914, 262–63.
124. Carpenter, "Above All": 51.
125. E.g. *BoC AR 1914*, Part 2, Bucks Asylum 30 October 1914, 200.
126. *BoC AR 1914*, Part 2, Brentwood Asylum 30 June 1914, 224.
127. Mercier, *Organisation*, 37.
128. Colney Hatch LCC/MIN/01007 Meeting, 12 July 1918 Between pp. 111–12, LMA.
129. *BoC AR 1914*, Part 2, Menston Asylum 14 May 1914, 330.
130. Mercier, *Organisation*, 37.
131. Mercier, *Attendant's Companion*, 64.
132. *BoC AR 1914*, Part 1, 27.
133. *BoC AR 1914*, Part 2, Salop Asylum 8 July 1914, 297.
134. Arthur Newsholme, *Hygiene: A Manual of Personal and Public Health* (London: George Gill and Sons Ltd, 1902); "The City of Coventry: Local Government and Public Services," 275–98, in *A History of the County of Warwick: Volume 8, the City of Coventry and Borough of Warwick*, ed. WB Stephens (London: Victoria County History, 1969).
135. Mercier, *Organisation*, 37.
136. Lomax, *Experiences*, 106–7; BoC, Memorandum for the Minister of Health on Mr. Montagu Lomax's book *The Experiences of an Asylum Doctor*, 21 September 1921 MH 58/222 TNA.
137. Cobb Inquiry, 23 March 1922 JR Smith (chairman, Prestwich VC) Q:1311, MH 58/219 TNA.
138. *BoC AR 1914*, Part 2, Wotton and Barnwood Asylums 17 October 1914, 231; Glamorgan Asylum 4 November 1914, 229.
139. LCC LCC/MIN/00583 Meeting, 30 April 1918, 522. Cobb Inquiry, 16 March 1922 Nurse Jane Dagg Q:983–44 and 991–93, MH 58/219 TNA.
140. *BoC AR 1914*, Part 2, Whittingham Asylum 28 February 1914, 254.

141. *BoC AR 1914*, Part 2, West Sussex Asylum 3 April 1914, 315–16.
142. Cobb Inquiry, 15 March 1922 Mr. Sale Q:728, MH 58/219 TNA.
143. Cobb Inquiry, 30 March 1922 Dr. Ogilvy Q:1898, MH 58/220 TNA.
144. Cobb Inquiry, 6 April 1922 WH Skevington Q:2607–8, MH 58/220 TNA.
145. *BoC AR 1914*, Part 2, Norwich City Asylum 10 June 1914, 368; Mercier, *Attendant's Companion*, 81, 90–91.
146. *BoC AR 1914*, Part 2, Long Grove Asylum 11 December 1914, 277; Horton Asylum 4 December 1914, 275.
147. *BoC AR 1914*, Part 2, Horton Asylum 4 December 1914, 275.
148. *BoC AR 1914*, Part 2, Prestwich Asylum 4 March 1914, 247.
149. *BoC AR 1914*, Part 2, Long Grove Asylum 11 December 1914, 278.
150. Cobb Inquiry, 30 March 1922 Dr. Ogilvy Q:1888–89, MH 58/220 TNA.
151. Cobb Inquiry, 15 March 1922 AM Donaldson Q:662, MH 58/219 TNA.
152. Charles Mercier, *A Textbook of Insanity* (London: George Allen and Unwin, 1914), 14.
153. *BoC AR 1914*, Part 2, Horton Asylum 4 December 1914, 275; Long Grove Asylum 11 December 1914, 277.
154. Riggall, *Reminiscences*, 23.
155. Riggall, *Reminiscences*, 9.
156. Berkshire Mental Hospital, "Interim Report of the House Sub-Committee on the Report of the Departmental Committee of Inquiry dated 1922 and the Recommendations of the Board of Control Resulting from the Inquiry. Berkshire Mental Hospital, 25 May 1923," MH 51/686 TNA; Claybury LCC/MIN/00945 Meeting, 20 August 2014, 178 LMA.
157. Hanwell H11/HLL/A/14/003/012/001 Letter book, including in-letters and copies of out-letters, statistics and other information 1915–1927, 86 LMA.
158. Hanwell LCC/MIN/01095 Meeting, 19 July 1915, 126 LMA.
159. Claybury LCC/MIN/00948 Meeting: 21 June 1917, 123; 11 October 1917, 219 LMA; Colney Hatch LCC/MIN/01006 Meeting, 4 May 1917, 170 LMA.
160. Napsbury H50/A/01/024 Meeting, 29 August 1915, 138–39 LMA.
161. BoC W/FM, 14 July 1915, 481 MH 50/43 TNA.
162. Napsbury H50/A/01/025 Meeting, 18 December 1915, 9–10; BoC letter to VC, 16 December 1915 LMA.
163. Lunacy Act 1890 section 41; *BoC AR 1914*, Part 2, Prestwich Asylum 4 March 1914, 245.
164. Cobb Inquiry, 30 March 1922 Dr. Ogilvy Q:1915, MH 58/220 TNA.
165. Lomax, *Experiences*, 71.

166. Anon. "Asylum Report," *JMS* 61 (1915): 288–321, 294.
167. Mercier, *Textbook of Insanity*, 14.
168. Sarah Chaney, "Useful Members of Society or Motiveless Malingerers? Occupation and Malingering in British Asylum Psychiatry, 1870–1914," 276–297, in *Work, Psychiatry and Society c. 1750–2015*, ed. Waltraud Ernst (Manchester: Manchester University Press, 2016), 291.
169. Chaney, "Useful Members": 280; Claybury, Female patient case notes 1917, Louise F, Redbridge Heritage Centre.
170. Lomax, *Experiences*, 105.
171. Mercier, *Attendant's Companion*, 71.
172. LCC LCC/MIN/00579 Meeting, 25 November 1913, 38 LMA; Claybury LCC/MIN/00948 Meeting, 13 September 1917, 193–94 LMA; Lomax, *Experiences*, 112–14.
173. *BoC AR 1914*, Part 2, Brecon and Radnor Asylum 6 May 1914, 199; Parkside Asylum 2 July 1914, 208.
174. Hanwell LCC/MIN/01095 Meeting, 7 June 1915, 66–67 LMA; Colney Hatch LCC/MIN/01004 Meeting, 18 June 1915, 124 LMA.
175. Mercier, *Organisation*, 2.
176. Andrew Scull, *The Most Solitary of Afflictions: Madness and Society in Britain, 1700–1900* (New Haven and London: Yale University Press, 1993), 289; Kathleen Jones, "The Culture of the Mental Hospital," 17–27, in *150 Years of British Psychiatry 1841–1991*, ed. German Berrios and Hugh Freeman (London: Gaskell, 1991), 21.
177. Carpenter, "Above All": 156, 158; *BoC AR 1914*, Part 2, The Chestnuts, Walthamstow, 28 October 1914, 228.
178. Chaney, "Useful Members": 278.
179. LCC LCC/MIN/00581 Meeting, 30 November 1915, 125 LMA.
180. Hanwell LCC/MIN/01096 Meeting, 23 October 1916, 214 LMA.
181. Claybury LCC/MIN/00948 Meeting, 1 March 1917, 41 LMA.
182. LCC LCC/MIN/00579 Meeting, 29 September 1914, 647 LMA.
183. Colney Hatch H12/CH/A/08/001 Reports to Sub-Committee 22 February 1918, 20; 12 July 1918, 74; Napsbury H50/A/01/025 Meeting, 22 January 1916. Between pp. 69–70, LMA.
184. Anon. "Happenings," *United Methodist*, 7 February 1916, 62; LCC LCC/MIN/00583 Meeting, 18 December 1917, 230 LMA.
185. BoC, letter and memorandum to superintendents, 9 July 1918 MH 51/239 TNA.
186. LCC LCC/MIN/00580 Meeting, 29 June 1915, 615–16; LCC/MIN/00581 Meetings: 21 December 1915; 29 February 1916, 395–96 LMA.
187. LCC LCC/MIN/00581 Meeting, 30 May 1916, 626 LMA.
188. BoC, letter to MSs, 19 January 1918 MH 51/239 TNA.

189. BoC W/FM, 21 October 1914, 221 MH 50/43 TNA; *BoC AR 1914*, Part 2, Hull City Asylum 12 October 1914, 358.

190. *BoC AR 1914*, Part 2, Hants Asylum 6 November 1914, 234.

191. Home Office—(Class II.—Vote 4). *Hansard* HC Deb, 23 July 1913, vol. 55, cc. 2061–132; BoC, "Increased Annual Death Rate in Asylums," 15 January 1919 MH 51/239 TNA.

192. BoC W/FM 2 September 1914, 177 MH 50/43 TNA.

193. UK Lunacy Patients Admission Register 1846–1912, https://www.anc estry.co.uk/search/collections/uklunpatadmreg/.

194. Colney Hatch LCC/MIN/01003 Meetings: 20 November 1914, 169; 12 February 1915, 287 LMA.

195. Mercier, *Organisation*, 85–87; Lomax, *Experiences*, 114.

196. LCC LCC/MIN/00583 Meeting, 29 January 1918, 270 LMA.

197. Cobb Inquiry, Dr. Shaw Bolton 7 April 1922 Q:2842, MH 58/220 TNA.

198. Lomax, *Experiences*, 112–14.

199. Mercier, *Organisation*, 86–87; Lomax, *Experiences*, 114.

200. Colney Hatch H12/CH/A/08/001 Reports to sub-committee 17 May 1918, 57 LMA.

201. MACA, Herbert G, SA/MAC/G.3/9 WL.

202. Hanwell LCC/MIN/01096 Meeting, 29 January 1917, 297 LMA.

203. Hanwell LCC/MIN/01096 Meetings, 5 June 1916, 83; 29 January 1917, 297 LMA.

204. LCC LCC/MIN/00583 Meeting, 30 April 1918, 501–2 LMA.

205. Claybury LCC/MIN/00949 Meeting, 25 April 1918, 47–48 LMA.

206. Lomax, *Experiences*, 68.

207. Jones, "Culture": 24.

208. *Office for National Statistics, Average Life Spans: Life Expectancy at Birth, Median Age at Death and Modal Age at Death, 1841 to 2010, England and Wales* (undated), https://www.ons.gov.uk/ons/rel/mor tality-ageing/mortality-in-england-and-wales/average-life-span/chd-fig ure-1.xls; Colney Hatch H12/CH/B/16/014 Case notes of female patients who died in 1936–1937; H12/CH/B/26/005 Civil register of patients 1916–1917 LMA.

209. Colney Hatch LCC/MIN/01007 Meeting, 29 November 1918, 197 LMA.

210. Lomax, *Experiences*.

211. Hilton, *Improving Psychiatric Care*, 9, 11, 14.

212. BoC, "Orders for Destruction of Documents," 31 March 1909 MH 51/723 TNA.

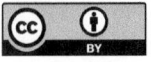

CHAPTER 7

Difficult Diseases: Tuberculosis and Other Infections

INTRODUCTION: ELSIE AND MOHAMMED

A Muslim couple, Elsie and Mohammed, arrived at Victoria Station, London, in January 1915. They were refugees fleeing war-torn Belgium. Born in 1883, Elsie was a dressmaker and "artistic worker". Her mental troubles began following the birth of her daughter:

> She was very depressed, weeping and covering her face with her hands. She kept getting out of bed and attempting to escape. She refuses her food at times. She has been in this depressed condition for some time and shows no improvement.

After two years in Hanwell she moved to Colney Hatch, the London County Council (LCC) asylum which admitted many patients born abroad and for whom English was not their mother tongue. At Colney Hatch, she could be alongside other Belgian refugees, which might provide a more favourable social and therapeutic environment for her than Hanwell. Elsie suffered an episode of dysentery in October 1917. A few weeks later physical examination revealed some weight loss and dullness in her left lung. She died of tuberculosis in April 1918.[1] The post-mortem noted "bed sores" (today, pressure sores or ulcers), which, according to psychiatrist Charles Mercier, were "a discredit to an attendant, and ought never be allowed in an asylum patient", a statement with which the asylums' Board of Control ("the Board") concurred.[2] Elsie's

© The Author(s) 2021   213
C. Hilton, *Civilian Lunatic Asylums During the First World War*,
Mental Health in Historical Perspective,
https://doi.org/10.1007/978-3-030-54871-1_7

weight loss could have been due to dysentery or tuberculosis or to her mental state. Tuberculosis was alarmingly frequent in asylums, and dysentery was "deplorably common",[3] although almost non-existent in the general population, to the extent that one asylum medical officer argued that fear of catching it reduced asylum admissions.[4]

Elsie's family arranged for a "Muslim priest" to officiate at her funeral.[5] A few weeks later, Mohammed wrote to the authorities:

> Kindly return to above address all belongings from late Elsie M—s. Should the Medical Superintendent, the Committee, etc., etc., think the belongings are not fit for discharge, they may do what they have done with Elsie M—s.

Mohammed's message reverberates with distress. The asylum sent him her belongings, a wedding ring and dress ring, by registered post. They forwarded her "plate of artificial teeth" to the Paddington Guardians, their rightful owners. Her clothes and other day-to-day items were asylum property.[6]

Deaths in asylums, particularly from infectious diseases, escalated during the war. The increase may have been related to the many wartime changes we have seen so far, including: vacating asylums to create war hospitals which resulted in overcrowding of those remaining; many inexperienced staff and low staff morale; and inadequate food, fuel, clothing, bathing routines and other basic amenities. In this chapter we shall explore aspects of medical and scientific knowledge concerning infectious diseases and how that knowledge was applied in the asylums. The various themes all relate to Elsie's story: death rates; post-mortems; tuberculosis; and other infectious diseases.

Death Rates and Post-mortems

In 1914, based on diagnosis during life plus post-mortem evidence, tuberculosis, general paralysis of the insane (GPI, brain syphilis), and the vague category of "senility" accounted for over one third of total asylum deaths in England and Wales.[7] GPI was discussed in Chapter 3, and aspects of the other two categories are discussed below. The overall annual asylum death rate of under ten per cent rose to 12 per cent in 1915–1916, leaped to over 17 per cent in 1917 (resulting in the LCC discussing paying overtime to asylum mortuary attendants[8]) and peaked in 1918 at 20 per cent

(Table 7.1).[9] There was little alarm, because the causes of death were the same as pre-war and the rise did not point to staff directly failing in their duty of care according to the Lunacy Act, resulting in suicide or injury. The total asylum population in England numbered around 100,000 and the national population over 32 million, but during the war half the total national increase in tuberculosis deaths occurred in the asylums.[10] Regarding the incidence and death rates of other acute infectious diseases, asylums compared unfavourably with the general population, including in London, where they remained comparatively low throughout the war.[11]

Table 7.1   Deaths in asylums: mortality per 1000 resident patients and total deaths

	1913	1914	1915	1916	1917	1918	1919	1920
Mortality per 1000 resident patients								
General Paralysis		15.7	16.5			17.5		13.6
Dysentery	2.2	2.5	4.0	5.0	10.0	9.0		2.6
Typhoid	0.3		0.6	0.5	1.2	1.1		0.4
Tuberculosis	17.0	12.5	19.0	23.0	37.0	51.8		15.8
Tuberculosis mortality per 1000 community residents, not age adjusted								
Tuberculosis	*1.35*		*1.51*	*1.53*	*1.62*	*1.69*		*1.13*
Total asylum deaths								
a. Total asylum deaths	10,075	10,594	12,710	12,888	17,130	18,330	11,217	7945
b. Total asylum patients	104,868	106,451	105,858	103,574	98,621	90,459	86,950	90,950
Deaths (a/b) per cent	9.6	9.9	12.0	12.4	17.4	20.3	12.9	8.7

Sources BoC, "Increased Annual Death Rate in Asylums," 15 January 1919, 532 MH 51/239 TNA; *Second Annual Report of the Board of Control, for the Year 1915* (London: HMSO, 1917), 12–13; *BoC AR 1918*, Appendix A, 27; *Seventh Annual Report of the Board of Control, for the Year 1920* (London: HMSO, 1921), 26; Drolet, "World War I and Tuberculosis": 690

Death rates provide important evidence about disease, but like other data, they are not infallible, they have limitations and require careful interpretation. They do not measure new occurrences the disease, neither how long it lasts nor how severely it incapacitates the sufferer. They are therefore somewhat crude measures of disease activity. Waltraud Ernst, in his study of death rates in asylums, noted problems of "the nature of the statistics on which they are based and the categorizations underlying them", associated with doubtful validity and reliability of the figures collected.[12] Caution is also needed when comparing rates of disease and death between asylums and community because figures may not be adjusted for different age distributions. Death rates, however, were not confounded by transferring seriously physically ill asylum patients to general hospitals or sanatoria as they were treated in-house. Also, comparing two relatively small asylums, in 1914, Northumberland Asylum to the east of the Pennines had the highest annual death rate nationally (38 per cent) and Cumberland and Westmorland to the west had the lowest (nine per cent),[13] suggesting that death rates were not directly related to asylum size.

A patient who died in an asylum was typically subject to a post-mortem examination.[14] Post-mortems indicated to the rest of the medical world that the care of lunatics was part of medical practice and that asylum doctors sought to improve their understanding of cause and pathology of the disorders from which their patients suffered, just as their colleagues in general hospitals. However, interpretation of post-mortem examinations and the terminology used in reports could be ambiguous.[15] Differences were likely to have been due to the skills and understanding of individual pathologists, as illustrated by the use of the terms derived from the word "senile".[16] "Senility" was often used synonymously with old age, when the body's organs shrink or "atrophy" in later life. Not only was there was no specified chronological age designating "old", but senility might affect only one part of the body, such as baldness, a type of "early local senility".[17] At Hanwell, reports from a consecutive sample of ten post-mortems of men age over 60 concluded that the main cause of death for all of them was "senile decay", of whom three were also labelled as having "senile dementia".[18] In contrast, in a similar series of ten at Colney Hatch carried out by a different pathologist, none mentioned senile decay. Only three included the term senile in any form, but each was used in a different way: senile debility, senile dementia and senility.[19] Drawing on all twenty of these post-mortems, three of the four whose cause of death was attributed to "senile dementia" had normal weight brains, making that conclusion unlikely. Overall, when incorporated into death certificates, imprecise senility-related terms lacked scientific or clinical meaning. The label was convenient, subjective and detracted from the need to acknowledge other pathology which might have more accurately explained the death. The post-mortem of James K age 64 demonstrates this. The pathologist found his brain to be normal but intestines "congested and inflamed", suggesting dysentery, but the report concluded that the primary cause of death was senile decay with dysentery secondary.[20] This sort of conclusion would under-estimate the number of deaths due to preventable infections.

Routine post-mortems were controversial, taking little account of their emotional significance for bereaved relatives. The Board advised seeking consent from a patient's relative at the time of admission to the asylum, to agree to a post-mortem in the event of their death. The request for consent appeared in the standard admission letter sent to the relative, alongside information on more immediate matters, such as visiting times. At the time of admission to an asylum, which portrayed itself as an institution offering hope of recovery and not as somewhere that patients were sent to die, the relative was more likely to be concerned about current problems and recovery, making them unlikely to pay attention to information about death. However, unless the relative objected in writing to the post-mortem, consent was inferred.[21] With the original notification long forgotten, a post-mortem could distress relatives who were under the impression that they had not consented to it.[22] Fulham Board of Guardians sharply reprimanded Hanwell asylum's "visiting" committee (VC) for neither informing a husband of his wife's death nor explicitly requesting consent at that time concerning performing a post-mortem. The VC discussed the Guardians' letter and replied that it would not change its practice.[23] As with other practices, the process reflected institutional convenience rather than the wellbeing of the patient or his family. The asylum did not have to respond in such a callous way. Pamela Michael and David Hirst described how customs and rules about communication concerning deceased patients at Denbigh Asylum in Wales were influenced by local culture.[24] Doing the same at Hanwell for a diverse urban population would have been more complicated, but feasible. The different approaches suggest that asylums interacted in different ways with the populations they served. The Denbigh leadership showed more compassion and flexibility in this matter than the Board recommended, or Hanwell VC applied.

TUBERCULOSIS

The wartime rise of asylum tuberculosis needs to be contextualised in its pre-war course and how the authorities responded to it. For over a decade, rates of asylum tuberculosis were approximately ten times higher than in the community.[25] There were two hypotheses to explain this: either insane people had an inherent predisposition to tuberculosis alongside their mental disorder in accordance with "degeneration" theories; or, asylum conditions predisposed to it.[26] Dr. Francis Crookshank, in 1899, blamed the asylums, "the fault lies with the institution harbouring the germs. It is no excuse that the person infected has 'family tendencies.'"[27] He attributed high rates to overcrowding, poor ventilation, lack of out-door activity, unhygienic wards and "a certain quality of diet."[28] To Crookshank, environmental and dietary remedies were needed, and were morally and economically justified on the grounds that improvements would enable long-term patients to work better and acute patients to recover faster. He also recommended segregating patients known to be infectious, and weighing all patients every three months since weight loss often accompanied early stages of tuberculosis.[29]

Soon after Crookshank's critique, the Medico-Psychological Association (MPA) appointed a Tuberculosis Committee to investigate. It concluded that high rates of tuberculosis in public asylums called for urgent measures.[30] It made recommendations, but implementation was hardly detectable. Psychiatrist William Stoddart blamed the asylum leadership, "underfeeding and overcrowding, enforced...by lay committees with excessively economical tendencies".[31] Psychiatrist and researcher Frederick Mott, based on his pre-war study of tuberculosis, stressed the importance of early diagnosis with a view to ensuring the patients' "isolation and treatment" and that they expectorated into "proper receptacles".[32] He also specified the need, with which the Board concurred, for asylums to provide wards with verandas deep enough to shelter beds for outdoor nursing (Fig. 7.1).[33] Mott reassured the LCC asylums that they were already taking adequate dietary and environmental measures to prevent tuberculosis,[34] which, in view of his standing regarding science and asylums, risked encouraging complacency even if his view was accurate and appropriate for some. The Board encouraged, and reiterated

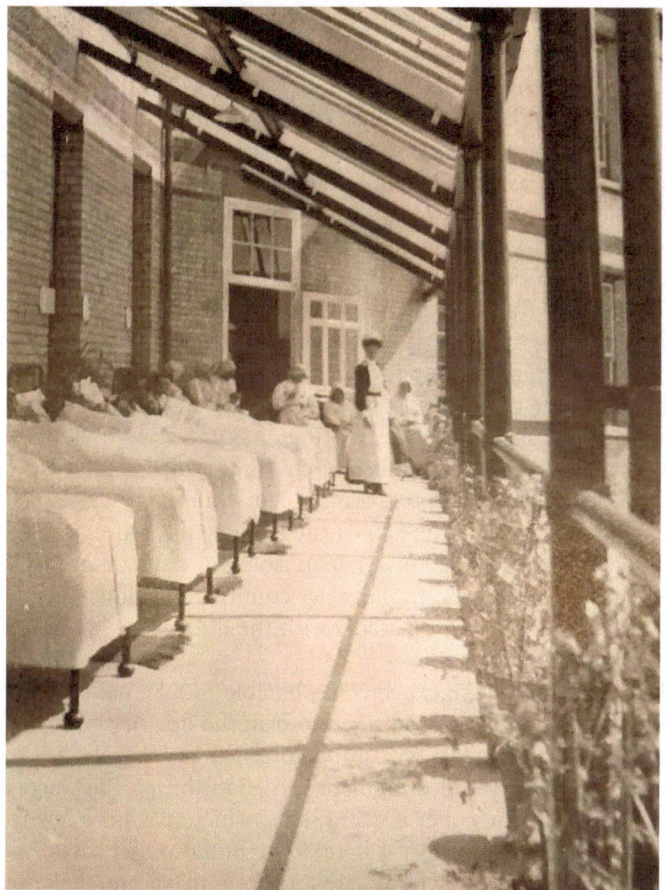

Fig. 7.1 Verandah for nursing patients with tuberculosis in the open air, at Horton Asylum. Given to Mott by the medical superintendent. Photographer unknown (Mott, "Tuberculosis in London County Asylums": opposite, p. 116)

during the war, the need to regularly weigh patients, as Crookshank and others had advised, but implementation varied.[35] Also in the war years, most experts recommended physical examination rather than X-ray screening to detect lung tuberculosis, but with medical staff shortages the standard three-monthly physical health checks for patients were abandoned, with the risk of overlooking new or emerging cases.[36]

In the community, many adults harboured the mycobacterium causing tuberculosis, so some asylum deaths would have included patients admitted with latent, smouldering, quiescent, or inactive disease which ripened into a full-blown, rapidly fatal condition activated by wartime asylum deprivations.[37] Some patients arrived in asylums suffering from tuberculosis, such as Lily R, whose story appears in Chapter 3. Others, such as Elsie M probably acquired it after admission. Numerous asylum practices, known to be unhygienic, risked spreading it and other infectious diseases. Practices included: treating healthy and infectious patients together in open wards; patients not washing their hands before meals or after using the lavatory; inadequate hand washing by people preparing food and working in the laundry; lack of measures to prevent inhalation of mycobacterium tuberculosis; and drying soiled underclothing in the ward to be worn again without washing.[38] Some asylum laundries used washing machines and the disinfectant chlorine, which could be produced by electrolysis of brine at the asylum,[39] but foul linen was handled too often, including counting items into the laundry to ensure accountability for losses. Many asylums had insufficient isolation wards, especially during the war, lacked laboratory facilities to confirm infectious diseases, and communicated poorly about patients with the disorders when transferring them between wards or asylums.[40]

Asylum ward staff were expected to be able to take patients' temperatures, identify physical symptoms and inform the doctor about them, and to be able to nurse patients with tuberculosis, including 24-hours in the open air.[41] Temporary and untrained ward staff during the war were less likely to have these and other nursing skills, which may have been a factor in Elsie M developing not just tuberculosis, but also bed sores.

The LCC instructed asylums late in 1914 to vacate their detached villas, including some in use as isolation wards, as they were required for war purposes. Infectious patients were moved back into the main buildings.[42] With inadequate isolation and an under-trained workforce, standards of infectious disease management fell. The LCC may have had patriotic intentions but it is less clear that it understood the health risks associated with the instructions it gave.

Although notification of new cases of tuberculosis to the local authority Medical Officer of Health (MOH) became mandatory from 1912,[43] not all asylums and MOHs complied. Some MOHs allegedly discouraged the asylums from notifying them. Even where asylums sent notifications, the

MOH did not always transfer them to the official responsible for treatment in the locality where the asylum was situated, forwarding them instead to the MOH of the area from which the patient was admitted.[44] The Board received copies of death notices, but not copies of new diagnosis notifications.[45] This could have affected the Board's perception of the situation, diminishing its concern and reducing the likelihood of it endeavouring to provide prophylactic measures or better treatment. Overall, nobody in authority had a comprehensive picture of tuberculosis in asylums, nor took responsibility to counter the rising rates. Without being informed about diagnoses, the Board was also unlikely to know that over 90 per cent of asylum tuberculosis occurred in the lungs rather than in other parts of the body, compared to 75 per cent of community tuberculosis.[46] This meant that asylum tuberculosis was transmitted disproportionately by inhalation, associated with poor hygiene and lack of ventilation, rather than by it being ingested in infected milk or meat.[47]

Psychiatrist and historian John Crammer attempted to unravel the underlying causes of high tuberculosis incidence and mortality in his analysis of wartime deaths at the Buckinghamshire Asylum. He noted that the escalating deaths received little attention from the Board or the VC.[48] Wartime understaffing of the Board meant that one, rather than two, inspectors carried out asylum inspections, often a lawyer unaccompanied by a doctor. It is questionable whether lawyers had enough medical knowledge to respond adequately on matters of disease and death, but the annual inspection box had to be ticked, and a lawyer's inspection ensured that this happened. In 1917, medical superintendents made their concerns known to the Board, attributing rising death rates to food restrictions which predisposed patients to succumb to infection.[49] The Board appeared complacent, but the LCC was sufficiently alarmed to commission Mott to re-investigate tuberculosis in its asylums, although the minutes do not report his conclusions.[50] The LCC commissioned its investigation over a year before the Board began its study.[51]

Crammer identified overcrowding and poor nutrition as important causes. Overcrowding may have contributed to spreading tuberculosis but did not relate directly to death rates which peaked at the same time in asylums with and without it.[52] Concerning food, Crammer focussed on the reduction in the bread allowance, and thus the calorie intake, causing slow starvation resulting in lethargy, apathy, lowered vitality and impaired resistance to infection. He argued that Scottish asylums had a less steep rise in tuberculosis than English because the former had better food.[53]

However, the picture was more complicated: the rise outside the asylums in Scotland was also smaller than in England.[54] Elsewhere, diet and tuberculosis mortality showed poor correlation: in Germany, for example, severe wartime malnutrition was unaccompanied by a proportional rise in tuberculosis.[55] Returning to England, asylum death rates diminished post-war before the diet improved (Table 7.1),[56] also suggesting factors other than diet contributed to the tuberculosis death rate.

Workhouses in England had dietary regimes similar to those in asylums but did not experience a parallel escalation of tuberculosis. Before the war, many workhouses had vacancies,[57] and full employment in wartime may have emptied them further. Thus, although workhouses were requisitioned for military purposes like the asylums, those which remained as civilian facilities, did not suffer the same degree of overcrowding. Also, physical activity was strictly enforced in workhouses. This gave some protection against tuberculosis due to exercise being associated with better lung expansion. By contrast, asylums encouraged, but did not enforce, activity for people with severe chronic mental disorders such as schizophrenia and melancholia, for whom physical inertia may have increased their risk.[58]

Staff also risked contracting tuberculosis, but Mott could not demonstrate conclusively that they acquired it from patients.[59] All new staff were examined physically when they entered the asylum service. Some may have had undetectable, quiescent disease when they joined, and others may have acquired the infection while working there.[60] Staff also continued to work if the doctor decided that their disease was inactive,[61] and occasionally they died from the disease while still in service.[62] This raises questions of how ill and infectious a staff member might be while working with asylum patients. The LCC (General Powers) Act 1910 permitted asylum staff to receive sanatorium treatment, but this was not an option for patients. Asylum patients remained in the institution if they developed tuberculosis, but resident staff only remained there if their disease was considered unlikely to benefit from sanatorium treatment. Treatment for staff was inequitable with that for asylum patients, a situation unjustifiable on medical and public health grounds, but one to which the Lunacy Act contributed, because sanatoria were not licenced to accept certified lunatics. When a Banstead Asylum attendant, John Johnson, was too unwell to travel by rail to a sanatorium, the asylum paid 25s (£1.25p) to transfer him by car, and agreed to pay 35s a week for his in-patient treatment.[63] This weekly fee was over twice the amount spent on a patient in an asylum, suggesting that staff were regarded as valuable to the community compared to mentally unwell people who were frequently perceived as a long-term burden on the state.

In September 1918, Board leaders met with chief medical officer Sir Arthur Newsholme, to discuss the high death rate. Newsholme promised his department's cooperation.[64] The Board delegated three of its medical members, Sidney Coupland, Arthur Rotherham and Robert Branthwaite, to investigate asylums with the highest death rates. The Board exempted them from all other duties, a major decision when it was short-staffed.[65] They examined data up to and including 1917, thus excluding confounding mortality figures from the 1918–1919 influenza pandemic. They visited 26 asylums and compiled a short report in January 1919. They acknowledged non-war factors including asylum administration. They reiterated previously identified theories about overcrowding and poor nutrition, and commented that staff were unable to recognise early stages of illness, nurse the patients, or have sufficient time to maintain ward cleanliness. They attributed inequitable food distribution to inexperienced or temporary attendants, although that is hard to believe: serving food was hardly a scientific or specifically nursing skill.[66] The Board acknowledged that War Office demands, such as transferring sick patients between asylums to create the war hospitals, could have contributed to the spread of infection.[67] It also considered relevant the effects of the bitterly cold winter of 1916–1917, coupled with unsuitable buildings, fuel shortages and inadequate ward heating, all causes outside the Board's direct control.[68] Overall, the Board's statements characteristically passed the buck, rather than arguing that it could have taken more responsibility for vulnerable people under its care. Some VCs ignored the Board's report.[69] However, the Board affirmed its faith in the VCs who had to deal with the many challenges, and stated that "Asylum Authorities are alive to these difficulties, and that, as far as possible, they will endeavour to improve existing conditions."[70] However, the long-term failure to implement changes to help control tuberculosis since Crookshank's paper, suggests that their hope was wishful thinking. Without the power to mandate changes or permit the asylums greater financial flexibility, the Board had little alternative but to trust the VCs.

Godias Drolet, a statistician, analysed patterns of death from tuberculosis during, before and after the war. He identified peaks of mortality in several European countries, including in Denmark, the Netherlands, Belgium, Ireland and the United Kingdom.[71] Tuberculosis mortality peaked in 1917–1918 in many countries whether or not involved directly in the conflict, and allowing for different methods of data collection and a degree of error.[72] After the war, community tuberculosis rates fell to a level which would have been predicted if the rise had not occurred. When the rate across England changed, so did that in the asylums. Why the death rate fell to below its pre-war level so rapidly is an unsolved mystery for which material changes do not fully account.[73]

Crammer argued that, in its zeal for the war effort, the Board "abandoned the patients whose care they were supposed to safeguard" and that it was responsible for the excess mortality.[74] Crammer focussed on nutrition, overcrowding and understaffing, but did not discuss many other factors including the neglected high rates of asylum tuberculosis pre-war; inadequate processes of, and responses to, disease notification; poor hygiene and ventilation; lack of heating and harsh winters; inexperienced and temporary staff; complacent leadership; tuberculosis epidemiology; and budgetary constraints. It is easy to blame the wartime authorities—the Board, VCs, MOHs, MPA and medical superintendents—who let much pass, but if blame is due, it also falls on those who for over a decade pre-war were complacent and failed to make any serious attempt to reduce asylum tuberculosis.

Tuberculosis at Claybury and Hanwell: Case Studies

Pre-war, Mott identified more tuberculosis at Claybury than in other LCC asylums, although figures were partly dependent on post-mortems for which interpretation varied between pathologists.[75] Despite Mott's evidence, Claybury's medical superintendent, Robert Armstrong-Jones, asserted in 1914 that during his two-decade leadership the "tuberculosis death-rate was smaller than that of most of the other London asylums".[76] Typically, the VC did not challenge their medical superintendent's analysis, which lessened the pressure on them to examine or improve asylum practices.

Mid-war, Claybury faced numerous senior staff changes. Armstrong-Jones retired in 1916 and the VC appointed a succession of acting medical superintendents. First, they promoted the senior assistant medical officer, Charles Ewart, but he died soon after. The second, Thomas Fennessy, also already on the staff, left to serve in the forces[77] and was killed when the steamer Leinster was torpedoed.[78] In mid-1917, the VC appointed Guy Barham from Long Grove Asylum. He had a broad clinical experience, having worked as resident medical officer in a general hospital and as emergency officer at the London Hospital, Whitechapel.[79] Other senior "acting" appointments included the head night attendant.[80] Matron Margaret Russell retired after 36 years' service,[81] and the steward left, suffering from mental problems.[82] The LCC research laboratories with their staff, including Mott, were relocated to the Maudsley Hospital.[83] The many changes of senior personnel may have destabilised asylum management, practices and monitoring, with adverse outcomes for patients.

Casting a new pair of eyes on Claybury, Barham noted some disturbing legacies from his predecessors suggesting low standards of care. Falls and "accidents" to patients were excessive, storage of dangerous drugs was unsafe, and observation of patients at risk of suicide was inadequate. In November 1917, he raised his concerns with the VC. A couple of months later, when an outbreak of dysentery caused 36 deaths, Barham took the unusual step, before seeking the VC's agreement, of asking the local authorities to suspend admissions temporarily.[84]

From late 1917, Claybury had almost 70 deaths each month (from all causes), compared to an average monthly death rate of 20 during the previous two decades.[85] In April 1918, the VC discussed an outbreak of typhoid and Barham announced that he was seeking advice from a public health expert, William Hamer, the LCC's MOH. Seeking external medical advice was rare: it might give the impression to the VC that a medical superintendent did not know how to do his job, making him vulnerable to criticism or dismissal. Barham and Hamer joined forces to investigate the deaths.[86] A lawyer, Lionel Shadwell, inspected Claybury in June 1918 on behalf of the Board, unaccompanied by a doctor. He noted the high death rate from "natural and ordinary" causes. He showed little concern about these deaths, noting that suicide and accident rates, which might require legal action, were acceptable. Overall, he described the asylum as "creditable".[87] Shadwell's comments give credence to the suggestion that legal Board members overlooked medical matters.

Deaths declined during the summer, attributed to the warmer weather. In September 1918, Barham warned that the temperature inside the building needed to be kept around 55–60 F (13–15°C), otherwise "a very high death rate may be expected."[88] A month later the VC minutes recorded: "With the approach of the cold weather, and the need for greater economy in the use of fuel even than last year, when the heating of the building was kept low, a continued high death rate seems inevitable."[89] Despite Barham's concern, the VC appeared blasé. Later in the year, Barham announced the recommendations from his and Hamer's study, largely reiterating those from earlier research which had been ignored. At the same meeting, the VC said that it would consider requesting up to 300 more tons of coal above the rationed level.[90] The war had just ended, but intense shortages persisted. No reasons for the VC's abrupt about-turn were stated, but Barham's and Hamer's report was likely to open the asylum to further scrutiny by the LCC.

Hanwell also appointed an acting medical superintendent in 1917: Alfred Daniel replaced Percy Baily who had been on the staff since 1890.[91] Like Barham at Claybury, Daniel challenged established customs and practices, and cautiously and humanely advocated for the needs of patients in a way which was not evident in the later years under Baily's control.[92] Increasing tuberculosis mortality at Hanwell (10 deaths in 1913, 49 in 1917) alarmed Daniel. He attributed this to insufficient ward ventilation ("the general stuffiness that prevailed today cannot be healthy"[93]), lack of time in the open air, and unhygienic habits: "they spit about the wards promiscuously, the sputum dries and is inhaled by the healthy."[94] Painted windows to comply with lighting restrictions prohibited opening them in the evenings, and lack of heating and insufficient bed linen discouraged opening them at night.[95] In April 1918 the VC and the asylum engineer agreed to Daniel's proposal to erect two "tuberculosis shelters" using scaffolding and tarpaulins, so at least some of the 58 known cases could sleep out of doors.[96]

For both recently appointed acting medical superintendents, Daniel at Hanwell and Barham at Claybury, their assertive proposals to improve conditions for patients did not fall on deaf ears. This raises questions about the asylums' leadership strategy. Lay VCs appeared overly respectful of the judgement and expertise of their own medical superintendents, who may, in their long-term jobs-for-life roles, have been "burnt-out", associated with apathy, at a time when confronted by additional wartime challenges.

OTHER INFECTIONS: DYSENTERY,
TYPHOID AND INFLUENZA

During the war, dysentery and other forms of infective diarrhoea increased in many, but not all, public asylums.[97] Advice about prevention and treatment included isolating patients, preferably in a separate building, disinfecting all items in contact with them, and prescribing small quantities of neat brandy orally and starch-and-opium enemas if diarrhoea was severe.[98] It is unclear whether the advice was followed at Colney Hatch in 1917 when 130 people caught dysentery, half of whom died.[99]

The Board was keen to discover why, according to Mott's records since 1902, some asylums had no dysentery, while in others it was endemic and in others intermittent.[100] In the community, dysentery was rare.[101] It was also rare in private mental hospitals,[102] pointing to the infection being a factor of the institution, rather than an intrinsic risk of mental disorder as proposed by degeneration theories of a single predisposition to both. Staff also caught it, including kitchen workers, with an alarming potential for transmitting it.[103] Dr. Shaw Bolton, subsequently medical superintendent and professor at Wakefield Asylum, learnt the hard way about its transmissibility while an assistant medical officer at Claybury:

> He had started his tea one afternoon in the medical officer's room, when he was sent for to go and see a patient who had suddenly collapsed, a woman. After seeing her he gave instructions for the usual treatment, and went back to finish his tea without first washing his hands. Five days later he had an unpleasant attack of dysentery. At Claybury, about 1900-1903, it was not the fashion to believe that sane persons could catch the disease![104]

The bacterium shigella was the usual causal agent of dysentery. Signs and symptoms included fever, stomach cramps, ulceration of the large intestine, haemorrhage and bloody diarrhoea.[105] In 1914, the Board funded research into its nature, prevention and treatment.[106] The research took place at Wakefield Asylum, then under Shaw Bolton's leadership, where dysentery had been endemic since the asylum opened in 1818.[107] The pathologist there, Harold Gettings, aimed to detect carrier status, preferably by a blood test since it was "impossible to get officers in large asylums" to test faeces, even where suitable laboratory facilities were available.[108] Gettings modelled his goal on other tests for detecting early infections and carrier states[109]: the tuberculin test for tuberculosis,

Wassermann test for syphilis, and Widal test for typhoid. Unfortunately, Gettings did not know that asymptomatic carrier status for dysentery was rare.[110] He also aimed to produce a vaccine to prevent the disorder, although a century on, this has still not been achieved.[111]

In 1915, the Medical Research Committee (MRC, predecessor of the Medical Research Council) criticised the Board for sponsoring Gettings' dysentery research, a physical illness. It did not understand the diversity and complexity of physical and mental conditions coexisting in the asylums, or that the Board wanted research to benefit patients directly and promptly. Around the same time, the War Office wanted the MRC to provide solutions for the crisis of dysentery affecting troops in the Dardanelles, so the MRC took over funding Gettings' research. This allowed the Board to use its resources for other projects with a more specific mental health focus. The Board and the MRC also created a longer-term plan of collaboration "to establish a wider national scheme for research into mental diseases".[112]

Typhoid (enteric fever), another infectious disorder, was also far more common in asylums than in the community.[113] As with tuberculosis and dysentery, typhoid affected staff and patients.[114] As with dysentery and tuberculosis, good hygiene and quarantining could help prevent transmission.[115] Typhoid carriers could be identified by the Widal test and immunisation was available, unlike the options for dysentery.[116] At risk patients, and staff such as laundry women dealing with foul linen, were offered and usually accepted immunisation, although occasionally one refused and succumbed to the infection.[117] Occasionally and unexpectedly, patients who were predicted to become long-stay, improved mentally after an episode of typhoid, allowing them to be discharged. This outcome reinforced the belief in overlapping aetiologies of mental and physical illnesses, giving rise to speculation about the effects of infection, inflammation and immunisation and the possibility of prevention and treatment of mental disorders.[118]

"Spanish" influenza, another devastating infection, added to wartime adversities. Influenza prevailed among soldiers on both sides of the conflict in spring 1918. In mid-1918, mortality from the disorder increased world-wide. The unusual summer timing of the first outbreak worried public health officials who predicted a second wave.[119] It came: the biggest and most fatal, in autumn 1918, and a third in spring 1919.[120] The magnitude and unexpectedness of the pandemic overshadowed the end of the war. The war took the lives of 10 million people, and the pandemic killed over 40 million world-wide. About 700,000 British soldiers were killed in the war, and 225,000 people died from 'flu in Britain, 70,000 in November 1918 alone.[121] The nation did its duty according to expectations inculcated into it during the war: it stoically "carried on". The Local Government Board in Whitehall, responsible for public health, did little apart from issuing an occasional memorandum.[122]

A combination of military and civilian hardships probably increased people's vulnerability to 'flu: insanitary trenches; overcrowded military ships and trains; women exhausted from war work plus their domestic chores; and a medical system largely geared to military needs. The 'flu was particularly lethal to young adults, but there was little association between mortality and social class or overcrowding in domestic dwellings. The Board was unable to explain the pattern of influenza incidence and mortality in the asylums. Eleven asylums had no deaths during the most devastating wave, including one asylum which otherwise had extremely high mortality rates.[123] In some, either men or women died, but not both.[124] At Claybury in November 1918, female staff were affected disproportionately more than male staff or patients and, along the lines of the example set by Barham at the time of the dysentery outbreak a few months earlier, the asylum took the precaution of suspending female admissions.[125] Some potentially harmful practices continued, such as certifying and transferring severely physically ill patients from the community and general hospitals to the asylums.[126] Some were so ill at the time of transfer that they died soon after. The Board advised against moving such patients, whose mental disturbances were probably due to delirium resulting from the 'flu. It used the opportunity to highlight the inadequacy of general hospital facilities, particularly for treating people with physical disorders whose associated mental impairment was likely to be temporary.[127]

Conclusions

Reflecting on the chronic high levels of asylum tuberculosis pre-war, and the tragedy of the devastation it caused during the war, psychiatrist Lionel Weatherly commented in 1919: "the death-rate of tuberculosis in our large asylums is a standing disgrace to our country, and I earnestly hope something will soon be done to mitigate this crying evil."[128] Managing infectious diseases in asylums was characterised by poor coordination, fragmented and poor communication and leadership indifference.

There were scientific uncertainties, but much was known and was not applied. The system was peppered with inequalities, unjustifiable on medical or public health grounds, such as providing sanatorium treatment for asylum staff but not for patients. This gives the impression of clinical decision-making being related to an individual's or a group's perceived social and economic value: staff were seen as workers who could contribute whereas mentally unwell people were a drain on resources. The focus on employment was compatible with the National Insurance Act 1911 which provided health insurance for breadwinners but not for their dependants.

Crammer asked why the Board failed to solve the problem of rising deaths. He answered that in its zeal for the war effort, the Board "did not try very hard" and it "abandoned" its patients.[129] The Board passed the buck on some health-related issues. It acted sluggishly on others. The culture was to make do and continue, to self-justify and not to seek more, although at some point that conflicted with the medical ethical principle of *primum non nocere*, first do no harm. The Board had a duty to ensure humane care in its asylums, but it appeared to lack the skills and assertiveness to tackle some of the tasks demanded of it. Its decisions at the beginning of the war may have been suitable for a short-term conflict—and many believed that was what it would be[130]—but evidence is lacking to suggest significant revision of plans in the context of a prolonged war. In addition, if Board inspections were to be meaningful, they needed to be undertaken by people who had sufficient clinical experience and judgement, otherwise they would fit the requirements of administrators rather than the needs of patients and staff.

Some well-established medical superintendents, despite their expertise, appeared complacent or burnt-out after two decades of consistently taking enormous responsibility. With complacent medical leadership, it is hardly surprising that the lay VCs ignored potentially relevant scientific findings which were difficult to weigh up and interpret. In contrast to the long-established medical superintendents at Claybury and Hanwell, their newly appointed replacements challenged the VCs and advocated more for their patients.

Excessive infections in asylums during the war were probably associated with a large pre-war reservoir of infective micro-organisms. This baseline helps explain their relative frequency and rise during the war compared to the same diseases in the general population. For tuberculosis, the authorities had failed to act on the advice of the MPA and others to attempt to reduce infection and mortality by any means known. Asylums knew what to do, but did too little, too late. Post-war, the Board made recommendations based on its report about asylum mortality, noting that war conditions alone did not account for the "alarming increase" in asylum sickness and that the asylums should improve their hygiene and public health measures.[131] It advised the asylums what to do, much as it and its predecessor, the Commissioners in Lunacy, had done unsuccessfully for over a decade pre-war. *Plus ça change, plus c'est la même chose.*

NOTES

1. Colney Hatch H12/CH/B/16/003 Case notes of female patients who died in 1918–1919 LMA.
2. Colney Hatch H12/CH/B/22/014 Autopsy book for female patients 1916–1918 LMA; Charles Mercier, *The Attendant's Companion: A Manual of the Duties of Attendants in Lunatic Asylums* (London: J and A Churchill, 1898), 76; *First Annual Report of the Board of Control, for the Year 1914 (BoC AR 1914)* (London: HMSO, 1916), Part 2, Hereford County and City Asylum 4 May 1914, 235.
3. William Stoddart, *Mind and Its Disorders* (London: Lewis, 1908), 424.
4. Stoddart, *Mind*, 421; Robert Branthwaite, *Some Observations on the Prevalence of Tuberculosis, Dysentery, and "Severe Diarrhoea" in Mental Hospitals* (London: HMSO, 1923); Patrick O'Doherty, "Some Features of the Recent Outbreak of Enteric Fever at Omagh District Asylum," *Journal of Mental Science (JMS)* 60 (1914): 76–81, 80.
5. Colney Hatch H12/CH/B/47/016 Letter to VC from Elsie's friend (name illegible), 30 April 1918 LMA.
6. Colney Hatch H12/CH/B/47/016 Reception orders, medical certificates, notices of death, discharge or removal and correspondence for female patients who died or were discharged or removed 1918, LMA.
7. *BoC AR 1914*, Part 2, Causes of deaths in all lunacy institutions, 87–98.
8. LCC LCC/MIN/00583 Meeting, 27 November 1917, 169 LMA.
9. *Sixth Annual Report of the Board of Control, for the Year 1919* (London: HMSO, 1920) (*BoC AR 1919*), Appendix A: 20.
10. John Crammer, "Extraordinary Deaths of Asylum Inpatients During the 1914–1918 War," *Medical History* 36 (1992): 430–441, 431.
11. Ayers Gwendoline, *England's First State Hospitals and the Metropolitan Asylums Board, 1867–1930* (London: Wellcome Institute of the History of Medicine, 1971), 230.
12. Waltraud Ernst, "The Limits of Comparison: Institutional Mortality Rates, Long-Term Confinement and Causes of Death During the Early Twentieth Century," *History of Psychiatry* 23 (2012): 404–18, 405.

13. *Fifth Annual Report of the Board of Control, for the Year 1918* (London: HMSO, 1919) (*BoC AR 1918*), Appendix B: 31–32.

14. *BoC AR 1914*, Part 2, Bucks Asylum 30 October 1914, 201.

15. Anon. *The LCC Hospitals: A Retrospect* (London: LCC, 1949), 105; Ernst, "The Limits of Comparison": 405.

16. Frederick Mott, "Tuberculosis in London County Asylums," *Archives of Neurology and Psychiatry from the Pathological Laboratory of the London County Asylums, Claybury, Essex* 4 (1909): 70–116, 84, 115; Jennifer Wallis, *Investigating the Body in the Victorian Asylum* (London: Palgrave Macmillan, 2017), 226; *Fourth Annual Report of the Board of Control, for the Year 1917* (London: HMSO, 1918) (*BoC AR 1917*), 15.

17. James Ritchie, "Hypertrophy and Atrophy," 217–23, in *Text-Book of General Pathology*, ed. MS Pembrey and James Ritchie (London: Edward Arnold, 1913), 219–20.

18. Hanwell H11/HLL/B/31/006 Post-mortem register, males, 1915–1917 LMA.

19. Colney Hatch H12/CH/B/23/013 Autopsy book for male patients 1916–1918 LMA.

20. Hanwell H11/HLL/B/31/006 Post-mortem register, males, 1915–1917 LMA.

21. BoC W/FM, 4 February 1920, 35 MH 50/48 TNA.

22. Claybury LCC/MIN/00948 Meeting, 26 April 1917, 88 LMA.

23. Hanwell LCC/MIN/01093 Meeting, 8 December 1913, 5–6 LMA.

24. Pamela Michael and David Hirst, "Recording the Many Faces of Death at the Denbigh Asylum, 1848–1938," *History of Psychiatry* 23 (2012): 40–51, 50.

25. Mott, "Tuberculosis in London County Asylums": 85.

26. Francis Crookshank, "The Frequency, Causation, Prevention, and Treatment of Phthisis Pulmonalis in Asylums for the Insane; Essay for Which Was Awarded the Bronze Medal of the Medico-Psychological Association, 1899," *JMS* 45 (1899): 657–83, 667.

27. Crookshank, "Frequency": 668.

28. Crookshank, "Frequency": 670.

29. Crookshank, "Frequency": 673–74.

30. William Menzies, "Some Points Connected with Tuberculosis in Asylums," *JMS* 51 (1905): 548–60.

31. Stoddart, *Mind*, 422.

32. Mott, "Tuberculosis in London County Asylums": 113, 116.

33. *BoC AR 1914*, Part 2, Upton Asylum 16 March 1914, 207.

34. Mott, "Tuberculosis in London County Asylums": 113, 116.

35. *BoC AR 1914*, Part 2, Salop Asylum 8 July 1914, 298; Plymouth Borough Asylum 22 May 1914, 374; BoC, "Food Allowances," 23 July 1918, 513 MH 51/239; John Murray, "Tuberculosis and World War

I," *American Journal of Respiratory and Critical Care Medicine* 192 (2015): 411–14, 413.

36. Murray, "Tuberculosis and World War": 411; BoC, letter to MSs, January 1915, MH 51/239 TNA.
37. Murray, "Tuberculosis and World War": 414; HL Rieder, *Epidemiologic Basis of Tuberculosis Control* (Paris: International Union Against Tuberculosis and Lung Disease, 1999).
38. *BoC AR 1914*, Part 2, North Wales Asylum 20 March 1914, 215; BoC, "Increased Annual Death Rate in Asylums," 15 January 1919 MH 51/239 TNA; Hanwell LCC/MIN/01098, 8 April 1918, 6–7 LMA; *BoC AR 1918*, 25.
39. *BoC AR 1914*, Part 2, Bexley Asylum 20 March 1914, 266; Northumberland Asylum 4 May 1914, 292.
40. *Third Annual Report of the Board of Control, for the Year 1916* (London: HMSO, 1917) (*BoC AR 1916*), 25–28.
41. Mercier, *Attendant's Companion*, 77–89. Anon. "Examination for Nursing Certificate," *JMS* 62 (1916): 644–45; *BoC AR 1914*, Part 2, Three Counties Asylum 16 June 1914, 195; Hants Asylum 6 November 1914, 233.
42. LCC LCC/MIN/00580 Meeting, 10 November 1914, 3 LMA.
43. Reginald Dudfield, "Reforms Needed in the Notification of TB," *Proceedings of the Royal Society of Medicine* (*Proc RSM*) 15 (1922): Section of Epidemiology and State Medicine, 75–92, 75.
44. Dudfield, "Reforms Needed": 78; Frank Spreat, *Report of the Medical Officer of Health for the Year 1914* (Friern Barnet Urban District Council, 1915), 3, 19.
45. Branthwaite, *Observations*, 3.
46. Public Health England, *Annual Tuberculosis (TB) Data for England and Wales, from 1913 Onwards* (2013), https://www.gov.uk/government/publications/tuberculosis-tb-annual-notifications-1913-onwards.
47. Branthwaite, *Observations*, 7–9.
48. Crammer, "Extraordinary": 430–31, 439.
49. *BoC AR 1917*, 23.
50. LCC LCC/MIN/00583 Meeting, 24 July 1917, 17 LMA.
51. BoC W/FM, 18 September 1918, 240–41 MH 50/46 TNA.
52. BoC, "Increased Annual Death Rate in Asylums," 15 January 1919, 532 MH 51/239 TNA.
53. Crammer, "Extraordinary": 437.
54. Godias Drolet, "World War I and Tuberculosis: A Statistical Summary and Review," *American Journal of Public Health and the Nation's Health* 35 (1945): 689–97, 692.
55. Murray, "Tuberculosis and World War": 413; Drolet, "World War I and Tuberculosis": 690.

56. BoC W/FM, 14 May 1919, 117 MH 50/47 TNA.
57. Peter Higginbotham, *The Workhouse: The Story of an Institution*, "The Workhouse in Wartime," http://www.workhouses.org.uk/wartime/.
58. Mott, "Tuberculosis in London County Asylums": 78.
59. Mott, "Tuberculosis in London County Asylums": 115.
60. Mott, "Tuberculosis in London County Asylums": 73.
61. Claybury LCC/MIN/00948 Meetings, 13 September 1917, 195–96; 3 January 1918, 286 LMA.
62. LCC LCC/MIN/00583 Meeting, 24 July 1917, 16 LMA.
63. LCC LCC/MIN/00583 Meeting, 24 July 1917, 5–7 LMA.
64. BoC W/FM, 18 September 1918, 240–41 MH 50/46 TNA.
65. BoC W/FM, 9 October 1918, 262 MH 50/46 TNA.
66. BoC, "Increased Annual Death Rate in Asylums," 15 January 1919, 532 MH 51/239 TNA; *BoC AR 1917*, 23; Colney Hatch LCC/MIN/01003 Meeting, 18 December 1914, 215–16 LMA.
67. *BoC AR 1914*, Part 1, 15–16.
68. *BoC AR 1917*, 23.
69. Crammer, "Extraordinary": 437–38.
70. *BoC AR 1919*, 35.
71. Drolet, "World War I and Tuberculosis": 692.
72. Drolet, "World War I and Tuberculosis": 689.
73. Murray, "Tuberculosis and World War": 414.
74. Crammer, "Extraordinary": 441.
75. Mott, "Tuberculosis in London County Asylums": 74, 115.
76. Robert Armstrong-Jones in discussion on Harold Gettings, "Dysentery Past and Present," *JMS* 60 (1914): 39–56, 51.
77. Claybury LCC/MIN/00948 Meeting, 5 July 1917, 134–35 LMA.
78. Claybury LCC/MIN/00949 Meeting, 7 November 1918, 215 LMA; Sinking of Leinster, 10 October 1918, http://rmsleinster.com/.
79. *The Medical Directory 1917* (London: J and A Churchill, 1917).
80. Claybury LCC/MIN/00948 Meetings: 19 July 1917, 167–68; 22 November 1917, 254 LMA.
81. Claybury LCC/MIN/00949 Meeting, 26 March 1918 LMA.
82. Claybury LCC/MIN/00948 Meeting, 19 July 1917, 169 LMA.
83. LCC LCC/MIN/00582 Meeting, 25 July 1916, 26 LMA.
84. Claybury LCC/MIN/00948 Meetings: 8 November 1917, 242–45; 3 January 1918, 290–91 LMA; Claybury LCC/MIN/00949 Meeting, 28 February 1918, 9 LMA.
85. Claybury LCC/MIN/00949 Meeting, 12 September 1918, 169 LMA.
86. Claybury LCC/MIN/00949 Meetings: 25 April 1918, 44–45; 20 June 1918, 86–88 LMA.
87. Claybury LCC/MIN/00949 Meeting, 20 June 1918, 86–88 LMA.
88. Claybury LCC/MIN/00949 Meeting, 12 September 1918, 169 LMA.

89. LCC LCC/MIN/00584 Meeting, 29 October 1918, 25 LMA.
90. Claybury LCC/MIN/00949, 5 December 1918, 233, 238, 239 LMA.
91. *The Medical Directory 1890* (London: J and A Churchill, 1890).
92. Hanwell LCC/MIN/01097 Meeting, 17 December 1917, 253–54; LCC/MIN/01098 Meeting, 16 December 1918, 202–4 LMA.
93. *BoC AR 1914*, Part 2, Durham Asylum 8 May 1914, 222.
94. Hanwell LCC/MIN/01098 Meeting, 8 April 1918, 6–7 LMA.
95. Hanwell LCC/MIN/01096 Meeting, 9 October 1916, 200 LMA; Committee on the Administration of Public Mental Hospitals (Chairman: Sir Cyril Cobb) (Cobb Inquiry), 15 March 1922 Mr. Sale Q:664, 731, MH 58/219 TNA.
96. Hanwell LCC/MIN/01098 Meeting, 8 April 1918, 6–7 LMA.
97. *BoC AR 1916*, 22, 25.
98. Stoddart, *Mind*, 426.
99. Colney Hatch LCC/MIN/01007 Meeting, 12 July 1918, 111–12 LMA.
100. Sidney Coupland in adjourned discussion on Gettings, "Dysentery," (1914): 43; *BoC AR 1914*, Part 1, 31; Branthwaite, *Observations*, 15.
101. Harold Gettings, "Dysentery, Past and Present," *JMS* 59 (1913): 605–21, 605.
102. Branthwaite, *Observations*, 18.
103. Colney Hatch LCC/MIN/01007, 1 November 1918, 175 LMA.
104. J Shaw Bolton in adjourned discussion on Gettings, "Dysentery," (1914): 53.
105. Stoddart, *Mind*, 426–27.
106. Sidney Coupland, BoC, "Report on Replies to Circular Letter re: Scientific Research," 1914 MH 51/81 TNA.
107. J Shaw Bolton application for funding for study by Dr. Gettings, December 1914, MH 51/83 TNA.
108. J Shaw Bolton in adjourned discussion on Gettings, "Dysentery," (1914): 55.
109. J Shaw Bolton application for funding for study by Dr. Gettings, December 1914, MH 51/83 TNA.
110. Myron Levine, Herbert DuPont, Mohammed Khodabandelou, and Richard Hornick, "Long-Term Shigella-Carrier State," *New England Journal of Medicine* 288 (1973): 1169–71.
111. W Morley Fletcher and BoC, Meetings, 27 July, 21 September 1915 MH 51/86 TNA.
112. W Morley Fletcher and BoC, Meetings, 27 July, 21 September 1915 MH 51/86, and correspondence, 26 February, 4 March 1915 MH 51/85 TNA.
113. *BoC AR 1917*, 39.
114. Colney Hatch LCC/MIN/01006 Meeting, 15 June 1917, 192 LMA.

115. *BoC AR 1919*, 30.
116. Claybury LCC/MIN/00948 Meeting, 21 June 1917, 125–26 LMA.
117. Colney Hatch LCC/MIN/01007 Meeting, 22 February 1918, 36 LMA; LCC LCC/MIN/00583 Meeting, 30 July 1918, 684 LMA.
118. O'Doherty, "Enteric Fever": 80.
119. Arthur Newsholme, "Discussion on Influenza," *Proc RSM* 12 (1919): General Reports, 1–18, 12.
120. NPAS Johnson, "The Overshadowed Killer: Influenza in Britain in 1918–19," 132–155, in *The Spanish Influenza Epidemic of 1918–19*, ed. Howard Phillips and David Killingray (London: Routledge, 2003), 132.
121. Johnson, "Overshadowed Killer": 132, 134.
122. Johnson, "Overshadowed Killer": 142, 150–51.
123. *BoC AR 1918*, 18.
124. *BoC AR 1919*, 31–32.
125. Claybury LCC/MIN/00949 Meeting, 5 December 1918, 241 LMA.
126. Claybury LCC/MIN/00948 Meeting, 3 January 1918, 286 LMA.
127. LCC LCC/MIN/00584 Meeting, 28 January 1919, 211–12 LMA; Tom Williams, "The Management of Confusional States with Special Reference to Pathogenesis," *JMS* 63 (1917): 389–400.
128. Lionel Weatherly, "The Incidence of Tuberculosis Amongst Asylum Patients," *Lancet* 6 September 1919, 456–57.
129. Crammer, "Extraordinary": 437, 441.
130. Imperial War Museum, "Voices of the First World War: Over by Christmas," (2018), https://www.iwm.org.uk/history/voices-of-the-first-world-war-over-by-christmas.
131. BoC, "Increased Annual Death Rate in Asylums," 15 January 1919, 532 MH 51/239 TNA.

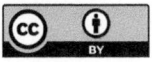

CHAPTER 8

Accidents, Injuries, Escapes and Suicides

INTRODUCTION: A CULTURE OF KINDNESS OR HARM?

"The asylum exists for the benefit of the patients" Charles Mercier reminded staff when he summarised the approach they needed to take: to be kind, courteous, sympathetic, tactful, and not overbearing or bullying; to "cheer the unhappy", "soothe the excited" and "make peace between the quarrelsome".[1] Staff must never threaten, tease or frighten, mock, jeer, insult, disparage or deceive a patient, lose one's temper with or strike a patient or punish one in any way.[2] Mercier spelled this out because he was aware of harsh practices. He instructed staff (bold in the original), that: **"under no circumstances whatever should a patient be knelt on**. More broken ribs and broken breastbones are due to this practice than to all other circumstances put together".[3] Staff struck patients, but according to one wartime staff member, "the attendant who knows his business seldom leaves a mark on the patient he abuses", a state of affairs also referred to by Louise Hide in her study of late-Victorian and Edwardian asylums.[4] One former patient reported that when he dared to criticise his attendants, they punished him with concealable torments, including giving him strong laxatives, placing a live earwig in his porridge and heavily over-salting his soup then laughing when he spat it out.[5] Another former patient who became an attendant, described his colleagues as unsympathetic and harsh. He noted their abusive language, which he attributed to them being "under the delusion that almost

© The Author(s) 2021
C. Hilton, *Civilian Lunatic Asylums During the First World War*,
Mental Health in Historical Perspective,
https://doi.org/10.1007/978-3-030-54871-1_8

everything in the universe was composed of blood", repeatedly using a word "which rhymes with ruddy": "You have read of Moses and the old time necromancers of Egypt turning water into blood. They could turn everything into blood."[6]

Rachel Grant-Smith wrote about her experiences as an asylum patient. She alleged brutality and degrading nursing practices. She described being "forced" to take laxatives, for her "bad behaviour", and unless she cooperated "it meant my being forcibly laid down and three or four nurses pulling my mouth open and pouring it down."[7] She observed distressing scenes:

> Fanny Black and Miss Hurd were made to sit out of bed on the chamber utensil many hours in the night, quite naked, often for an hour at a time. Miss Hurd has lately died from consumption. A young nurse, named Green, promised me, after I had spoken to her about ill-treating patients, that she would not do it again, and subsequently told me that she would get into trouble for not kicking a patient, Mrs. Beverley, to keep her quiet when told by Nurse Rooke to do so.[8]

The British periodical *Truth* published a summary of Grant-Smith's report in July 1914.[9] Conveniently for the authorities, it disappeared from the public agenda when national priorities supervened.

The terms "rough handling" and "rough usage" appeared frequently in minutes and reports of the asylums' Board of Control ("the Board").[10] However, with reports from staff and patients usually given credence in a hierarchical fashion, if a patient alleged rough handling and a staff member denied it, the patient was rarely believed.[11] Staff expected each other to conform to their unwritten peer group rules of loyalty to colleagues, which included collusion in the event of a complaint. Inconsistencies in reports between patients and staff, and often agreement between ward staff of the same grade, suggest that loyalty to colleagues took precedence over patients' wellbeing.[12] Some of these issues, and some others, are illustrated by an incident in the life of Edith B, a 42-year-old schoolteacher admitted to Colney Hatch in 1913 (Fig. 8.1).[13] Edith had a psychotic illness and her "certified cause of insanity" was "religious mania".[14] In July 1915, her doctor wrote:

Fig. 8.1 Edith B, soon
after admission
(Photographs of female
patients at Colney
Hatch 1908–1918
H12/CH/B/18/003
LMA)

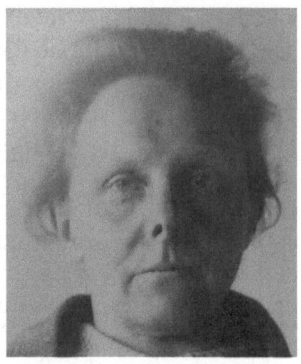

She is very grandiose and exalted and believes that she is the Virgin Mary
and that the archangel has visited her and greeted her with "Hail, Mary,
full of grace." She states that she had a child afterwards. She is excitable,
garrulous and spiteful and entirely irrelevant in conversation. She is in fair
health.

Sometimes she "could feel the Holy Child leave her womb." Edith's clinical notes recorded ups and downs. Occasionally they mentioned injuries,
allegedly inflicted by other patients, on one occasion a black-eye, and on
another, cuts which required stitching. Later she had scabies, a skin condition associated with an unhygienic environment. Her delusions persisted,
and she gradually became "demented, solitary, unemployable."[15]

In 1916, Edith reported that Nurse H hit her. Edith had a bruised
face. Clear that something had happened, the visiting committee (VC)
investigated. The nurse denied hitting Edith but admitted to pushing her
in the lavatories (a common location for displays of anger, out of sight of
others[16]) and Edith hit her face on one of the partitions. Nurse H apol-
ogised and said that she "did not mean to be rough". Nurse K, a more
senior staff member, witnessed the incident, and gave another account,
that Nurse H took hold of Edith by her neck in a very rough manner but
did not strike her. Each person told a different story.

The VC insisted that Nurse H resign although it could have dismissed
her.[17] Resignation was less harsh than dismissal. It was less damaging
to her reputation if she sought another job, and it did not entail
her forfeiting her superannuation contributions. The minutes did not
mention her previous work record and her apology appears to have been

taken as an admission of guilt rather than an indication of remorse. The same VC adjudicated over allegations about another nurse in similar circumstances a few months later. In that case, the VC cautioned her as they were sure that she "had no intention of being unkind to the patients but that she must, in future, on such occasions be most careful in handling the patients".[18] The VCs' inconsistency in dealing with misdemeanours contributed to staff insecurity and their lack of trust in the leadership.[19]

Edith's story demonstrates some of the challenges faced by asylum authorities when trying to deal with untoward incidents, whether "accidents" or injuries, escapes or suicides. This chapter aims to bring together components of asylum life—the patients, senior and junior staff, the public, the law, the Board and the VCs—to create a broad picture about what happened when things went wrong. There are drawbacks, in that much of the material is necessarily anecdotal with inconsistencies and contradictions. However, cases provide enough evidence to identify patterns of attitudes, behaviours and decision making, from which conclusions can be drawn.

ABUSE IN THE ASYLUMS: ALLEGATIONS AND OUTCOMES

Most VC members had no specific training to help them evaluate allegations of abuse or maltreatment, although a few could draw upon their experience as magistrates. The VCs were often bewildered by inconsistent, contradictory and vague evidence, particularly from patients who changed their original statements.[20] They attributed this inconsistency to their mental disturbance being all-encompassing, a medically acceptable perspective. According to Mercier, "they are out of their minds and not responsible for what they do or say", even when their delusions and hallucinations were unrelated to the subject in hand.[21] Allegations made on their behalf by relatives or friends were considered similarly contaminated because of their source.

Evidence has not come to light that VCs or superintendents raised the possibility that inconsistent reports from patients were associated with them fearing repercussions from the staff they accused. Indications that this happened include a newspaper report, some years before the war, about the inquest into the death of Charles Andrews who sustained rib fractures while a patient at Colney Hatch. It stated that he had told his wife that he "had 'been knocked about' for an act which he could not help, but he would not tell her by whom" suggesting that he feared retribution if he exposed maltreatment by staff.[22] Patients' fear was also likely to have been a factor in the VC's investigations into allegations that Attendant Frampton indecently assaulted young male patients in his charge. The patients had to give evidence in front of the accused. Evidence was conflicting, with some allegations "forgotten". The confusing picture led the VC to conclude that the allegations were false.[23] Shortly after, Frampton was arrested and charged with indecent exposure to some boys in Finsbury Park. The similarities between the behaviours supported the reality of the patient' allegations, but only then was Frampton dismissed from asylum employment. Scandalous allegations by patients, especially when accompanied by contradictory evidence, were particularly unlikely to be believed.[24]

Staff as well as patients might "forget" incidents. When allegations arose about Attendant Orton hitting and injuring a patient, both parties "forgot" what happened. Orton absconded from Colney Hatch, resulting in automatic dismissal and forfeit of his superannuation contributions.[25] Police traced him to Portsmouth, with the result that the asylum wrote to him about their concerns: the return of his uniform and keys. Nothing further was heard from him until he reappeared at Colney Hatch, seeking repayment of his superannuation. He maintained that he had no memory of any misdemeanours.[26] Sir John Collie, medical examiner for the London County Council (LCC) and author of a book on malingering, examined Orton and declared his memory loss genuine, thus salvaging the superannuation.[27] Other incidents did not end so well for the alleged perpetrator.

In addition to patients' words lacking credibility, so too did those of junior staff who were placed only just above patients in the asylum hierarchy. In consequence, after an untoward event, juniors were more likely to be disciplined than the seniors under whom they worked. This can be illustrated by the events around Mrs. I, a patient at Colney Hatch who was "under continuous observation because of suicidal tendencies." A probationer nurse, new to the ward that morning, was delegated to look after Mrs. I when the ward's qualified staff went to breakfast, but Mrs. I managed to break the glass door of a medicine cupboard and took a fatal dose of camphor. At the investigation, the qualified staff said they had told the new nurse specifically to look after Mrs. I, although there were no witnesses to that from outside their circle. The asylum informed the Board, which concluded that the new nurse was "careless and incapable", and recommended to the VC that it "terminated her engagement."[28] There is no record about whether the Board questioned the appropriateness of the established staff in delegating responsibility to a probationer, or what they actually told her about Mrs. I. Staff closed ranks, and the words of those more senior prevailed, as if trustworthiness and judgement automatically increased with status.

Asylums provided different degrees of detail about their investigations into untoward events. However, minutes hint at clandestineness, such as when the VC at Colney Hatch decided to inform the Board about an incident only if asked directly. If that happened, it would report that the asylum had dispensed with the nurse's services, and "as all the corroborative evidence has been by patients, it is doubtful whether a conviction would be obtained."[29] Despite the recurring pattern of institutional secrecy in some cases of ill treatment, "wilful neglect" or allowing a patient to escape sometimes prompted the Board to contact the Director of Public Prosecutions.[30] Penalties for a member of staff found guilty of a misdemeanour under the Lunacy Act 1890 included imprisonment or a fine of up to £20.[31] This was a hefty punishment considering that a ward attendant's salary (after deductions for uniform and "living in") was under £40 a year.[32] If a case went to court, publicity was almost inevitable, risking criticism about the asylum and its leadership and creating a "blot on the copy book for what the asylums sought to provide".[33] Mercier emphasised that a lapse in staff vigilance could result in "catastrophe": injury or death to those under their care, and disaster to their own career.[34] For many male staff who lived in tied cottages with their families this was a huge concern, as dismissal or imprisonment would also wreck the lives of their family. Fear of the consequences probably contributed to staff perpetuating cultures of secrecy and dishonesty.[35]

Another mechanism of concealment occurred after altercations when attendants failed to follow instructions to "report the occurrence immediately to the Medical Officer" even if "in the attendant's own opinion no injury had been caused to the patient."[36] Sometimes in these circumstances the patient died, the injury being more serious than the attendant surmised. A doctor's examination of the patient soon after an incident could help clarify the course of events. The patient's words might be believed if they were compatible with the clinical findings, and while superficial injury such as red marks, bruises or scratches were still in evidence, they could indicate the recent timing of the injury. Without that early assessment, possibly fatal internal injuries identified later were unlikely to be attributed to a particular attendant or shift, providing a degree of immunity for the perpetrator.

Despite secrecy around episodes of rough handling, patients could be remarkably up to date with asylum news which might then spread further afield, creating gossip and disrepute about the asylum and its leadership.[37] Short visiting times, ward staff reading patients' out-going letters, and most new junior staff being required to live-in helped guard against this. In addition, with time, both patients and staff could become institutionalised, moulded into the system and minimising protest, although, unlike the patients, staff who were uncomfortable with the regime were free to leave. Occasionally someone contacted an external body, placing an asylum's reputation on a knife edge of publicity, as at Colney Hatch in the case of a 33-year-old Spanish patient, Juan R, recorded as dying from "rupture of intestine caused by falling against a table."[38] Officially categorised as an accident, this seems an unlikely explanation since, in a fall, reflex contraction of powerful abdominal muscles would help protect internal organs from blunt trauma, a matter learnt, if not in anatomy classes at medical school, then on the sports field. There was no mention of loss of consciousness preceding the injury, which might have prevented reflex muscle action. If the patient had lost consciousness, the alleged perpetrators would probably have mentioned it in their defence. A patient-witness stated that two attendants had treated Juan roughly, but the attendants denied it, and staff words over-rode those of patients. However, someone wrote to the Spanish Consul General, asserting that a Spanish patient had been murdered in the asylum, prompting the consul to contact the asylum. The VC minutes only tell us that the medical superintendent was due to meet the consul, and in common with documentation of other complaints, they lack detail of the discussion and outcome.[39] It is likely that the superintendent reassured the consul that patients' were unreliable witnesses and that his attendants were, in words similar to those of the Board, "as humane and deserving a body of workers as can be found".[40]

In contrast to assumptions that staff were humane, patients were assumed to be irresponsible, untrustworthy and sometimes dangerous, requiring stringent safety precautions. Some precautions were obvious, such as ensuring the safe keeping of brooms, broken chairs, fire pokers and roller towels which could be used as weapons against self or others.[41] Others limited the freedom of patients, many of whom did not require the measures but were subject to them nevertheless. They could be condescending, such as routinely counting patients in and out when being escorted between ward and work-place.[42] The value of others which were demeaning were debated, such as staff searching patients' clothes every night to check for concealed home-made weapons, perhaps a stone or other hard object in a sock, stocking or handkerchief.[43] When implemented as blanket precautions, rather than protecting patients and staff, they could hinder patients' self-confidence, self-esteem and (re)building of healthy social relationships necessary for achieving the best possible quality of life, whether inside or outside the asylum. The Board, however, supported many of these practices, erring on the side of caution, even though, for some patients, this contradicted its stated objective of providing as near normal a life as possible.

The authorities were alert to the problem that abuse and injury was not all one-way, and that, from time to time, staff sustained injuries at the hands of patients.[44] Most injuries to staff were minor but occasionally they could be life threatening, news of which sometimes reached the local or national press.[45] Newspaper reports could reinforce and perpetuate stereotypes of dangerous lunatics who needed to be confined to asylums, alongside gratitude and admiration of the asylums and their dedicated staff who endured such treatment. Some staff lost their jobs following injury, such as a probationer nurse who sustained a detached retina after being hit by a patient because "the loss of sight to an eye precludes the employee from being an efficient nurse".[46] Another nurse was too nervous to return to work after a patient injured her ear. She sought compensation, for which the asylum was liable under the Workmen's Compensation Act 1897.[47] No details are given of the ear injury, but "compensation neurosis" or "trauma neurosis", was recognised pre-war, including minor physical injury triggering mental symptoms which recovered on securing a financial settlement.[48] In contrast, the psychological consequences of physical abuse of patients appeared to be disregarded.

Louise Hide commented that it was impossible to quantify how often physical altercations occurred on the wards, among patients, between patients and staff, and among staff. Minor incidents which were resolved at ward level were unlikely to reach the ears of the VC, let alone the Board.[49] Nevertheless, the Board admitted to having to deal with allegations of brutality inflicted by attendants "almost daily and sometimes had to prosecute."[50] This comment was made in the context of the Board's response to concerns about asylums practices which Leonard Winter, a temporary wartime attendant, had raised with the Society of Friends and the National Council for Lunacy Reform. The response indicated that the Board knew about ill-treatment and that it proposed disciplinary measures, a "bad apple" approach, removing individual staff who were considered undesirable in order to prevent spread of sub-standard practice to others.

Brutality towards vulnerable individuals was (and is) never acceptable, but if "almost daily" meant five times in a working week, that amounted to 250 incidents a year known to the Board affecting an asylum patient population of 100,000. This estimate may be the tip of the iceberg, but it also fits with anecdotal evidence given by former patients to the Cobb Inquiry into asylum practices. They described their attendants' behaviours in a variety of ways which suggest that physical abuse was neither an inevitable nor daily part of a patient's asylum experience. One patient recalled that he "never saw the attendants use more force on a man than was absolutely necessary for the way the man was acting".[51] Another described them as "decent Englishmen who do their best for everybody".[52] Others noted variable degrees of benevolence:

> some I found good,...did what they thought best for the patients; they are the salt of the institution. Then there is a second class who...do as little work as possible and do anything to make it a comfortable job....And the third class, who are frankly brutal.[53]

The middle group were the majority, more likely to demonstrate "indifference and callousness" rather than malice.[54] Overall, it appears reasonable to conclude that most patients were not physically victims of brutality most of the time. However, it is harder to be conclusive about the extent of the emotional harm caused to them by experiencing, witnessing or hearing about abuse. It is still harder to determine the frequency of non-physical bullying and infringements of human dignity, such as bad language from staff ("I heard more filthy language in the asylum than in the slums of Liverpool and London"[55]). Bad language was unlikely to have been used in the presence of seniors and left no visible scratches or bruises.

Broken Bones and Cauliflower Ears: Facts and Fictions

In the contested narrative of harm to patients and the reputation of asylums, theories of fragile bones, haematoma auris (popularly termed "cauliflower ear") and status lymphaticus (discussed in Chapter 3) emerged to explain injury and sudden death. For two of the conditions, Latin names added authority; fragile bones did not acquire one, probably because "fragilitas ossium" was already used to describe a hereditary syndrome which presented in childhood.[56] Injuries sustained by patients demanded explanations which, from the perspective of staff and leadership, preferably laid the responsibility for them on patients rather than staff. Scientific theories assisted with this.

Emerging concepts of accident proneness and hypotheses that insane patients had generally fragile bones gained ground in the late nineteenth century, helping to deflect blame from staff accused of heavy-handed restraint or deliberate injury to patients.[57] Well-reasoned explanations, at a time of enthusiasm about scientific medical breakthroughs, could convince professionals and public. The fragile bone hypothesis was timely, coinciding with other discoveries about bone abnormalities, such as the effects of poor diet and lack of sunshine,[58] but distinguishing between science and supposition was tricky, partly due to research and statistical methodology. Not all authorities concurred that asylum patients had fragile bones.[59] Charles Macnamara, a medically qualified polymath writing in the late nineteenth and early twentieth centuries, was unconvinced by fragile bone theories accounting for injuries. His investigations into bone strength failed to identify anything to support increased fragility compared to sane people of the same age:

> It seems to me more probable that when several of the ribs are found to be fractured during life, or after death, in the case of lunatics, it is not impossible that the injury has been caused by the attendants kneeling on the patients' chests to keep them from moving [and it was] just as likely to happen…to a person in sound health as to one in an insane condition.[60]

Psychiatrist Lionel Weatherly also expressed scepticism of the fragility hypothesis alongside outrage about insufficient penalties imposed on attendants found to have broken a patient's ribs. He remarked scathingly: "We have Societies for the protection of children, cats, dogs and horses;

they are sent to prison. We find an attendant is fined £2 for breaking the ribs of a patient".[61] One late-nineteenth century newspaper report proposed that, in the absence of direct evidence of any other cause, asylum deaths associated with rib fractures should incur an automatic manslaughter charge against the attendant.[62] Jennifer Wallis commented that the Scottish physician, William Lauder Lindsay, argued that the disappearance of mechanical means of restraint during the nineteenth century had increased the risk of injury due to attendants single-handedly trying to restrain patients or convey them into a seclusion room.[63] Lauder's conclusion was cited by a colleague in France: "if England *is* the country of non-restraint, it is also the country of broken ribs".[64]

Regarding training for medical students and doctors in the subject of fractures and other injuries associated with insanity, one textbook of psychiatry which discussed physical conditions to which insane people were considered liable, mentioned neither fragile bones nor haematoma auris.[65] Similarly, some general textbooks of medicine and surgery did not mention them.[66] Other textbooks, such as Norman Barnett's surgical compendium, warned that "Lunatics are subject to fractures without marked cause, attendants often being wrongly blamed for having caused them." It gave reasons why asylum patients might have fragile bones, such as tuberculosis and syphilis.[67] However, neither caused generally fragile bones, and their circumscribed lesions were rare in ribs and would have been detectable at post-mortem.[68] Overall, there is little evidence that tuberculosis or syphilis would have accounted for the frequency of fractures.[69] Later, Edward Hare, a mid-twentieth century psychiatrist, recalled his experience of working with patients with brain syphilis (general paralysis of the insane, GPI): he "never met one with fractured ribs and [did not] recall reading or being told that this was a complication to be looked for."[70] If rib fractures were even a rare direct complication of GPI, it is likely that some echoes of them would have continued to appear in textbooks as something about which practitioners should be aware. More likely, GPI caused disturbed behaviours which made the patient liable to excessive force which was used punitively or during manual restraint by insufficiently trained and exasperated staff.

It is hard to believe that the deaths of Henry M at Portsmouth Asylum, attributed to a fracture of the wrist, or of Lucy R at Bristol, with a fractured forearm following a struggle with a nurse, told the whole story.[71] These relatively minor injuries were unlikely to have been fatal, unless complications ensued, such as untreatable infection. Should that have happened, it is likely that staff or VCs would have referred to it as an exonerating factor. The practice of not informing the asylum doctor about an altercation soon after it happened, plus reduced numbers of post-mortems during the war, may have resulted in only obvious injuries being recorded and more serious internal injuries remaining undetected. The fragility hypothesis allowed VCs to acknowledge that struggles took place between patients and staff, but to draw the conclusion that injury was due to physical vulnerability associated with insanity, and that the force used was appropriate to the degree of disturbed behaviour caused by their mental state.[72] The Board probably over-trusted VCs' analyses about injuries and failed to probe objectively. If a VC set out a convincing case, coroners tended to concur, recording a verdict of death by misadventure rather than manslaughter.[73]

Haematoma auris was another condition directly attributed to insanity. As Russell Barton, a medical superintendent in the 1960s, described:

> when I introduced the course for senior charge nurses I explained to them the curious condition known as auris haematoma, which was a big red swelling of the ear which usually occurred a little while before the patient died, and it was thought to be the blood pushed out of the brain. And so I explained this...
> the big market where they sold cattle and stuff. You see when they move a calf from one stall to another - 'e don't go calm like! So ya' grab 'im ba' the ears and ya pull 'is tail and then e's gotta go where ya' push 'im – and 'e does!
> And of course it immediately rang a bell.[74]

Haematoma auris occurred more commonly on the left than the right, suggesting that it was caused by the right hand of a person facing the patient and giving a blow, or using that hand to lead them by the ear. Hare explained that the disorder was most common in patients with the most disturbed behaviours. He referred to one asylum where attendants were held responsible for it and the condition disappeared.[75]

True accidents could happen, manual handling of patients could be inadvertently harsh, but excessive force could also be applied deliber-ately, disproportionate to the patient's needs. Too often the leadership turned a blind eye to the possibility of malicious injury. Medical-scientific explanations attributing injury to a patient's inherent predisposition were acceptable to public and professionals and allowed the asylum leader-ship to exonerate staff, reassure the public of the adequacy of the care provided, and preserve the reputation of their institution, even when treatment was detrimental to the patients.[76]

ESCAPES

Patients discussed how to escape from asylums. At Hanwell, rumours were rife that the easiest way was to take advantage of low lighting levels at night while the main door was unlocked in order to enable evacuation in the event of a direct hit in an air raid. Only one patient, Alice B, was reported to have escaped this way, almost two years after the unlocked door policy began.[77] Montagu Lomax discussed issues around escape and patients' freedom of movement, noting that in some mental hospitals in other countries, many patients had "parole" of the grounds. Patients with parole seldom abused the privilege and, as at Hanwell, unlocked doors did not equate with attempted mass exodus. Lomax argued that the freedom of parole was "a restorer of hope and self-confidence to minds sadly in need of both" and that "It is not those patients who are most trusted who attempt to escape, it is those who despair of ever getting out, and who are reckless in consequence."[78] Lomax agreed with Mary Riggall, that patients on parole felt their discharge imminent so did not want to endanger its realization. In her own case, she was aware that any actions deemed misbehaviour could be misconstrued as part of her insanity and jeopardise her discharge, so she decided against trying to escape.[79]

The term "escape" was used in the Lunacy Act 1890 which stipulated:

> If any manager, officer, or servant of an institution for lunatics wilfully permits, or assists, or connives at the escape or attempted escape of a patient, or secretes a patient, he shall for every offence be liable to a penalty not exceeding twenty pounds nor less than two pounds.[80]

The Act also required an asylum to search for its missing patient for 14 days, after which time, if still at liberty, the patient was declared not insane and could no longer be detained under the original order.[81] Without outside help, such as advice, plans or money,[82] dressed in asylum clothes, almost penniless, and miles from home, a successful escape suggested that the patient was desperate alongside having courage, ingenuity and organisational skills. One patient climbed down a ward stack-pipe after throwing his bundle of clothes outside, another removed a window pane and lowered himself to the ground on knotted sheets.[83]

Mr. K helped his wife Elizabeth to escape, by walking out from Colney Hatch with her at the end of visiting time. He posted her asylum-owned clothes back to the asylum from Peterborough, with an address-less covering note explaining that she was doing well.[84] Possibly inspired by Elizabeth's success, two months later, Bertha B absconded with her visitor. She too went to a secret location.[85]

Some escapees were "recaptured", a word usually applied to criminals or animals, with language reinforcing notions that patients were dangerous.[86] Napsbury noted that of its eight escapees in 1914, four were recaptured within the 14-day time limit.[87] Often, a local person, sometimes a child, brought them back. Local people accepted the patients as needing help, although the expectation of a half-a-crown (12½p) reward might have encouraged them to assist. A sympathetic local acceptance of asylum patients was inconsistent with a more negative wider public understanding about them. VCs, however, had different concerns when patients escaped: one VC was less bothered about the escapee's wellbeing than about the asylum clothing he wore at the time, listing each item, including under-garments, which would have to be replaced.[88]

Escapes from asylums were uncommon, the Board's data indicating that a dozen or so of 100,000 detained patients escaped each week.[89] During the war, one medical superintendent commented that it was "extraordinary that accidents and escapes are so few in number seeing that our temporary staff are by no means in the prime of life, many in fact are elderly".[90] In addition to using the term "accidents" to mean "injuries" which the authorities deemed to be accidental, the statement indicated that asylums preferred to employ younger staff, partly because of their physical abilities. This gives insight into the leadership's perceptions of acceptable ways of managing disruptive patients. The possibility that older male staff, or women nurses working on male wards, could use non-physical methods successfully to manage disturbed patients, received little consideration. Neither did the low rate of escapes prompt an honest review of the feasibility of unlocking more doors. In the conservative and risk-averse culture of the asylum leadership, the easiest course was to not ask too many questions or make suggestions which might rock the boat. Occasionally, an escape ended in suicide,[91] an outcome which the authorities could use to further justify their caution.

SUICIDES

Before the war, the suicide rate for England and Wales was approximately one in 10,000 of the general population (all ages), about 3500 people a year.[92] In 1914, of around 100,000 patients certified under the Lunacy Act, there were 34 suicides nationally, about three in 10,000.[93] Twelve of these took place after certification, mainly in workhouse infirmaries, before transfer to an asylum.[94] Two occurred when on trial leave and two after escape, leaving 18 who were patients within the asylums at the time,[95] a figure little more than in the general population outside.

If asylum suicide rates were as low as reported, we need to understand how people of high risk of suicide were managed in the asylums. Anne Shepherd and David Wright's study of two asylums to the west of London revealed that between one quarter and one third of patients were classified as suicidal on admission. Vigilance was the main treatment, or sedation, particularly in understaffed asylums.[96] Mercier advised that "a suicidal patient must never be allowed out of sight" although the Board disputed this, recognising that a balance had to be achieved as constant supervision could also be detrimental to recovery.[97] Some of the practical aspects of observing patients were discussed in Chapter 6, such as the absence of doors on lavatories. However, to facilitate observation, adequate communication between staff was essential, as in the case of Mrs. I. To this end, asylums were expected to implement a standard procedure. Each "suicidally disposed patient" would have a separate "caution parchment" which the staff member responsible for observing the patient was expected to read, understand and sign, handing it on to the colleague taking over at the end of the shift or if the patient was moved to another location.[98] Textbooks also provided valid advice: if the patient was melancholic, "Favourite hours for suicides to make their attempts are the early hours"[99] and "the experienced nurse is always suspicious of the happy smiling face that conceals a heavy heart. Be especially watchful over such patients and also over convalescent patients".[100]

Suicide and "attempted suicide" were criminal acts until 1961.[101] This legal status could lead to concealment of the act, which could not only affect statistics, but more importantly would impact on the help sought by and offered to distressed and despairing people. The criminal designation of attempted suicide meant that the Home Office delegated to the police the responsibility for ensuring that the offence was not repeated. The police did not want this responsibility and considered it a medical duty;

the asylums did not want the person if they had physical injuries; neither did the general hospitals, on the grounds that they lacked the skills to calm a disturbed patient. These disputes about responsibility overlapped with financial concerns, as close observation was also costly.[102] Each organisation tried to pass the buck and responded in a way which was detrimental to the wellbeing of the troubled human being who required help.

In contrast to the police view, William Norwood East, a forensic psychiatrist during the war years, regarded conviction for attempted suicide as an effective way to secure appropriate treatment: for people not sufficiently insane to be certified, a prison hospital could provide rest, good food, quiet, and medical attention. It also provided a fixed period of detention, unlike Lunacy Act certification which risked an indeterminate period in an asylum. Once a prisoner, a second court appearance would precede release, allowing review of the situation. Another advantage was that more philanthropic resources were available to criminals released from prisons than lunatics discharged from asylums, including material assistance and help to secure employment.[103] This philanthropic provision fitted with Jose Harris's analysis that "late Victorian lower classes preferred to be thought bad rather than mad",[104] and that for the suicidal person and his family, a criminal record balanced favourably against the stain of lunacy certification. According to East, very few of those convicted returned except for malingerers and alcoholics, suggesting successful interventions, although other outcomes, such as suicide or death from other causes, rather than improvement in mental wellbeing, could have contributed to his statistics.[105]

The rehabilitative role of prison hospitals, as East advised, was compatible with other theories, notably those of Émile Durkheim who viewed suicide as a social, rather than psychiatric issue. Durkheim was reluctant to accept psychiatrists' claims that most instances of suicide were a consequence of insanity, an opinion based on their experience in the asylums with limited professional responsibilities in the wider community.[106] Durkheim regarded suicide as a social phenomenon, due to the interaction between the actor and society. He argued that each society had a collective inclination towards suicide and that, despite looking like a highly individual and personal phenomenon, suicide was explicable through social structures and functions.[107] This hypothesis fitted with lower suicide rates internationally during the war, a time of intense emotional pressure together with greater social cohesion.[108]

Although in the community attempted or successful suicide was designated a criminal act, within the asylum the rule of law focused on staff in immediate charge of the patient.[109] For those staff, William Stoddart spelt out a terrifying image of the worst scenario:

> a suicide in an asylum is regarded throughout the lunacy world as more or less of a disgrace, and the staff of a particular institution is in a state of depression and anxiety for days or weeks after the occurrence, even among those who did not know the patient. [Should a member of staff's] carelessness lead to such a catastrophe....[he] is discharged from the asylum without a character and reported to the Board of Control, which enters his name in a black book, so that he may never more be engaged in mental nursing, and he is prosecuted in a court of law for criminal carelessness, and may be sentenced to a term of imprisonment.[110]

In contrast, even when a VC failed to implement the Board's safety recommendations to prevent suicide,[111] the leadership was not implicated directly or likely to be prosecuted. The onus fell on the staff of the lowest ranks who interacted with the patients face to face.

CONCLUSIONS

Ward staff were undervalued as individuals, paid at the level of unskilled workers and had little training in therapeutic methods. They were expected to work in a pressurised and stressful, overcrowded and under-staffed, almost impossible situation, under an authoritarian regime where seniority was seen to equate with superior personal attributes. The style of leadership induced distrust between lower ranks of the workforce and their masters who also had the right to dismiss them summarily, for disobedient, or otherwise aberrant, behaviours. These systemic tensions prohibited lower ranks from verbalising their workplace difficulties to those in authority. If work became intolerable, the emotional fragility, vulnerability and frustration of staff could be expressed physically, typically against those with even less power than they themselves had. Expressing one's emotions in this way has acquired different labels at various times, from "kicking the cat" to "Munchausen's by proxy" and "displaced aggression".

According to Lomax, attendants failed to make patients their prime concern:

It is the injury to themselves that most attendants are thinking of, much more than the possible injury to the patient....I don't suppose an attendant really cares twopence if a lunatic commits suicide or escapes, provided the blame for either cannot be brought home to himself.[112]

Within the asylum's hierarchical management structure, staff at the same level would rely on each other for support, including concealing, and thus perpetuating, each other's misdemeanours. The Board indicated that it knew about asylum rough handling, but apart from taking disciplinary measures it did not identify systemic problems which might require attention. Punishment of staff was used as a deterrent and to weed out supposedly "bad apples" to prevent contamination of the batch. The "resignation" or dismissal of the accused staff member appeared to satisfy the Board that the VC had done its duty, and the Board did not probe matters further.[113]

The asylum leadership demonstrated to staff that harsh and punitive methods were acceptable to control people considered to be of lower status if their actions deviated from what was expected. Rigid discipline, obedience and punishments, may have been exaggerated during the war, reflecting a more military style leadership. However, military methods which fostered discipline and taught aggressive tactics were unlikely to nurture kindness, emotional support and respect of the sort required in healthcare institutions with the objectives of providing, in the words of the Lunacy Act, "care and treatment". The Board, like the VCs, did not link harsh practices to their own authoritarian management style, but at its worst, the patients and ward staff had to cope with a punitive system characterised by a sanctimonious leadership, dysfunctional communication, distrust, dishonesty, secrecy and fear.

NOTES

1. Charles Mercier, *The Attendant's Companion: A Manual of the Duties of Attendants in Lunatic Asylums* (London: J and A Churchill, 1898), 72.
2. Mercier, *Attendant's Companion*, 3.
3. Mercier, *Attendant's Companion*, 31.
4. Committee on the Administration of Public Mental Hospitals (Chairman: Sir Cyril Cobb) (Cobb Inquiry), 15 March 1922 AM Donaldson Q:607, MH 58/219 TNA; Louise Hide, *Gender and Class in English Asylums 1890–1914* (Basingstoke: Palgrave Macmillan, 2014), 158.

5. Cobb Inquiry, 15 March 1922 Mr. Cox Q:403, 408, 413, MH 58/219 TNA.

6. Cobb Inquiry, 15 March 1922 AM Donaldson Q:614, 640–42, MH 58/219 TNA.

7. Rachel Grant-Smith, *The Experiences of an Asylum Patient* (London: George Allen and Unwin Ltd, 1922), 85.

8. Grant-Smith, *Experiences*, 85.

9. Grant-Smith, *Experiences*, 9.

10. Colney Hatch LCC/MIN/01006 Meeting, 13 July 1916, 207–8 LMA.

11. Colney Hatch LCC/MIN/01007 Meeting, 9 August 1918, 131 LMA.

12. Russell Barton, "Foreword," ix–xi, in Barbara Robb, *Sans Everything: A Case to Answer* (London: Nelson, 1967).

13. Colney Hatch H12/CH/B/18/003 Photographs of female patients admitted and discharged 1908–1918 LMA; Census 1911 https://www.ancestry.co.uk/cs/uk1911census.

14. Colney Hatch LCC/PH/MENT/04/016 Lists of patients admitted, died and recommended for discharge, 1911–1917 LMA.

15. Colney Hatch H12/CH/B/16/012 Case notes of female patients who died in 1933–1934 LMA.

16. Hide, *Gender and Class*, 158; Erving Goffman, *Asylums: Essays on the Social Situation of Mental Patients and other Inmates* (1961; Harmondsworth: Penguin, 1980), 99.

17. Colney Hatch LCC/MIN/01005 Meeting, 24 May 1916, 103–4 LMA.

18. Colney Hatch LCC/MIN/01006 Meeting, 18 May 1917, 179 LMA.

19. Hanwell LCC/MIN/01096 Meeting, 26 February 1917, 324–25 LMA.

20. Hanwell LCC/MIN/01093 Meeting, 27 April 1914, 189–90; Colney Hatch LCC/MIN/01003 Meeting, 4 December 1914, 198 LMA.

21. Mercier, *Attendant's Companion*, 2.

22. Anon. "London Gossip," *North-Eastern Daily Gazette* (Middlesbrough, England), 3 March 1887.

23. Colney Hatch LCC/MIN/01001 Meeting, 7 November 1913, 309–10 LMA.

24. Colney Hatch LCC/MIN/01002 Meeting, 21 November 1913, 12 LMA.

25. Hanwell LCC/MIN/01093 Meeting, 6 July 307–8 LMA.

26. Hanwell LCC/MIN/01094 Meetings: 20 July 1914, 10; 14 September 1914, 59–60 LMA.

27. John Collie and Arthur Spicer, *Malingering and Feigned Sickness* (London: E Arnold, 1913); Hanwell LCC/MIN/01094 Meeting, 26 October 1914, 103–4 LMA.

28. *First Annual Report of the Board of Control, for the Year 1914* (London: HMSO, 1916) (*BoC AR 1914*), Part 1, 28.

29. Colney Hatch LCC/MIN/01001 Meeting, 9 May 1913, 75–79 LMA.

30. Lunacy Act 1890 sections 322–24; BoC W/FM 17 March 1920, 80 MH 50/48 TNA.
31. Lunacy Act 1890 section 322.
32. Colney Hatch H12/CH/C/04/004 Male attendants' wages book 1917–1918 LMA.
33. Mercier, *Attendant's Companion*, 124.
34. Mercier, *Attendant's Companion*, 1.
35. Montagu Lomax, *The Experiences of an Asylum Doctor* (London: Allen and Unwin, 1921), 89.
36. *Fifth Annual Report of the Board of Control, for the Year 1918* (London: HMSO, 1919), 29, 31.
37. Cobb Inquiry, "Reports of Visits to Mental Institutions: Mrs. Munn," 1922, MH 58/221 TNA.
38. Civil Registration Death Index, England and Wales, 1916–2007, https://www.ancestry.co.uk/search/collections/onsdeath93/.
39. Colney Hatch LCC/MIN/01005 Meeting, 14 July 1916, 218 LMA.
40. Cobb Inquiry, 16 February 1922 Mr. Trevor Q:1, MH 58/219 TNA.
41. Mercier, *Attendant's Companion*, 23–24; BoC W/FM 29 August 1917, 253 MH 50/45 TNA.
42. Mercier, *Attendant's Companion*, 12.
43. Mercier, *Attendant's Companion*, 24; Jane Hamlett and Lesley Hoskins, "Comfort in Small Things? Clothing, Control and Agency in County Lunatic Asylums in Nineteenth- and Early Twentieth-Century England," *Journal of Victorian Culture* 18 (2013): 93–114, 105.
44. *BoC AR 1914*, Part 2, Kesteven Asylum 27 January 1914, 262.
45. Anon. "A Homicidal Attack on Dr Hetherington, Medical Superintendent, District Lunatic Asylum, London-Derry," *Journal of Mental Science* (*JMS*) 61 (1915): 169, citing *Belfast Evening Telegraph* 26 November 1914.
46. LCC LCC/MIN/00584 Meeting, 26 November 1918, 98 LMA.
47. LCC LCC/MIN/00583 Meeting, 14 May 1918, 572 LMA.
48. William Thorburn, "The Traumatic Neuroses," *Proceedings of the Royal Society of Medicine* 11 (1914): Neurological Section, 1–14; Ryan Hall and Richard Hall, "Compensation Neurosis: A Too Quickly Forgotten Concept?" *Journal of the American Academy of Psychiatry and the Law* 40 (2012): 390–98.
49. Hide, *Gender and Class*, 157.
50. National Council for Lunacy Reform, minute book 1920–1921, 30 September 1920, Report of Mr. Parley, SA/MIN/A/1 WL.
51. Cobb Inquiry, 15 March 1922 Mr. Sale Q:693, MH 58/219 TNA.
52. Cobb Inquiry, 16 March 1922 Charles McCarthy Q:825, MH 58/219 TNA.

53. Cobb Inquiry, 30 March 1922 Edward Mason Q:2027, 2040, MH 58/220 TNA.
54. Cobb Inquiry: 30 March 1922 Edward Mason Q:2050; 6 April 1922 WH Skevington Q:2666, MH 58/220 TNA.
55. Cobb Inquiry, 30 March 1922 Edward Mason Q:2055, MH 58/220 TNA.
56. Anon. "Fragilitas Ossium (Osteopsathyrosis)," *Lancet* 13 December 1902, 1645–46; Russell Howard, *The Practice of Surgery* (London: Edward Arnold, 1914), 516–17.
57. Jennifer Wallis, *Investigating the Body in the Victorian Asylum: Doctors Patients and Practices* (London: Palgrave Macmillan, 2017), 101–30; SWD Williams, "On Fractured Ribs in the Insane," *Lancet* 3 September 1870, 323–24.
58. Theobald Palm, "Etiology of Rickets," *BMJ* 1 December 1888, 1247.
59. Wallis, *Investigating the Body*, 102–3; Anon. "A Death in a Lunatic Asylum," *Lancet* 8 January 1870, 58.
60. Charles Macnamara, *Lectures on Diseases of Bones and Joints* (London: J and A Churchill, 1887), 253.
61. Cobb Inquiry, 24 March 1922 Lionel Weatherly Q:1672, MH 58/219 TNA.
62. Anon. "London Gossip."
63. See Chapter 3 for discussion on different methods of restraint; also, Wallis, *Investigating the Body*, 105.
64. William Lauder Lindsay, cited in T Christian, "On the Alleged Fragility of the Bones of General Paralytics," *JMS* 31 (1886): 453–59, 457–58.
65. William Stoddart, *Mind and Its Disorders* (London: HK Lewis, 1908), 421–31.
66. e.g. William Osler, *The Principles and Practice of Medicine* (London and New York: Appleton, 1912).
67. H Norman Barnett, *The Student's Textbook of Surgery* (London: Heinemann, 1916), 200.
68. A King and R Catterall, "Syphilis of Bones," *British Journal of Venereal Diseases* 35 (1959): 116–28; James Miller, *Practical Pathology Including Morbid Anatomy and Post-Mortem Technique* (London: Adam and Charles Black, 1914), 260.
69. E.g. Hanwell H11/HLL/B/31/006 Post-mortem register, males, 1915–1917 LMA.
70. Edward Hare, "Old Familiar Faces: Some Aspects of the Asylum Era in Britain," 82–100, in *Lectures in the History of Psychiatry*, ed. Robin Murray and Trevor Turner (London: Gaskell, 1990), 90.
71. BoC W/FM 1 April 1914, 4; 3 June 1914, 81; 23 December 1914, 286 MH 50/43 TNA.
72. *BoC AR 1914*, Part 2, Derbyshire Asylum 8 July 1914, 216.

73. Hare, "Old Familiar Faces": 90; Colney Hatch LCC/MIN/01007 Meeting, 9 August 1918, 131 LMA.

74. Russell Barton, Oral history interview by Diana Gittins GC/244/2/19, 54 WL.

75. Hare, "Old Familiar Faces": 86.

76. W Sullivan, "Haematoma Auris in the Insane," *JMS* 53 (1907): 192–93.

77. Hanwell LCC/MIN/01097 Meeting, 13 March 1917, 11 LMA.

78. Lomax, *Experiences,* 224–25.

79. Mary Riggall, *Reminiscences of a Stay in a Mental Hospital* (London: Arthur Stockwell, 1929), 15.

80. Lunacy Act 1890 section 323.

81. Lunacy Act 1890 section 85.

82. Lomax, *Experiences*, 67, 69.

83. Colney Hatch LCC/MIN/01001 Meeting, 29 August 1913, 214; LCC/MIN/01002 Meeting, 24 April 1914, 213 LMA.

84. Colney Hatch LCC/MIN/01003 Meeting, 15 January 1915, 238–39 LMA.

85. Colney Hatch LCC/MIN/01004 Meeting, 12 March 1915, 7; 26 March 1915, 31 LMA.

86. E.g. Hanwell LCC/MIN/01096 Meeting, 29 January 1917, 297 LMA.

87. Napsbury H50/A/01/024 Meeting, 22 May 1915, 12 LMA.

88. Colney Hatch LCC/MIN/01005 Meeting, 25 February 1916, 90 LMA.

89. BoC W/FM, reported at each meeting, MH 50/43-48 TNA.

90. Hanwell LCC/MIN/01097 Meeting, 16 July 1917, 135 LMA.

91. BoC W/FM 23 December 1914, 286 MH 50/43 TNA.

92. W Norwood East, "On Attempted Suicide, with an Analysis of 1000 Consecutive Cases" *JMS* 59 (1913): 428–78, 434.

93. *BoC AR 1914*, Part 1, 27.

94. *BoC AR 1914*, Part 2, Durham Asylum 8 May 1914, 223.

95. *BoC AR 1914*, Part 1, 27.

96. Anne Shepherd and David Wright, "Madness, Suicide and the Victorian Asylum: Attempted Self-Murder in the Age of Non-Restraint," *Medical History* 46 (2002): 175–96, 193.

97. Mercier, *Attendant's Companion*, 6; *Fourth Annual Report of the Board of Control, for the Year 1917* (London: HMSO, 1918), 37.

98. *BoC AR 1914*, Part 2, Lancaster Asylum 22 July 1914, 247; Mercier, *Attendant's Companion*, 22.

99. Mercier, *Attendant's Companion*, 10.

100. William Stoddart, *Mental Nursing* (London: Scientific Press Ltd, 1916), 31.

101. Until the Suicide Act 1961 (England and Wales).

102. Christopher Millard, "Re-inventing the 'Cry for Help': 'Attempted Suicide' in Britain in the Mid-Twentieth Century c.1937–1969" (PhD thesis, Queen Mary University of London, 2012) 46–48.
103. East, "Attempted suicide": 430–31.
104. Jose Harris, *Private Lives, Public Spirit: A Social History of Britain 1870–1914* (Oxford: Oxford University Press, 1993), 57.
105. East, "Attempted Suicide": 430–31.
106. Émile Durkheim, *Suicide. A Study in Sociology* (tr. John Spaulding and George Simpson) (London: Routledge and Kegan Paul, 1979), 62.
107. George Simpson, "Introduction," 13–32, in Durkheim, *Suicide*, 16.
108. Maurice Halbwachs, *The Causes of Suicide* (tr. Harold Goldblatt) (1930; London: Routledge and Kegan Paul, 1978), 213–14.
109. Lunacy Act 1890 sections 322–24.
110. Stoddart, *Mental Nursing*, 27.
111. *BoC AR 1914*, Part 1, 27; Part 2, Salop Asylum 8 July 1914, 297.
112. Lomax, *Experiences*, 89.
113. E.g. BoC W/FM 14 October 1914, 209 MH 50/42 TNA.

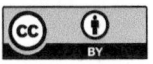

CHAPTER 9

Shackles and Chains: Some Concluding Thoughts

THEN AND NOW

The past has continuity with the present and the future. The present can assist in formulating questions to help investigate the past, and the past can shed light on current policy, practice and culture, and inform debate on future health services.[1] Iron shackles and chains, once used to restrain mentally disturbed patients in asylums in England, were replaced by leather and strong cloth many years before the First World War. Today's shackles and chains are metaphorical, like heavy-duty polymer threads, nearly invisible but resistant to breakage. They limit the lives of people with severe enduring mental illness who live in the community. They also tie government, public and professionals to concepts and values from the past, such as the acceptability of resourcing mental health and social care services which barely reach the levels needed, and rarely exceed them. Threads also link research challenges past and present: neuroscience has still not disclosed answers to allow us to prevent or cure schizophrenia, bipolar (manic-depressive) and other disabling psychiatric disorders, despite an ever-increasing grasp of their underlying causative mechanisms. These age-old challenges continue to spur on researchers, to overcome obstacles and to achieve scientific, pharmacological and clinically significant breakthroughs. Psychiatrists and others supporting patients over the last century have worked amid ongoing clinical and scientific uncertainty. They have aimed to identify the best pathways to

© The Author(s) 2021   263
C. Hilton, *Civilian Lunatic Asylums During the First World War*,
Mental Health in Historical Perspective,
https://doi.org/10.1007/978-3-030-54871-1_9

alleviate their patients' suffering while grappling with shifting concepts, hypotheses and disease classifications, in the context of practice shaped by national and local events and government policy endeavours. Historians and clinicians need to be wary of disparaging our forebears' practices and understanding of scientific evidence through our lens of hindsight, just as we hope that future generations will analyse dispassionately the strengths and deficits of our less than perfect knowledge and its clinical application.

Other continuities bind past and present. Asylums had walls of stone, bricks and mortar and patients lived communally in barrack-like buildings segregated by gender. The system of community care since the asylums closed lacks physical walls, but metaphorical ones exist. People with severe chronic mental illness today have more privacy, personal autonomy and independence than those a century ago, and many respond well to new medical, psychological or social treatment approaches. But many are unemployed, have poor physical health, receive inadequate social welfare payments and insufficient support from suitably trained staff, and are separated from their families and from broader community involvement. Asylum care had, and community care has, downsides and upsides. Both need to be understood in the distinct cultural frameworks of their times and in the broader context of societal values, including about institutions, illness, treatment, care, autonomy, independence, risk and protection.

The Board of Control ("the Board") and some individual psychiatrists, notably Charles Mercier, William Stoddart and Lionel Weatherly,[2] advocated gold standards of humane treatment leading at best to recovery, otherwise to a fulfilling life for those with the most severe chronic mental disorders who were unable, according to clinical reasoning and lunacy law at the time, to leave the asylums. Best practice was recognised, but emulated insufficiently, and asylums spanned a range of standards from admirable to appalling, as community care does today. Despite shared ideals between the asylums and community care, particularly the importance of people with chronic psychiatric disorders having as near normal lives as possible, some constructive asylum practices have been lost in the community care system. To take the example of employment: paid or unpaid meaningful occupation has long been considered helpful in the context of mental disorders to build confidence and self-esteem and improve health and wellbeing. In praiseworthy asylums up to 90 per cent of patients were engaged in some sort of daily work in 1914[3] which could be linked to the skills they acquired pre-admission.[4] By comparison, in 2013, when the UK working-age employment rate was 71 per cent,[5] only 10–15 per cent of people with schizophrenia were in employment although many more could, and wanted to, work.[6] This is a modern tragedy.

By the First World War, model asylum practices embracing humane and individually focussed psycho-social treatment had waned and care had become increasingly custodial, but even then, patients recovered and were discharged. Asylums were too often overcrowded, understaffed, unhygienic and warehouse like. This social warehousing was a consequence of long-term legal and financial constraints linked to values, knowledge and attitudes of professionals, policy leaders and the general public. Once it became accepted as normal, it perpetuated as a convenient way to proceed, unquestioned by most people. Similarly, when standards worsened, associated with wartime austerity, too often the state of affairs was accepted as the new normal and created little protest. When Lionel Shadwell, for example, inspected Claybury and noted high death rates, he was not alarmed as they were from "natural and ordinary" causes of the sort prevalent pre-war.[7] The continuation of pre-existing trends could be ignored, in contrast to the response when something unexpected appeared, whether shell-shock, or the Covid-19 pandemic as I write. Something new demands attention, but concurrently can expose the realities faced by vulnerable people living in deprived circumstances, whether pauper lunatics in the asylums of the past, or people living in poverty, or under community care, or in institutions today. At a time of crisis, long-lasting deficits temporarily become newsworthy.[8] The risk is that, after the crisis, in a period of reconstruction, the deficits fall back to their pre-crisis low priority. This happened to the asylums, perpetuating injustices and inequalities. We are yet to see what will happen after the Covid-19 pandemic.

The wartime asylums, and limitations of community care today, demonstrate provision of health and social care services which fail to meet the needs of many of those whom they are meant to serve. During the war, the asylum leadership waited as long as they dared, arguably too long, before asking for more resources to prevent deterioration in disastrously poor asylum standards. Today, despite admirable campaigning by patient-led groups, voluntary organisations, the Royal College of Psychiatrists and others, in the present climate of austerity the needs of some of the most seriously mentally ill people are side-lined.[9] Dangers exist when complacency prevails within a mental health service system, then and now. As Adrian James wrote in his forward to this book: "Continued self-reflection and challenge are vital. We could still do so much more."

LEADERSHIP: ATTITUDES AND STANDARDS

At the beginning of the war, speculation and hope that victory would be within easy reach informed asylum planning. Decisions made on that basis for a short-term national emergency may have been justifiable, but as time went on without compensatory adjustments for the prolonged duration, the asylum environment became harsher. Food declined in quality and quantity; care was more custodial and less rehabilitative; fewer and less well-trained staff were employed, often on temporary contracts; and many patients were moved from their "home" asylum to other overcrowded asylums at a distance, to make way for military casualties. The Board claimed at the beginning of the war that compromises in the asylums would not be detrimental to patients' well-being. This did not hold.

Despite the Board "policing" the asylums, it only had authority to advise and persuade medical superintendents and "visiting" committees (VCs) to make improvements. Responses of VCs fluctuated, arguably associated with insufficient knowledge about health and illness and the full purpose and intricacies of asylum function. Their level of activity appeared to be that which was the minimum required to conform to the Lunacy Act or other mandatory or closely monitored directives. They frequently attributed inactivity to financial constraints, which became more burdensome associated with wartime price rises. The asylum system was torn between how it assisted with wartime objectives and how it provided for the patients' needs. For the leadership, the war took priority. It was simpler to demonstrate patriotism and to go with public and government sentiment, rather than advocate for patients who were not valued by society.

At all levels, staff defended and justified their decision making, or passed the buck up or down the ladder, deflecting responsibilities away from themselves. The Board passed its dilemmas to the Home Office, War Office, Ministry of Food and other Whitehall bodies. The VCs passed theirs to the Board or medical superintendent, or to lower ranks of staff, who passed their discontent onto the patients. Risk of dismissal deterred low ranks of staff from criticising the asylum,[10] and some took out their frustration on patients by "rough handling" them, and then justifying their actions as being reasonable responses to the patients' needs.

Theories about patients being inevitably unreliable due to their insanity, and being susceptible to physical injury, such as by having fragile bones, helped staff avoid punishment for their heavy handedness. Complaints made by patients concerning their care, or by their relatives on their behalf, were typically ignored, interpreted as signs of mental derangement. Patients who reported maltreatment were liable to retribution. For them, it came in the form of further physical or psychological abuse from the staff on the wards. If VCs paid attention to the complaints, investigations were likely to be undertaken behind closed doors within the institution by senior people with potential conflicts of interest.[11] Rough handling was not unique to the wartime asylums: abuse by staff in hospitals and other residential institutions caring for vulnerable people has continued through the twentieth century and into the twenty-first.[12]

According to Adolph Meyer, the "rigidly moralising attitude" of "Anglo-Saxon" communities aimed to regulate and remove, rather than understand, mental disorders.[13] Removing mentally disturbed people to asylums placed them out of sight and out of mind, minimising community conscience and public interest and any sense of responsibility towards them as fellow human beings. Removing them also assisted with concealing institutional inadequacies and revealing as little as possible to the public. Little external oversight, interest and communication enshrined the asylum system, protected the reputations of institutions and leadership, and added to public perceptions of stigma and fear of asylums, of insanity and of those suffering from it. Theories of degeneration or hereditary predisposition to insanity added to overall negativity (but did not necessarily deter doctors from treating patients so labelled). It is unsurprising, amid the secrecy, fear and negativity, that the Boards of Guardians, who took decisions on behalf of their local communities, were reluctant to pay more to the asylums for the patients' care.

In contrast to a rigid asylum management system, there was flexibility for clinical debate. In the context of scientific uncertainty and needing to evaluate the murky waters of neuroscience hypotheses and research, discussion and debate were strengths which could help ensure a diversity of approaches with no single new method of clinical treatment being able to dominate practice. It could, however, contribute to the leadership's over-caution and conservatism verging on complacency about making changes. Combined with paternalism, a preoccupation with budgets, obedience to higher authorities and to the lunacy legislation, the style of leadership contributed to sluggish responses in the face of changing needs and circumstances.

The Board kept its head down, usually complied with demands from above and only rarely advocated for patients in its asylums. Despite some openness from the leadership about science and psychiatry, it is hard to conclude with a contextualised and respectful analysis of the asylum management system. It was secretive, self-protective, shady, patronising, rejecting of ideas from outside (except from seniority or science), censorious of staff lower in the hierarchy, and neglectful of patients, despite care and treatment of those patients being the stated rationale of the asylums.

PATIENTS, OUTCOMES AND AUSTERITY

Providing appropriate individualised care and treatment was influenced by powerful stakeholders who held diverse values and objectives and too often cut corners and services. Ongoing frugality in asylum management culture was particularly evident in the context of competing priorities associated with wartime austerity. The wartime asylums were characterised by a decline in standards rather than a cliff-edge change. Many defects pre-war became increasingly hazardous as the war progressed. Food, nutrition, fuel, hygiene, overcrowding, understaffing, staff discontent, and medical attention to patients were some of the aspects which deteriorated. The result was disastrous from the point of view of patient wellbeing.

Clinical notes reveal severe mental and physical illness in asylum patients which caused much suffering and disability. Some people entered asylums with rapidly fatal diseases, some were discharged (whether or not fully recovered), and others stayed as patients until they died months or years later, too often from potentially preventable infectious diseases. Despite recent popular fiction featuring women incarcerated for no other reason than giving birth to an illegitimate child, this was rare.[14] Neither did asylums seek to admit people purely because they were socially "impossible, inconvenient or inept" to create "Warehouses of the Unwanted", as Andrew Scull described.[15] Some troublesome people were dumped by families who had done all they could and had reached a point of despair, coping with an impossible domestic situation with insufficient guidance and support, but this does not mean that the patients were "unwanted". Others were dumped from within the healthcare system, particularly patients who had serious physical illness complicated by hallucinations, delusions and disturbed behaviours, likely to have been due to delirium.[16] Transferring these physically ill patients to asylums from other institutions, particularly workhouse infirmaries or general hospitals, was medically illogical. The practice reflected the ongoing attitudes of many non-asylum doctors, to get a "hopeless" patient, especially if perceived as senile or delirious, off their hands as rapidly as possible.[17]

Despite the total number of asylum patients declining, mainly due to high death rates and fewer admissions, overcrowding worsened, associated with more custodial care and fewer discharges, linked to reduced bed availability for civilian patients due to asylums being converted into war hospitals. The reduced admission rates were multifactorial, likely to have been associated with: greater social cohesion in the face of national adversity; reduced alcohol intake; some men being admitted without certification to military mental hospitals; and awareness by the magistrates and doctors who oversaw admissions that there were fewer beds and standards had dropped.[18]

As opposed to aiming for prolonged detention, discharging patients from asylums as soon as possible was vital, to vacate beds to allow admission of new, acutely unwell, patients. Around 40 per cent of patients were discharged within a year of admission in the late Victorian era, but this rate declined when asylums filled up with many long-term, chronically ill people, and custodial care replaced more active, individualised treatment. By 1918, the discharge rate had fallen by one third.[19] The chronic course of many severe mental disorders, insufficient rehabilitative treatment combined with the Lunacy Act's cumbersome bureaucratic discharge procedures, and an excessively cautious approach to determining whether a patient might still be dangerous to themselves or to others, all contributed to obstructing discharge. With vague disease classification, and the Board's annual report for 1918 preoccupied with causes of death rather than of admissions, it is not possible to determine whether there were any significant changes in the types of mental disorder for which patients were admitted (except related to alcohol intake) which might have affected outcomes during the war. From the evidence available, it is likely that overcrowding and understaffing worsened from their pre-war levels and did not allow sufficient therapeutic attention to promote recovery. Other factors which contributed to custodial batch-living, rather than active and rehabilitative treatment, included poor staff morale and questionable methods of placing patients on wards according to their behaviours, for organisational convenience, rather than linked to identified cause, or likely treatment requirements, or expected prognosis.

There was also a lack of after-care. One argument used against providing it was that former patients would not want any assistance which might reveal their asylum admission and pauper lunatic status to their local community, as it might lead to them being ostracised. This opinion, from some of the leadership, was convenient and in line with maintaining the *status quo*, but the Mental After Care Association's (MACA) papers suggest that the argument was flawed. MACA's archives may be biased in their own favour, but they nevertheless reveal that patients valued MACA's support, and that the charity had to turn people away as demand exceeded means. Generalisations by the asylum leadership about patients' views revealed their own negativity and lack of understanding of insanity. Concerning after-care, even if a patient's judgement was assumed to be inevitably impaired while they were mentally unwell, by definition, at the time of discharge their judgement would have recovered alongside their sanity, and their views should have been attended to. Negative attitudes towards insanity, not listening to patients, and a persistent desire to minimise short-term expenditure, were hardly ideal qualities for management teams supposedly working in the patients' best interests.

The way in which the asylum authorities dealt with the rising death rate from potentially preventable infections is also disturbing. Guidance was circulated to asylums for over a decade pre-war, based on scientific and public health evidence about what ought to be tackled to minimise the spread of infections, particularly tuberculosis, but implementation was neglected. At the beginning of the war, the asylum annual death rate from all causes hovered around 10 per cent. In 1915 the Board showed no inclination to investigate when deaths had risen to an unprecedented high of 12 per cent (Table 7.1). By the end of the war the death rate was 20 per cent, with relatively little of that due to the influenza pandemic. The general population, despite poverty and hardship, did not suffer the high rates of infectious diseases of patients in the asylums, before or during the war. The huge peak of tuberculosis deaths in the wartime asylums was multifactorial,[20] but included neglect.

Overall, patients suffered not just because of the disorders which led to their admission but because of the way the institutions were managed before and during the war. No doubt many people did their best, despite ambiguous science for mysterious and frightening mental disorders which often ran a chronic course. However, the leadership's negative attitudes towards the people they were meant to serve, and, among other things, their rigidity, complacency and penny-pinching, impaired their patients' health and wellbeing, with death rates from preventable disorders far in excess of those in the community. Fighting the war was a necessity, but it is questionable whether the degree of asylum neglect was necessary, justifiable or compatible with basic principles of medical ethics.[21]

Failure to prevent and treat physical disorders suffered by mentally unwell people was not just a feature of the Edwardian era and the First World War: it happens today. As a century ago, diet, lifestyle and late diagnosis of physical disorders continue to contribute to inequalities in life expectancy for people with serious chronic mental illnesses.[22] The physical disorders in 2020 are primarily cardiovascular disease and diabetes,[23] different from those a century ago. It is conceivable, as some of our forebears argued, that people with severe mental illnesses also have a biological susceptibility to life-shortening disorders, but it is unlikely, as the types of disorders over time are so different. It is more likely that the acquisition of the various physical problems were, and are, associated with poverty, deprivation, lifestyle and other external risk factors, whether in the asylum or community. In 2018, a study of physical health problems in people with bipolar disorder and schizophrenia concluded that the mortality gap between them and the general population was widening.[24] There is recognition that people with these mental disorders can benefit from support to make healthy lifestyle changes,[25] but during the last decade of austerity, the increasing mortality gap suggests that resources are insufficient or ineffective. It is disturbing that any parallels can be drawn between the potentially preventable physical diseases experienced in First World War asylums and in mental healthcare in 2020.

MAKING CHANGE

Public support for mentally disturbed soldiers was heartening. It initially helped the soldiers receive more dignified standards of care than those provided for mentally disturbed civilian patients, and it had the potential to encourage good care for all patients with mental disorders. During the war, public support extended to civilian patients as far as assisting the London County Council to change the designation of its institutions from "asylum" to "hospital".[26] This was an important symbolic step towards how the leadership intended the asylums to function, as well as indicating the effect which the public could have on the authorities for making change. Public opinion, however, was not always welcome: in the judgement of those in authority, including the Board, trained personnel with scientific, clinical and legal knowledge already knew what to do and how to do it.

Shell shock reinforced earlier understanding that mentally disturbed people could recover and that benefits could be derived from early treatment, although the Lunacy Act obstructed that for civilians. Shell shock also encouraged new psychological methods of treatment, but those were only accessible to people who could afford private care because they required staff time, impractical in overcrowded and understaffed asylums. Having shell shocked patients in the asylums highlighted inadequacies of provision for their civilian counterparts, but the soldiers' special status, clothing and privileges also caused problems. These could detract from plans to improve the lives of civilian patients, such as by the gambling, jealousy and theft associated with soldier patients receiving half-a-crown a week, discouraging the authorities from introducing cash remuneration for working patients. This study points to the importance of pre-war ideals and psycho-social, cultural, administrative, financial, clinical and other factors arising from inside the civilian asylum system during the war, as slowly, but erratically, leading to changes in asylum culture and practice. Post-war, rather than changing asylums for the better, shell shock was swallowed up into it, with many long-term civilian and soldier patients treated similarly, side by side in the asylums.[27]

Reduced asylum bed occupancy after the war, particularly when the war hospitals began to revert to their pre-war use, diminished any sense of urgency to provide more or better facilities or to expand services, such as after-care, to meet civilian patients' needs. Post-war inflation also detracted from improving standards in the asylums. The cost of treating a patient in an asylum in 1921 was more than double that in 1914, necessitating lifting the Lunacy Act's cap on charges payable by the Boards of Guardians.[28] This rise mainly covered costs of higher staff salaries, reduced hours of work, and improved working conditions. Undoubtedly, these measures had the potential to improve care for patients. However, that was not their purpose. They were a response to the National Asylum Workers' Union (NAWU) campaign since 1918, cotemporaneous with the increased influence of trade unions on workers' lives. Spending more of the asylum budget on staffing risked reducing the amount spent directly on patients.

The Board was initially ambivalent towards establishing a Ministry of Health, partly as it was concerned about protecting its own role. Nevertheless, it eventually welcomed its transfer, and that of the asylums, from the Home Office to the new Ministry in 1919.[29] The Board reasonably expected the move to help "dispel prejudices which often arise against Lunacy authorities and administrations, and which often affect injuriously, patients under treatment or even after recovery."[30] Whether it did that, or to what degree, is outside the scope of the present study, but the move brought mental and physical illnesses closer together for administrative purposes. Alongside changing "asylum" to "hospital", it was another important step on the long path towards "parity of esteem", to fund services for people with mental and physical illnesses in proportion to the morbidity which they cause, a goal still not achieved.[31] Despite the move to the new Ministry, other branches of healthcare—public health, maternal and child health, medicine and surgery—remained priorities on professional, public and government agendas, as judged by recurring themes in the *Lancet*[32] and the concerns of the Reconstruction Committee. In 1920, the Minister of Health, Christopher Addison, introduced a bill into parliament covering a diversity of health-related needs, one of which was to permit voluntary admission to public asylums. The bill was rejected by the Lords, much to the disappointment of the Board.[33]

A tricky situation was that the Board only had the authority to recommend change rather than to enforce it. The Board suggested, cajoled, named and shamed, and used any other technique it could to persuade asylums to raise standards. Tactics of persuasion could succeed but were most likely to do so with the most motivated. Too often, the Board's informal approach, trusting the VCs and medical superintendents to do what was asked in the interests of the patients, did not work. The Board, for example, had repeatedly prompted the VC at Prestwich to replace patients' earth closets with water closets. This was only implemented when the deficit came under public scrutiny at the Cobb Inquiry in 1922, as a result of Montagu Lomax's book about his wartime asylum experiences.[34]

Witnesses at the Cobb Inquiry revealed many defects in asylum care, treatment and facilities, but the inquiry report concluded that "the care and treatment of the insane is humane and efficient" and "compares favourably with that in any other country". The first of these statements is incompatible with much evidence presented at the inquiry by former patients and lower tiers of staff. The second is relative and raises questions about how it was derived, since the inquiry did not evaluate international evidence. Notwithstanding the report's reassurance, it also stated that there were "certain directions in which improvements and developments could be effected with advantage. It is of course obvious that these would involve increased expenditure", for which the community had responsibility.[35] It was good that Cobb acknowledged the importance of the public for making changes, but it was unfortunate that the country was in the midst of a financial crisis and that greater involvement would require major organisational and culture shifts by the public and the leadership, neither of which were on the horizon.

Cobb's report was not alone in its pattern of negating evidence from patients and lower ranks, reassuring the responsible authorities of the adequacy of their leadership, and then countering its own conclusions by arguing for improvements. In particular, it resembled the responses of the committees of inquiry into the *Sans Everything* allegations of scandalous care of elderly people in National Health Service long-stay geriatric and psychiatric wards four decades later.[36] Ultimately, the *Sans Everything* inquiries led to many improvements. Similarly, follow-up of the Cobb Report included a Royal Commission which led to the more patient-focussed Mental Treatment Act 1930.[37]

Forty years after the Lunacy Act and 25 after the first parliamentary attempt to reform it, the Mental Treatment Act permitted early and voluntary admission to the mental hospitals in line with long-term psychiatric understanding of its likely health benefits. This achievement and its implications meant that, more directly than psychological and clinical understanding derived from shell shock or from research into psychiatric disorders, Lomax's book stimulated processes which ultimately liberalised rules on admission and shaped treatment for patients in mental hospitals across the country.

FINAL WORD

It is easy to imagine a nurse or attendant a century ago expressing sentiments similar to those of an anonymous mental health nurse in the *Guardian* in 2019:

> I'm a mental health nurse. There are no good decisions, only least bad ones. I often feel I'm letting my patients down, but I do this job because

I believe in the healing power of small acts of kindness.... My day off. I go to the pub and see my friends, who make effort to give me space to talk about work. My answers are scant, because it would drain us all to go into detail, and I just want to enjoy my pint. I work in close proximity to so much suffering that I can never quite find the language to explain it all.[38]

Despite the problems in the asylums we must remember much care and many kindnesses. Kindness from staff members was assumed so it was not noteworthy. It was rarely mentioned specifically in official records, only coming to light in the context of some other pressing matter. Within the asylums we know about Nurse H's remorse for injuring Edith B, compassion shown to Louise F at Claybury, Eliza Maidman's loyalty to her asylum, and acting medical superintendents Guy Barham and Alfred Daniel who spoke up to provide better treatment for their patients. Colney Hatch sought to provide for the religious, language and cultural needs of the East End Jewish community, Belgian refugees, prisoners of war and others. Some patients had a sense of community with meaningful relationships within their asylum home, and maintained strong bonds with their families.

Outside the asylums, the Home Office refused permission to deport Mayer L, MACA pioneered individualised rehabilitation programmes, parliamentarians in both Houses challenged the government about inadequate provision for civilian patients with mental disorders, and Mercier, Stoddart, Weatherly and others advocated forcefully and repeatedly for humane and therapeutic treatment and lunacy law reform. We must be grateful too to the lower ranks of staff and the patients who stood their ground to say what needed to be said, especially at the Cobb Inquiry, and to a handful of patients, such as Mary Riggall, James Scott and Rachel Grant-Smith, who revealed their personal stories of asylum life, good and bad, with a view to encouraging change for the better.

NOTES

1. Rab Houston, "Past and 'Pastism' in the History of Psychiatry," *Lancet Psychiatry* 6 (2019): 206–8.
2. E.g. Charles Mercier, *The Attendant's Companion: A Manual of the Duties of Attendants in Lunatic Asylums* (London: J and A Churchill, 1898); William Stoddart, *Mental Nursing* (London: Scientific Press, 1916); Lionel Weatherly, *A Plea for the Insane: The Case for Reform in the Care and Treatment of Mental Diseases* (London: Grant Richards Ltd, 1918).

3. *First Annual Report of the Board of Control, for the Year 1914* (*BoC AR 1914*) (London: HMSO, 1916), Part 2, Brecon and Radnor Asylum 6 May 1914, 199.
4. Diane Carpenter, "'Above All a Patient Should Never Be Terrified': An Examination of Mental Health Care and Treatment in Hampshire 1845–1914" (PhD thesis, University of Portsmouth, 2010), https://researchportal.port.ac.uk/portal/files/5877161/Diane_Carpenter_PhD_Thesis_2010.pdf, 156, 158; *BoC AR 1914*, Part 2, The Chestnuts, Walthamstow, 28 October 1914, 228.
5. SANE, *Schizophrenia and Employment: Putting the Lived-Experience of Schizophrenia at the Heart of the Employment Agenda*, 2013, http://www.sane.org.uk/uploads/schizophrenia_employment_web.pdf; Office for National Statistics, *Statistical Bulletin: Labour Market Statistics*, April 2013, http://www.ons.gov.uk/ons/dcp171778_305051.pdf.
6. Schizophrenia Commission, *The Abandoned Illness*, 2012: 6, https://www.rethink.org/media/514093/TSC_main_report_14_nov.pdf.
7. Claybury LCC/MIN/00949 Meeting, 20 June 1918, 86–88 LMA.
8. Mental Health Foundation, *The COVID-19 Pandemic, Financial Inequality and Mental Health*, 2020, https://www.mentalhealth.org.uk/sites/default/files/MHF-covid-19-inequality-mental-health-briefing.pdf.
9. House of Commons Committee of Public Accounts, *Improving Access to Mental Health Services*, Sixteenth Report of Session 2016–2017, HC 80, https://publications.parliament.uk/pa/cm201617/cmselect/cmpubacc/80/80.pdf.
10. Colney Hatch LCC/MIN/01001 Meeting, 23 May 1913, 95–96 LMA; Napsbury H50/A/01/024, Meeting, 5 November 1915, 249 LMA.
11. Claire Hilton, *Improving Psychiatric Care for Older People: Barbara Robb's Campaign 1965–1975* (London: Palgrave Macmillan, 2017).
12. John Martin with Debbie Evans, *Hospitals in Trouble* (Oxford: Blackwell, 1984); Louise Hide and Joanna Bourke, "Cultures of Harm in Institutions of Care: Introduction," *Social History of Medicine* 31 (2018): 679–87.
13. Adolph Meyer, "The Aims of a Psychiatric Clinic," 1–11, in *XVIIth International Congress of Medicine, London 1913. Section XII Psychiatry. Part 1* (London: Henry Fowde, Hodder and Stoughton, 1913), 1–2.
14. E.g. Sebastian Barry, *The Secret Scripture* (London: Faber and Faber, 2008); Maggie O'Farrell, *The Vanishing Act of Esme Lennox* (London: Headline Review, 2006).
15. Andrew Scull, *The Most Solitary of Afflictions: Madness and Society in Britain, 1700–1900* (New Haven: Yale University Press, 1993), 370.

16. Claybury LCC/MIN/00948 Meeting, 3 January 1918, 286 LMA.
17. Tom Arie, "Dementia in the Elderly: Diagnosis and Assessment," *BMJ* 1 December 1973, 540–43, 541.
18. *BoC AR 1914*, Part 1, 10; *Sixth Annual Report of the Board of Control, for the Year 1919 (BoC AR 1919)* (London: HMSO, 1920), 10; *Seventh Annual Report of the Board of Control, for the Year 1920 (BoC AR 1920)* (London: HMSO, 1921), Appendix A, 87.
19. *BoC AR 1919*, Appendix A, 22–23.
20. John Murray, "Tuberculosis and World War I," *American Journal of Respiratory and Critical Care Medicine* 192 (2015): 411–14.
21. John Keay, "Presidential Address on the War and the Burden of Insanity," *Journal of Mental Science* 64 (1918): 325–44.
22. King's Fund, *Mental Health: Our Position*, 2019, https://www.kingsfund.org.uk/projects/positions/mental-health.
23. NHS England, *Improving the Physical Health of People with Serious Mental Illness: A Practical Toolkit*, 2016, https://www.england.nhs.uk/mentalhealth/wp-content/uploads/sites/29/2016/05/serious-mental-hlth-toolkit-may16.pdf.
24. Joseph Hayes, Louise Marston, Kate Walters, Michael King and David Osborn, "Mortality Gap for People with Bipolar Disorder and Schizophrenia: UK-Based Cohort Study 2000–2014," *British Journal of Psychiatry* 211 (2017): 175–81.
25. Sarah Barber and Graham Thornicroft, "Reducing the Mortality Gap in People with Severe Mental Disorders: The Role of Lifestyle Psychosocial Interventions," *Frontiers in Psychiatry*, 28 September 2018, https://doi.org/10.3389/fpsyt.2018.00463.
26. LCC LCC/MIN/00583 Meeting, 18 December 1917, 234–36 LMA.
27. Peter Barham, *Forgotten Lunatics of the Great War* (New Haven and London: Yale University Press, 2004), 297.
28. *Eighth Annual Report of the Board of Control, for the Year 1921* (London: HMSO, 1922), 27–28.
29. Ministry of Health Act 1919 section 3.
30. *BoC AR 1920*, 1.
31. Claire Hilton, "Parity of Esteem for Mental and Physical Health Care in the United Kingdom: A Hundred Years War?" *Journal of the Royal Society of Medicine* 109 (2016): 133–37.
32. E.g. Anon. "Cerebellar Syndrome Following Heat Stroke," *Lancet* 26 October 1918, 561–62; Anon. "Lethargic Encephalitis and Poliomyelitis," *Lancet* 28 December 1918, 888; Anon. "Standardisation of Pathological Methods," *Lancet* 26 October 1918, 563; Anon. "Botulism

Due to Canned Vegetables," *Lancet* 16 November 1918, 677; Walter Spencer, "Caesarean Section Three Times on the Same Patient," *Lancet* 7 December 1918, 778–79.

33. Ministry of Health (Miscellaneous Provisions) Bill. *Hansard* HL Deb 14 December 1920 vol 39 cc119-49; *BoC AR 1920*, 2.

34. Committee on the Administration of Public Mental Hospitals (Chairman: Sir Cyril Cobb) (Cobb Inquiry); Montagu Lomax, *The Experiences of an Asylum Doctor* (London: Allen and Unwin, 1921).

35. Ministry of Health, *Report of the Committee on Administration of Public Mental Hospitals* Cmd. 1730 (London: HMSO, 1922), 80.

36. Mental Health Service. *Hansard* HC Deb 19 March 1965, vol. 708 cc.1645–1719; Ministry of Health, *Findings and Recommendations Following Enquiries into Allegations Concerning the Care of Elderly Patients in Certain Hospitals* Cmnd. 3687 (London: HMSO, 1968); Claire Hilton, *Improving Psychiatric Care for Older People: Barbara Robb's campaign 1965–1975* (London: Palgrave Macmillan, 2017).

37. Hilton, *Improving Psychiatric Care*; Report of the Royal Commission on Lunacy and Mental Disorder Cmd. 2700 (London: HMSO, 1926).

38. Anon. "I'm a Mental Health Nurse: There Are No Good Decisions, Only Least Bad Ones," 11 November 2019, https://www.theguardian.com/society/2019/nov/11/mental-health-nurse-no-good-decisions-patients.

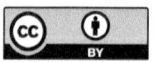

INDEX

© The Editor(s) (if applicable) and The Author(s) 2021
C. Hilton, *Civilian Lunatic Asylums During the First World War*,
Mental Health in Historical Perspective,
https://doi.org/10.1007/978-3-030-54871-1